THE COMPLETE PATIENT HISTORY

MAURICE KRAYTMAN, M.D.

Associate Professor
of Clinical Medicine
University of Brussels

The Complete Patient History

McGRAW-HILL BOOK COMPANY

New York
St. Louis
San Francisco
Auckland
Bogotá
Düsseldorf
Johannesburg
London
Madrid

Mexico
Montreal
New Delhi
Panama
Paris
São Paulo
Singapore
Sydney
Tokyo
Toronto

NOTICE

Medicine is an ever-changing science. As new research and clinical experience broaden our knowledge, changes in treatment and drug therapy are required. The editors and the publisher of this work have made every effort to ensure that the drug dosage schedules herein are accurate and in accord with the standards accepted at the time of publication. Readers are advised, however, to check the product information sheet included in the package of each drug they plan to administer to be certain that changes have not been made in the recommended dose or in the contraindications for administration. This recommendation is of particular importance in regard to new or infrequently used drugs.

THE COMPLETE PATIENT HISTORY

34567890 DODO 8765

This book was set in Helvetica by Kingsport Press, Inc. The editors were J. Dereck Jeffers and Irene Curran; the designer was Judith Michael; the production supervisor was Milton J. Heiberg.
The printer and binder was R. R. Donnelley & Sons Company.

Library of Congress Cataloging in Publication Data

Kraytman, Maurice.
    The complete patient history.

    Includes index.
    1. Medical history taking. I. Title.
[DNLM: 1. Medical history taking—Handbooks.
WB290 K91c]
RC65.K73   616.07′5   78–16107
ISBN 0–07–035421–9

CONTENTS

PREFACE

Correct diagnosis is based on the history of the development of symptoms, connected with the detailed physical examination and the rational use of laboratory testing. History taking is undoubtedly the most important and difficult part of the clinical examination. This book is intended as an aid to medical personnel (medical students, residents, general practitioners, physician assistants, nurse practitioners) in the taking of a patient's history. It is divided into three parts.

Part One delineates the sequential steps in history taking, stressing possible technical and psychological pitfalls and their avoidance. This part also emphasizes the respective place of nondirective and leading questions in the interview.

Part Two contains 49 chapters devoted to specific complaints. Each chapter includes seven sections: (1) definition and pathophysiology of the complaint to be investigated; (2) etiology, with tables of differential diagnosis, including a paragraph about the iatrogenic causes of the complaint; (3) a series of questions centered around the complaint, with the possible clinical and/or pathophysiological meanings of a positive response; (4) physical signs pertinent to the complaint and their possible clinical interpretation; (5) laboratory tests relevant to the complaint with the diagnostic possibilities of the results; (6) reminders and clinical hints of diagnostic significance; (7) selected references.

Part Three deals with inquiries which apply to every patient regardless of his or her particular problem: evolution of the illness; its effects on the patient; complete personal and family medical history; review of systems; personal and social profile.

The reader will notice that the formulation of the Questionnaires is generally directive and that many questions can be answered with a simple "yes" or "no." The author is aware of the criticism such wording can raise. He knows that the taking of a history should start with having the patient give an account of the illness, then proceed with nondirective questions, and finally with specific, leading questions, until all necessary information is obtained. He also knows that the questions should be put in words understandable to the patient and that the interviewer should try to use the patient's own words. It is technically impossible to present open-ended questions in lay language that could apply to every patient and be accompanied by their possible meanings. Therefore, the questions had to be put in a directive form. They should be considered as being addressed to the reader as reminders of what information must be collected to explore and understand the patient's illness. It is up to the reader to adapt the questions to the actual patient being interrogated and to rephrase them first in a nondirective form or, if necessary, in a directive form.

For each question, the most likely meanings of the response are given. It is evident, however, that a positive answer to a question could have several meanings and suggest several diagnostic possibilities. In a patient who complains of problems breathing when lying down at night, left-heart failure is a distinct possible etiology, and it is presented as such. However, psychogenic dyspnea, asthma, or even such an arcane entity as sleep apnea cannot be excluded. Also, the significance of the responses might well be qualified by the patient's feelings toward the illness. Thus the correct diagnosis will be based on the full analysis and characterization of the patient's complaint and personality, as well as on the physical examination and laboratory results. For all these reasons, the most important term in the heading "Possible meaning of response" might well be the adjective "possible," which appears in boldface type in the text to remind the reader that the suggested diagnoses are not exclusive of other clinical entities. More extensive etiologic possibilities are to be found in the tables of differential diagnosis and in the sections "Useful Reminders and Diagnostic Clues."

Rather than containing lengthy lists of innumerable diseases, the tables of differential diagnosis present the most frequent causes. These are arranged, whenever possible, according to pathophysiological mechanisms. Similarly, no attempt has been made to cite all drugs capable of eliciting a given complaint. Instead, the most frequently used medications have been mentioned. The sections "Physical Signs Pertinent to the Complaint" and "Laboratory Tests Pertaining to the Complaint" are intended to complement the clinical information derived from the history taking. They list the most salient features of common diseases. Laboratory investigations have been limited to the most common and useful ones, and some of them are tagged with the reference mark * (= if appropriate) to remind the reader that diagnostic procedures should be ordered discriminately and economically. Problem-centered history taking inevitably results in the fragmentation of the various components of clinical syndromes under separate headings. The Glossary of Clinical Manifestations reassembles the main symptoms and signs mak-

.ing up disease entities, which are thus reconstructed according to their classical description.

Frequent causes of complaints are <u>underlined</u>. Characteristic clinical features and crucial differentiating questions are *italicized*. Potentially life-threatening or urgent conditions are in **boldface** type.

The aim of this book is not to propose branching diagnoses or algorithms. Rather, it attempts to aid the interviewer's interrogation of the patient and to help the interviewer correlate the patient's responses with possible disease entities.

It is the author's hope that readers of this book will find it useful in their daily medical practice.

ACKNOWLEDGMENTS

I wish to express my appreciation to the medical students who critically discussed the manuscript. I am particularly grateful to D. R. Gens, A. Gibson, T. S. Hope, B. Lepolstat, W. A. Lerner, L. Liebman, A. L. Miles, D. L. Newfield, and A. R. Rosenstock for their painstaking reading and their constructive comments. I am indebted to Dr. C. Delhaye who kindly reviewed the chapters "Abnormal Vaginal Bleeding" and "Amenorrhea" and offered many useful criticisms and suggestions. Finally, I would like to thank Mr. J. D. Jeffers and Ms. I. Curran of the McGraw-Hill Book Company for their helpful and skillful editorial guidance.

Maurice Kraytman

THE COMPLETE PATIENT HISTORY

PART ONE

The Sequential Steps in History Taking

The importance of history taking in the process of making a differential diagnosis cannot be overemphasized. It has been estimated that the history allows a correct diagnosis in over 50 percent of internal diseases. However, history taking is not just a process of collecting information on the onset and evolution of an illness. It must also give an insight into the patient's personality, the ability of the patient to cope with the medical problem, and the effects of the problem on the patient. It serves as the basis for the relationship between patient and interviewer.

Whenever possible, the interview should take place in privacy. The patient should be put at ease and assured that there will be time enough to discuss fully any matter of concern. When confronted with a confused patient or a patient who minimizes, denies, or conceals symptoms, it is essential to interview a reliable relative or friend.

1. The first step in history taking is to invite the patient to express the reason for seeking medical advice. In order to obtain the patient's chief complaint, a question of a general nature, such as, "What can I do for you?" or "Please tell me about your trouble," is frequently necessary. Avoid asking the patient, "What is wrong with you?" as the answer might be, "That's why I came to you!"

The patient should then be asked to give, in the patient's own terms, a full account of his or her illness. All facts believed associated with the complaint should be brought out, and the patient should be encouraged to give his or her feelings about the symptoms. Except in case of rambling, the patient should be allowed to discuss problems uninterrupted as they come to mind.

Do not disregard too rapidly details which seem irrelevant or even bizarre, or which do not fit with your initial hypothesis. *All* facts mentioned by the patient must be taken into account; they should be carefully analyzed before being eventually discarded.

When the patient seems to come to a stop, prompting with nonspecific questions, such as, "And then?" or "Are there any other problems?" is indicated.

A patient who has several complaints should be asked which one seems the most important.

2. After having afforded the patient the opportunity to describe his or her illness, the interviewer should then proceed methodically to analyze the complaint within the following framework: mode of onset and chronology; location and, if applicable, radiation of the symptom; character (or quality) of the symptom; intensity (or quantitative aspects) of the complaint; precipitating or aggravating fac-

tors; relieving factors; accompanying symptoms; iatrogenic factors; environmental factors; personal and relevant family medical history pertaining to the complaint; evolution of the illness and its effects on the patient.

The exploration of these features need not be done in a rigid sequence. For instance, when dealing with a pain problem, the first step should be to locate exactly the site of discomfort. With other complaints, such as fatigue or vertigo, the interviewer should first try to define exactly what the patient means, i.e., the character (or quality) of the complaint should be assessed first. Flexibility in the order of the questions is also required to avoid inhibiting any beneficial association of thoughts by the patient.

Inquiry into each of these topics should begin with nondirective questions, such as, "Does the discomfort remain localized? Does it move?" Asking a patient with chest pain on exertion, "Does the pain disappear rapidly when you stop walking?" is bad technique. The very formulation of the question may influence the patient. In a desire to be cooperative, the patient may provide information that the interviewer appears to want. The significance of "rapidly" may be quite different to the patient than to the interviewer. Finally, this type of question is too complex. It actually contains two separate questions: (1) "Does the pain disappear when you stop walking?" and (2) "Does the pain disappear rapidly?" Questions must explore one item at a time. The correct sequence would be "When you stop walking, does it affect your discomfort?" and, if so, "In how much time does the pain disappear?"

Some patients will give a clear, lucid description of their illness, and satisfactorily answer the interviewer's questions. However, in the majority of patients, verbosity, limited vocabulary, and/or forgetfulness will eventually force the interviewer to guide the patient by asking specific, directive questions to help clarify the subject. For example, with a patient complaining of lower back pain, the interviewer should first ask, in a neutral manner, "Does the pain move anywhere?" If the response is not explicit, the interviewer should specify, "Does the pain radiate to the buttock? the calf?"

Nondirective as well as directive questions must be concise and easily understandable by the patient. Avoid medical terms and technical expressions. Use the patient's own words ("trouble," "discomfort," etc.). This way you will not distort the patient's thoughts and substitute your own interpretation. Sometimes, it is useful deliberately to repeat the question (perhaps phrased differently) later in the interview if the original response appears doubtful.

The different aspects of the full analysis of a complaint will now be briefly discussed.

Mode of onset and chronology   The exact manner in which the illness began must be defined: what was the patient doing at the time of onset? where was the patient? what were the precise circumstances of the onset? Many patients believe that their illness began later than it actually did. If the patient has difficulty in recalling precisely the date of onset of the illness, the interviewer can help by referring to chronological landmarks, such as seasons or holidays: "How were you feeling during the summer vacation? the Christmas holidays?" Another useful reference point is the patient's last thorough medical examination for employment or insurance. Time relationships must be established by date. If the complaint is intermittent, ask the patient to specify the periodicity and frequency of the symptom, and to describe fully a typical episode.

Location and radiation of symptom   The patient should be invited to point (with a finger if possible) to the site of the discomfort and to its eventual radiation. He or she should also locate the depth at which the abnormal sensation seems to arise.

Character (or quality) of symptom   Generally, a patient will have difficulty describing this aspect of the complaint and will often resort to comparisons. For example, a patient with tension headache might say, "I feel as if my head were in a vise." The interviewer may aid the patient by presenting various descriptive terms or phrases. If the symptom is a pain, the question might be: "What sort of pain is it? dull? burning? constrictive?" The interviewer should be careful not to emphasize one descriptive term or one comparison more than another.

Intensity (or quantity) of symptom   Any complaint that lends itself to quantification should be defined in some measurable way. Diarrhea must be expressed in the number of stools per day, dyspnea or intermittent claudication in terms of level blocks walked before it is felt.

Precipitating, aggravating, and relieving factors   Some patients will spontaneously tell the interviewer that their complaint becomes better or worse under certain circumstances. For instance, a patient may indicate that a pain in the calves appears on walking and disappears on stopping. However, the interviewer generally must ask specific questions. For example, the interviewer, knowing that the pain of a peptic ulcer appears within hours after a meal and subsides after eating, will specifically ask about these circumstances. Again, the questions should be worded to avoid influencing the answers. Thus it is better to ask, "What effect does eating have on your pain?" rather than, "Does eating relieve your pain?"

Accompanying symptoms   Most often, the patient's complaint is only part of a constellation of symptoms grouped into clinical syndromes. Some patients frequently fail to realize that other symptoms they are presenting are related to the chief complaint, and they may even fail to mention the other symptoms, having become accustomed to them. For instance, a man complaining about edema in the lower extremities may not volunteer that he has been short of breath when walking and has been sleeping with two pillows for months. The interviewer must anticipate the missing symptoms in the patient's account of the illness and must inquire, in a directive manner, about associated phenomena that the patient may have failed to mention.

Iatrogenic factors   In this era of universal polypharmacopeia, the interviewer should never omit to have patients give a full account of all drugs they are currently taking. Many patients taking sleeping pills, tranquilizers, analgesics, laxatives, oral contraceptives, may become so accustomed to these medications that they do not consider them as drugs. It is not enough to ask the patient, "Do you take any medications?" Questions should be specific: "Do you take aspirin? sleeping pills? laxatives?" It is wise to ask the patient whether the drugs were prescribed by a physician or bought over the counter. Knowing that a patient uses drugs indiscriminately enables the physician to anticipate poor compliance with his or her own prescriptions.

Environmental factors   The patient's environment, job, hobbies, domicile, travels are all possible etiologic factors. It is important to know that the patient with cough and sputum of recent onset has a parrot at home, or that the present fever and recurrent chills appeared after a travel in a malaria-infested area. Direct questioning is imperative here.

Personal antecedents and family medical history pertaining to the complaint   The patient's personal antecedents and the family medical history may provide useful information on the present illness. For instance, it is important to learn that a jaundiced patient with acute pain in the right hypochondrium has a history of anemia and that relatives have undergone splenectomy to cure an anemia. What might have initially been interpreted as gallbladder colic now seems likely to be cholelithiasis complicating hereditary spherocytosis. Do not accept at face value the patient's version of past diagnoses by other physicians. Patient's terms such as "pneumonia," "heart attack," "pleurisy," must be critically analyzed. For instance, the details of a past "gallstone attack" should be elicited: "Where was the pain located? Did the color of the skin and/or urine change? Was there fever, chills?" etc.

Evolution of the illness and its effects on the patient   The interviewer should ask the patient a series of questions aimed at exploring the evolution of the illness and its overall effects on the patient's normal activities. A useful question always to be asked is "Why did you select this particular time to seek medical advice?" It occasionally brings out an important recent change in symptoms that the patient has omitted. Never forget to inquire about the patient's opinion regarding the illness: this question may reveal the patient's fears, apprehensions, or fantasies.

3. After full characterization of the symptom, the following areas are explored: complete personal and family medical history; review of systems; and finally the personal and social profile.

Personal past medical history   Information about previous illnesses, operations, and accidents should be obtained, preferably in chronologic order, with the dates and locations of occurrence, the names of the physicians involved, and the treatments applied. Specific questions will need to be asked of the patient. Again do not forget that the diagnoses reported by the patient may not be correct because of misinterpretation or misdiagnosis. On the other hand, diagnoses made by previous physicians should not be discarded lightly.

Family medical history   The health of family members should be ascertained. Diseases with hereditary or environmental factors should be mentioned specifically. Knowledge of the ethnic origin of the parents and of any consanguinity may be important.

Review of systems   In this part of the history taking, the interviewer specifically checks each system, from head to extremities, to make certain that neither physician nor patient has overlooked any symptom or sign of significance. Direct questions have to be asked.

Whenever a positive answer is obtained, the interviewer should clarify the newly elicited symptom by shifting back to nondirective questions and encouraging a description of the symptoms in the patient's own terms. If ambiguity still persists, leading questions should be asked. Chronology of events must be delineated. When a patient responds positively to nearly every question, a multisystem disease or a psychologic illness should be suspected.

Personal and social profile   The patient's ethnic, familial, educational, and social background, employments, habits, and moods should be explored. These features may play an important role in the health problem and may help evaluate the personality of the patient. For example, multiple jobs in a short period of time are suggestive of psychological difficulties; alcoholics are liable to certain diseases such as cirrhosis, acute pancreatitis, neurologic disorders. Some patients are reluctant to discuss their personal problems. Questions about these matters should initially be general and not probe too deeply so that the patient is not put on the defensive. When highly private problems are being discussed, it is better for the interviewer to lay aside his or her pen, as note taking may have an inhibitory effect on the patient.

At the end of the interrogation, the interviewer should always inquire whether the patient has questions to ask or anything to add: previous hidden anxieties may be revealed.

The above suggested sequence need not be rigidly adhered to; each patient demands an individual procedure. Particularly, patients who so wish should be allowed to speak freely about emotional problems at any time during the interview. However, it is psychologically wise to close the interview with the personal and social profile. In this way, inquiry about more intimate matters is postponed until after the medical aspects have been explored and sufficient time has elapsed to create a satisfactory patient-interviewer relationship.

PART TWO

Problem-centered History Taking

Cardiorespiratory System

1
Cough and Expectorations

DEFINITIONS AND GENERAL CONSIDERATIONS

Cough an explosive expiration which provides a means of clearing the tracheobronchial tree of mucus and foreign material.

Expectoration ejection, by coughing and spitting, of fluid or semi-fluid matter from the lungs and respiratory passages.

The afferent pathways of the cough reflex are in the trigeminal, glossopharyngeal, superior laryngeal, and vagus nerves. The efferent pathways lie in the recurrent laryngeal nerve, which causes closure of the glottis, and in the phrenic and spinal nerves, which cause contraction of the thoracic and abdominal musculature. The nerve endings in the airway passages are sensitive to contact with foreign material and inflammatory, mechanical, thermal, and chemical stimuli. The acinar units have no nerve supply; material from those areas has to move up into larger airways into the presence of nerve endings to initiate coughing. A cough may also occur as a result of stimulation of the parietal pleura and of afferent pathways originating in other viscera.

The normal adult produces about 100 mL of mucus from the respiratory tract in a day. It takes about 30 to 60 min for mucus and/or foreign material to be swept from the levels of the respiratory bronchioles up to the mouth. When excess mucus is formed, the normal process of removal may be ineffective and accumulation of mucus may occur, so that the mucous membrane is stimulated and the mucus coughed up as sputum.

ETIOLOGY

Inflammation: acute pharyngitis; acute laryngitis; acute tracheo-bronchitis (viral, bacterial); chronic bronchitis; bronchiectasis; lobar pneumonia; bronchopneumonia; lung abscess; pulmonary tuberculosis; fungal infections; parasite lung disease; pleuritis

Cardiovascular disorders: pulmonary edema; pulmonary infarction; pleural effusion; aortic aneurysm

Trauma, chemical, and physical agents: foreign bodies; cigarette smoke; chemical fumes; beryllium granulomatosis

Neoplasms: primary bronchogenic carcinoma; metastatic lung tumors; bronchial adenoma; alveolar cell carcinoma; primary mesothelioma; mediastinal tumors

Allergic disorders: bronchial asthma

Other causes: sarcoidosis; Wegener's granulomatosis; diffuse idiopathic interstitial fibrosis; alveolar proteinosis; atelectasis

QUESTIONNAIRE

* In this questionnaire and all succeeding ones, items in *italics* are characteristic clinical features; items in **boldface** type are potentially life-threatening or urgent conditions; and underscored items are common causes of complaint.

Possible *meaning of response*

1 Duration and mode of onset

1.1 How long have you had
   • a cough?
   • expectorations?

Up to 3 weeks: acute process: viral acute tracheobronchitis; bacterial bronchopneumonia
More than 3 weeks: process becoming chronic: pulmonary tuberculosis; pulmonary neoplasm
2 years or more: chronic bronchitis; bronchiectasis

1.2 Was the onset of cough acute?

If dry cough: inhalation of a foreign body; irritant substance; acute bronchitis, pneumonia (viral); pulmonary embolization

2 Intensity of the complaint

2.1 Do you cough and/or expectorate	
• daily?	<u>Chronic bronchitis</u>
• *for at least 3 months of 2 consecutive years?*	Characteristic of <u>chronic bronchitis</u>; bronchiectasis

2.1*a* Can you estimate the amount of your expectorations?

• 1 or 2 spits per day?	Reliable: very small amounts
• a teacupful per day?	Very large amounts
• *daily small quantities (usually mucoid)?*	Simple chronic bronchitis
• copious and purulent sputum?	Chronic mucopurulent <u>bronchitis</u>; bronchiectasis; lung abscess
• copious and clear secretions?	Alveolar cell carcinoma

3 Character of cough and/or expectorations

3.1 Do you have a chronic nonproductive cough?	Endobronchial tumor; extrinsic pressure on the trachea or on a bronchus; diffuse pulmonary infiltration or fibrosis; early heart failure with pulmonary congestion; nervous habit

3.1*a* Is the cough

• dry and persistent?	Pharyngitis
• "hacking": short, dry, often repeated?	Cough originating in the upper respiratory tract; chronic post-nasal drip
• dry, very irritating, often occurring in spasms?	Early symptom of left-heart failure
• "barking," harsh, painful?	Acute laryngitis; epiglottal involvement
• loud, "brassy"?	Tracheal or major airway involvement

• deep, "loose"?

Cough originating in bronchi or lung parenchyma: <u>acute bronchitis</u>; pneumonia (most dry coughs, if sufficiently prolonged, eventually become productive)

3.2 Does the cough occur
• in prolonged paroxysms
  • culminating in the production of sputum?

Chronic bronchitis

  • without expectorations?

In chronic bronchitis: exhausted patient abandons attempts to clear the bronchi of secretions ("unfinished cough"); asthma

3.3 In case of productive cough, is the sputum
• clear? white?

Mucoid sputum: viral infection; foreign substances (smoke, atmospheric pollution); any form of long-standing bronchial irritation; alveolar cell carcinoma (mucoid massive sputum)

• frothy and pink-tinged?

Pulmonary edema

• sometimes black, with soot particles?

Chronic bronchitis; coal miner's sputum may contain coal dust

• thick and yellowish, or greenish?

Purulent: infection in the tracheobronchial tree or lung; bronchiectasis; bacterial pneumonia; lung abscess; <u>chronic or recurrent mucopurulent bronchitis</u>

• gelatinous and rusty?

Pneumococcal pneumonia

• similar to currant jelly? tenacious?

Friedländer (*Klebsiella*) pneumonia (in only 25 to 50 percent of patients)

• containing threads?

Casts of the bronchial tree (inspissated mucus); bronchitis; bronchial asthma

• blood-streaked?

Tuberculosis; <u>bronchiectasis</u>; <u>lung tumor</u>

3.3*a* Is your expectoration difficult to eliminate?

Mucoid sputum is more viscous than purulent sputum and therefore often more difficult to cough up; asthma

3.4 Has your expectoration an offensive odor?

3.4*a* Does it taste or smell bad? ("rotten eggs")

Bronchiectasis; infection from fusospirochetal or anaerobic organisms; lung abscess

3.5 Do you cough and/or expectorate

• *mostly early in the morning?*

Accumulation of secretions during the night in the larynx and trachea: chronic bronchitis; bronchiectasis; chronic sinusitis

• all day?

Active and/or persistent underlying process

• at night?

Left-heart failure (dry cough); bronchial asthma

4 Precipitating or aggravating factors

4.1 Does the cough occur

• *with, or shortly after, ingestion of food?*

Tracheoesophageal fistula; hiatus hernia; esophageal diverticulum

• after exposure to irritant substances?

Causes of acute dry cough

4.2 Is your cough and/or sputum provoked or worsened by

• *a change in position?*

Localized area of bronchiectasis; lung abscess

• sudden changes in temperature?

Chronic bronchitis

• smoke? fumes or dust?

Bronchial irritants; chronic bronchitis

• exertion? laughter?

Chronic bronchitis: sudden increase in the depth of ventilation

4.2*a* Does the cough worsen during the night?

<u>Bronchiectasis</u>; chronic sinusitis with postnasal drip (pooled secretions)

5 *Relieving factors*

5.1 In case of nocturnal (and dry) cough, is it relieved
- *if you sit up? if you use more than one pillow?*

Pulmonary edema

6 *Accompanying symptoms*

6.1 Do you have
- fever? headaches? pain in your muscles?

Early symptoms of acute bronchitis or pneumonia (especially of viral origin)

- a sore throat? a running nose?

Upper respiratory infection

- night sweats?

Pulmonary tuberculosis

- chest pain?

Chest muscle pain associated with infection of the upper respiratory tract, with dry paroxysmal cough

-   *worsened by inspiration?*

Pleuritic pain: pneumonia; lung abscess; lung tumor with pleural involvement

- shortness of breath?

Chronic bronchitis with or without congestive heart failure; chronic asthma

-   *having preceded the chronic cough?*

Chronic obstructive lung disease, predominant emphysema

-   *having appeared after a long period of chronic cough?*

Chronic obstructive lung disease, predominant bronchitis

- a loss of weight?

<u>Bronchogenic carcinoma</u>; tuberculosis

• hoarseness?	Bronchogenic carcinoma involving the recurrent laryngeal nerve; laryngeal tumor; secondary laryngeal lesions in pulmonary excavated tuberculosis; viral laryngotracheobronchitis
• wheezing?	Acute or chronic bronchitis; asthma
• stridor?	Intrinsic or extrinsic **obstruction to the upper respiratory passages**
• loss of consciousness during a coughing fit?	"Cough syncope": in chronic bronchitis (in obese patients who smoke and drink heavily); also in neoplastic or vascular cerebral lesions

7   Environmental factors

7.1 Do you smoke? Do you inhale?	Heavy cigarette smokers are liable to chronic bronchitis and lung tumor
7.2 Have you ever • worked in a coal mine? uranium mine? • been exposed to beryllium? asbestos? rock dust? irritant substances?	Occupational chronic lung disease; (asbestosis and exposure to radioactive materials predisposes to bronchogenic carcinoma)
7.3 Do you have any pets? birds? pigeons?	Psittacosis
7.4 Have you ever been exposed to someone with tuberculosis?	

8   Personal antecedents pertaining to the complaint

8.1   Have you ever had a chest x-ray? a tuberculin skin test? a bronchoscopy? a bronchography? lung test? When? With what results?

8.2   Do you have

• frequent episodes of lung infection?	Chronic bronchitis; bronchiectasis; mitral stenosis; immunodeficiency diseases
• a heart condition?	Congestive heart failure with (nocturnal) cough
• allergy?	Bronchial asthma
• tuberculosis?	
• sinusitis?	A common accompaniment of diffuse bronchiectasis; may cause postnasal drip with cough

9   Family medical history pertaining to the complaint

9.1 Does anyone in your family have a lung disease?	In several members of a household: acute bronchitis of epidemic infectious origin; tuberculosis; mucoviscidosis; alveolar microlithiasis

PHYSICAL SIGNS PERTINENT TO THE COMPLAINT

Finding	**Possible** *significance*
Inspiratory stridor; wheezing	Laryngeal disease
Inspiratory and expiratory rhonchi	Tracheal and major airway involvement
Coarse, subcrepitant, crackling inspiratory rales	Involvement of terminal bronchioles; interstitial fibrosis and/or edema
Coarse rales altered by coughing	Secretions in the smaller airways; chronic bronchitis; bronchiectasis
Fine crepitant end-inspiratory rales	Fluid accumulation in alveoli: pneumonitis; pulmonary edema
Pharyngitis; normal chest examination	Upper respiratory infection
Fever; localized dullness; increased breath sounds; rales, wheezes	Bacterial and *Mycoplasma* infection

Prolonged expiration; hyperresonant lung fields; distant breath sounds; scattered rhonchi or wheezes	Chronic obstructive lung disease
Localized wheezing; atelectasis; supraclavicular lymphadenopathy; clubbing	Bronchogenic carcinoma
Fever; weight loss; posttussive crepitant rales; apical rales	Tuberculosis
Bilateral basilar moist rales; gallop rhythm; hepatomegaly; ankle edema	Congestive heart failure
Sinus tenderness	Chronic sinusitis accompanying bronchiectasis
Foul breath (halitosis)	Bronchiectasis; lung abscess

LABORATORY TESTS PERTAINING TO THE COMPLAINT

Procedure	*Finding*	*Diagnostic possibilities*
Sputum Gram's stain	Polymorphonuclear leukocytes	Infectious process
Acid-fast stain	Positive	Tuberculosis
Wright's stain	Eosinophilia	Asthma
Culture	Positive	Bacterial, mycoplasmal, fungal infection
Cytology	Positive	Bronchogenic carcinoma
Blood RBCs	Anemia	Lung cancer; tuberculosis; lung abscess

| WBCs | Leukocytosis | Infectious process |
| Cold agglutinin | Positive | Mycoplasmal pneumonia |

Pulmonary function tests

| Forced expiratory volume in 1 s/ vital capacity (FEV$_1$/VC) | Reduced | Chronic obstructive lung disease |
| | Normal or high | Restrictive lung disease |

Procedure	*To detect*
Chest x-ray ⎫ Tomography ⎭	Pneumonic lesion; tuberculosis; tumor; infiltrative lung disease; bilateral hilar adenopathy: sarcoidosis, lymphoma
Fiberoptic bronchoscopy with biopsy and/or brushing	Possible obstructed bronchus; carcinoma; foreign body; granulomatous lesions; lung abscess
Bronchography	Bronchiectasis; obstruction in distal bronchi; tracheobronchial distortion or malformation
ECG	Right ventricular strain pattern in chronic lung disease
Skin tests	Tuberculosis; histoplasmosis; coccidioidomycosis; blastomycosis
Mediastinoscopy*	Involvement of lymph nodes in the mediastinum
	Indications
Transtracheal puncture	Nonproductive cough; sputum contaminated by oropharyngeal flora or nonrepresentative of pulmonary secretions

* If appropriate.

USEFUL REMINDERS AND DIAGNOSTIC CLUES

Misleading Factors

Cough may be initiated by irritation of the external auditory meatus and outer aspect of the eardrum, which receives a nerve supply from the vagus.

It is risky to assume that the cough among cigarette smokers is due merely to cigarette smoking; the chest should be x-rayed to exclude underlying lesion.

Some patients deny cough while admitting to the presence of sputum, saying that they bring it up merely by "clearing the throat."

Female patients are inclined to swallow their sputum, even when it is being produced in large quantities. The character of the cough, if it is loose or moist, may indicate that sputum is present.

Diagnostic Considerations

Any changes in the character of a chronic "cigarette" cough may indicate bronchogenic malignancy, just as a change in bowel habit may indicate carcinoma of the colon.

Observation by the physician of the patient's sputum is mandatory.

Cough associated with a normal chest roentgenogram may occur in diseases of the:

Lung parenchyma (diffuse granulomatous and fibrotic diseases: sarcoidosis, scleroderma, diffuse interstitial fibrosis)

Pleura (acute pleuritis)

Airways (irritants, chronic bronchitis, asthma, partially obstructing endobronchial masses, acute tracheobronchitis, bronchiectasis, otorhinolaryngeal conditions).

SELECTED BIBLIOGRAPHY

Mitchell RS, Pierce JA: Cough, in Mac Bryde CM, Blacklow RS, *Signs and Symptoms,* 5th ed, chap 17, pp 328–336, Philadelphia: Lippincott, 1970

2
Cyanosis

DEFINITION AND PATHOPHYSIOLOGY

Cyanosis   a bluish discoloration of the skin, the mucous membranes, and nail beds resulting from an increased amount of reduced hemoglobin or of abnormal hemoglobin pigments in the blood and in the tissues of those areas.

Peripheral cyanosis is a result of diminished peripheral blood flow and vasoconstriction. Blood flow is slow, each red cell remains in contact with the tissue for a longer period, more oxygen is extracted from normally saturated arterial blood, and more unsaturated hemoglobin is present in the venous blood. Peripheral cyanosis is usually observed in peripheral tissues, central tissues such as the mucous membranes of the mouth or beneath the tongue being spared.

Central cyanosis is caused by arterial unsaturation. This results from impaired pulmonary function (alveolar hypoventilation, ventilation-perfusion abnormality, impaired oxygen diffusion), or from right-to-left shunts inside the heart (septal defect), between the great vessels (patent ductus arteriosus), or in the lungs. Cyanosis may also be produced by circulating abnormal hemoglobin derivatives (methemoglobin, sulfhemoglobin).

Cyanosis becomes apparent at a mean capillary concentration of 5 g reduced hemoglobin, 1.5 g methemoglobin, or 0.5 g sulfhemoglobin per 100 mL. In patients with severe anemia and marked arterial desaturation, cyanosis may be absent because the absolute amount of reduced hemoglobin is small. Conversely, patients with marked polycythemia will be cyanotic at higher levels of arterial oxygen saturation than patients with normal hemoglobin values.

ETIOLOGY

Peripheral cyanosis
Vasoconstriction: exposure to cold
Low cardiac output: congestive heart failure; shock

Peripheral vascular disease: arterial obstruction; venous obstruction
Acrocyanosis; livedo reticularis

Central cyanosis
Decreased arterial oxygen saturation
　Decreased atmospheric pressure: high altitude
　Impaired pulmonary function: alveolar hypoventilation; perfusion of nonventilated or underventilated lung; impaired diffusion of oxygen
　Anatomic right-to-left shunts: certain types of congenital heart disease (tetralogy of Fallot, patent ductus arteriosus); multiple small intrapulmonary shunts
Hemoglobin abnormalities (rare): methemoglobin (hereditary, acquired); sulfhemoglobin (acquired)

Iatrogenic Causes of Methemoglobin

Antipyretic drugs: acetanilid, phenacetin; benzocaine, lidocaine; chlorates; nitrites, nitrates; primaquine; quinones; certain sulfonamides: sulfathiazole, sulfapyridine (not sulfadiazine)

QUESTIONNAIRE

Possible *meaning of response*

1　Mode of onset and duration

1.1　Has the cyanosis been present since birth?

Congenital heart lesion, right-to-left shunt; hereditary methemoglobinemia (rare)

1.2　If the cyanosis has recently appeared, has the onset of the cyanosis been
　• acute (within hours)?

Severe respiratory infection; upper-airway obstruction by a foreign body; **massive pulmonary embolus; pneumothorax; cardiovascular collapse** (following myocardial infarction); **acquired methemoglobinemia**

• gradual? (weeks to months)	Severe (<u>chronic obstructive</u>) <u>lung disease</u>

2   *Location of cyanosis*

2.1   Is the cyanosis
• localized?	Peripheral cyanosis: decreased rate of blood flow
• to the lower limbs?	<u>Peripheral vascular disease</u>; "differential cyanosis" in patients with patent ductus arteriosus, pulmonary hypertension, and right-to-left shunt; livedo reticularis
• to the head, neck, and upper limbs?	Superior vena cava obstruction (bronchogenic carcinoma)
• to the hands and feet?	Acrocyanosis (without special age or sex incidence): constant, painless cyanosis
• generalized?	Central cyanosis; peripheral cyanosis: shock

3   *Precipitating or aggravating factors*

3.1   Does the cyanosis occur or worsen
• during exertion?	Congenital heart disease; central cyanosis due to arterial oxygen unsaturation: increased extraction of oxygen from the blood by the exercising muscles; diffuse pulmonary infiltration and fibrosis with diffusion abnormalities
• after ingestion of certain drugs?	Hereditary methemoglobinemia, heterozygous; acquired methemoglobinemia

3.1*a* Is the cyanosis present at rest? constant?

Central cyanosis due to arterial unsaturation; <u>cardiac failure</u>, low-output varieties; <u>chronic pulmonary lesion</u>: perfusion of nonventilated areas of the lung; congenital heart lesion, right-to-left shunt; hemoglobin abnormalities (rare)

3.2 In case of cyanosis located in the upper limbs, does it occur
- *in cold weather?*
- *when immersing the hands in cold water?*

Raynaud's disease or phenomenon: cyanosis may appear alone or follow initial pallor

4 *Accompanying symptoms*

4.1 Do you have
- headaches?

In methemoglobinemia: indicates concentrations of 20 to 50 percent methemoglobin

- shortness of breath?

<u>Chronic pulmonary disease</u>; <u>congestive heart failure</u> with peripheral cyanosis (may be secondary to a congenital heart disease)

- *relieved by squatting?*

Right-to-left shunts: tetralogy of Fallot

- a chronic cough? expectorations?

Central cyanosis due to impaired lung function, chronic obstructive lung disease, <u>chronic bronchitis</u>

- easy bruising?

In some patients with cyanotic congenital heart disease (high hematocrit, low fibrinogen concentration)

- intestinal, nose bleeding?
- bloody expectorations?

Hereditary hemorrhagic telangiectasia associated with pulmonary arteriovenous fistula

5   *Iatrogenic factors*   see Etiology

6   *Environmental factors*

6.1   Have you been
  • exposed to chemicals?
  • drinking well water?

Aniline dyes ⎫
May be high in ⎬ causing methe-
nitrates ⎭ moglobinemia

6.2   What is (was) your present (former) occupation?

Arc welders may inhale nitrous gases (methemoglobinemia secondary to industrial exposure to chemical is declining); occupational causes of chronic respiratory disease: silicosis, asbestosis, berylliosis; bagassosis

7   *Personal antecedents pertaining to the cyanosis*

7.1   Do you have
  • a cardiac condition?

Reduced cardiac output with peripheral cyanosis; congenital heart disease

  • chronic bronchitis? emphysema? asthma?

Central cyanosis due to impaired lung function: alveolar hypoventilation, perfusion of unventilated areas of the lung, impaired oxygen diffusion

  • a blood disease?

Polycythemia vera, or secondary to chronic pulmonary disease or congenital heart disease: contributes to, or may produce, cyanosis

8   *Family medical history pertaining to the complaint*

8.1   Do your parents also have skin with a bluish tint?

Hereditary methemoglobinemia associated with abnormal hemoglobin M (autosomal dominant trait)

8.1*a*   If not, do your siblings?

Reduced nicotinamide-adenine dinucleotide-methemoglobin reductase deficiency (recessive)

PHYSICAL SIGNS PERTINENT TO THE COMPLAINT

Finding	**Possible** *significance*
Bluish color of the skin and mucous membranes	Central cyanosis
Bluish color of the skin sparing mucous membranes	Peripheral cyanosis resulting from vasoconstriction and diminished peripheral blood flow: shock; congestive heart failure; cold exposure; peripheral vascular disease
"Red cyancsis"	Polycythemia vera: to be distinguished from true cyanosis
Cherry-red coloration of the skin	Carbon monoxide poisoning
Abnormal percussion; rales, wheezes	Severe lung disease with impaired pulmonary function and central cyanosis
Heart murmur	Cyanotic congenital heart disease with central cyanosis; tetralogy of Fallot
Cardiomegaly; distended jugular veins; hepatomegaly; edema	Severe congestive heart failure with low cardiac output, cutaneous vasoconstriction, and peripheral cyanosis
Telangiectases on skin and mucosae	Hereditary hemorrhagic telangiectasia with pulmonary arteriovenous fistulas
Cyanosis of an extremity with	
• coldness; absent pulses	Arterial obstruction with diminution in blood flow not sufficient to cause blanching of the skin
• edema; varicose veins; ulcers	Venous obstruction
Cyanosis and swelling of head, neck, upper extremities; superficial venous collateral vessels	Superior vena caval syndrome: bronchogenic carcinoma; primary mediastinal tumor; aneurysm

Clubbing   Central cyanosis; certain types
                                              of congenital cardiac disease;
                                              chronic pulmonary disease; lung
                                              abscess; pulmonary arteriove-
                                              nous shunts

LABORATORY TESTS PERTAINING TO THE COMPLAINT

Procedure	*Finding*	*Diagnostic possibilities*
Blood RBCs	Polycythemia	Secondary to arterial unsaturation in central cyanosis
Arterial oxygen tension (N*: 80 to 100 mmHg)	Normal Decreased	Peripheral cyanosis Central cyanosis
Arterial CO_2 tension (N: 35 to 45 mmHg)	Elevated	Central cyanosis due to chronic alveolar hypoventilation
Spectroscopic analysis of blood	Abnormal hemoglobin pigments	Methemoglobinemia; sulfhemoglobinemia
Pulmonary function tests FEV_3/VC	Reduced Normal or high	Chronic obstructive lung disease (COLD) Restrictive lung disease
Procedure	*To detect*	
Chest x-ray	Congenital heart diseases; pulmonary diseases; pulmonary arteriovenous fistula	
ECG	Congenital heart disease; right ventricular strain pattern in COLD	

Cardiac cathe- ⎫
terization   ⎬ Congenital heart disease; pulmonary arterio-
Pulmonary angi- ⎭ venous fistula
ography

* N = normal value.

USEFUL REMINDERS AND DIAGNOSTIC CLUES

Misleading Factors

Patients previously treated with silver salts may have a bluish skin (argyria), not to be confused with cyanosis.

In general, cyanosis is rarely recognized with confidence in white skins until the arterial saturation is 85 percent or less; in pigmented races, the arterial saturation has to drop far lower before one can be certain.

Livedo reticularis, a bluish mottling of the skin on the lower legs occurring predominantly in young females, should not be confused with cyanosis; it may be primary or secondary to systemic lupus erythematosus, polyarteritis nodosa, cryoglobulinemia, cholesterol embolization, Cushing's syndrome, or amantadine hydrochloride administration.

Diagnostic Considerations

If cyanosis is present when the patient is warm, it is more likely to be of central origin and not the result of reduced flow.

In many types of chronic pulmonary disease with fibrosis and obliteration of the capillary vascular bed, cyanosis is absent because of relatively little perfusion of underventilated areas.

Tetralogy of Fallot is the most common cyanotic heart defect seen in the adult. Approximately 70 percent of all cyanotic adults have a tetralogy of Fallot.

Cyanosis in congenital heart disease appears in patients with normal hemoglobin if the venous-arterial shunt exceeds 38 percent of the cardiac output of the heart.

Central cyanosis with arterial oxygen unsaturation may be observed in patients with cirrhosis (portopulmonary venous shunts or pulmonary arteriovenous shunts).

When cyanosis is not readily explained by malfunction of the circulatory or respiratory systems, abnormal hemoglobin derivatives should be suspected.

In case of	*Suspect*
Cyanosis without clubbing	Peripheral cyanosis; abnormal hemoglobin pigments; acutely developing central cyanosis
Clubbing without cyanosis	Subacute bacterial endocarditis; ulcerative colitis; occupational (jackhammer operators); lung cancer
Cyanotic patients who are "more blue than sick"	Hereditary methemoglobinemia

SELECTED BIBLIOGRAPHY

Braunwald E, Kahler RL, and Wintrobe MM: Cyanosis, hypoxia, and polycythemia, in Thorn GW et al (eds), *Harrison's Principles of Internal Medicine*, 8th ed, pp 170–176, New York: McGraw-Hill, 1977.

Lukas DS: Cyanosis, in Mac Bryde CM, Blacklow RS (eds), *Signs and Symptoms*, 5th ed, chap 20, pp. 358–368, Philadelphia: Lippincott, 1970

3
Dyspnea

DEFINITIONS AND PATHOPHYSIOLOGY

Dyspnea   the patient's subjective awareness of respiratory discomfort.

Tachypnea   increased rate of breathing.

Hyperpnea   increased depth of breathing.

Polypnea   rapid, shallow breathing.

Orthopnea   dyspnea that appears when the subject lies down and is relieved by sitting.

Platypnea   dyspnea assumed in the upright position and relieved by a recumbent one.

Dyspnea can be induced in healthy subjects by strenuous exertion and should be regarded as abnormal only when it occurs at rest or at a level of physical activity which would not normally be expected to cause respiratory discomfort.

As indicated by the above definition, dyspnea, i.e., difficult or painful breathing, is a subjective state. It includes different types of discomfort. The healthy subject who has just run 100 yd under 10 s, the cardiac patient after mild exertion, and the patient with emphysema will all complain of shortness of breath, but they are experiencing different sensations.

Dyspnea may be due to an increase in airway resistance, in the stiffness of the lung, in exercise ventilation, or, most commonly, to a combination of these factors. It can be viewed as an imbalance between the ventilating stimulus and the capacity to respond to the stimulus. It has been suggested that proprioceptive mechanisms in the respiratory muscles and thoracic cage create an awareness of disproportion between muscular effort and the level of ventilation produced.

Shortness of breath either during exercise or at rest is a common manifestation of many forms of pulmonary and cardiovascular disease. In the patient with obstructive lung disease (e.g., emphysema, asthma), the dyspnea is primarily related to the reduced capacity to respond to the ventilatory stimulus. In conditions where the lungs or thorax are stiffer than normal, dyspnea is a prominent symptom, because the inspiratory muscles have to develop greater tension to produce the same tidal volume. Dyspnea in pure left ventricular failure is primarily due to the increased stimulus from the congestion, which also causes some increase in stiffening of the lungs. The way in which breathlessness is described may have diagnostic value. Patients with obstructive lung disease generally complain about difficulty moving air in and out of the lungs. By contrast, patients with restrictive lung disease are short of breath on slight exertion. Patients may use the term "shortness of breath" when the discomfort is actually an abnormal awareness of breathing resulting from anxiety states.

ETIOLOGY

Table 3-1 Obstructive Disorders of the Lung (reduced VC with reduced FEV$_1$/VC ratio)

Upper-airway obstruction	*Lower-airway obstruction*
Acute	*Acute (or recurrent)*
Diphtheria	Asthma
Acute laryngopharyngitis	Inhalation of toxic vapors
Laryngeal edema (allergy)	Acute pulmonary embolism
Foreign-body aspiration	Carcinoid syndrome
Retained secretions	Polyarteritis nodosa
Retropharyngeal abscess	
Retraction of the tongue	
Laryngospasm (hypocalcemia)	
Chronic	*Chronic*
Tumor of larynx or trachea	Chronic bronchitis
Mediastinal tumor or nodes	Emphysema
Aortic aneurysm	Late complication of pulmonary
Scarring of trachea (from previous	fibrosis (pneumoconiosis, tuberc-
tracheostomy or trauma)	losis, sarcoidosis, scleroderma)

**Table 3-2   Restrictive Disorders of the Lung
(reduced VC with normal or high FEV$_1$/VC ratio)**

Interstitial lung diseases
Infection: bacterial (miliary tuberculosis), fungal, viral, parasitic
Diffuse interstitial fibrosis (Hamman-Rich syndrome); rheumatoid arthritis; scleroderma; idiopathic pulmonary hemosiderosis; sarcoidosis
Chemical and physical irritants:
   inorganic dusts: pneumoconiosis; asbestosis; berylliosis
   organic dusts: bagassosis; byssinosis
   chemical irritants (inhalational): silo-filler's lung; lipoid pneumonia; kerosene; phosgene; paraquat
   radiation
Diffuse alveolar diseases
Pulmonary edema
Pneumonia; uremic pneumonia
Pulmonary infarction; Goodpasture's syndrome
Alveolar proteinosis; lipoid pneumonia; desquamative interstitial pneumonia
Hypersensitivity: eosinophilic pneumonia; reactions to drugs; farmer's lung; bagassosis
Neoplastic: alveolar cell carcinoma; hematogenous metastatic malignancy; lymphangitic carcinomatosis; leukemia
Replacement of pulmonary parenchyma by nonventilating tissue
Atelectasis; bullae
Pneumonectomy
Compression of lung by space-occupying intrathoracic lesions: large tumors
Miscellaneous
Disorders of the pleura: pleural effusion; pleural fibrosis (with or without calcification); pneumothorax
Pericardial effusion

**Table 3-3   Neurologic, Chest-wall, and Respiratory-muscle Disorders
(restrictive pattern)**

Central nervous system: drug effect; infection and postinfection; trauma; primary or idiopathic alveolar hypoventilation (Ondine's curse)
Peripheral nervous system: amyotrophic lateral sclerosis; poliomyelitis; toxic neuropathy; infectious neuronitis (Guillain-Barré syndrome); miscellaneous severe neuropathies
Involvement of respiratory muscles: muscular dystrophy; amyotonia; myasthenia gravis
Thoracic cage limitations: kyphoscoliosis; obesity; trauma; surgery; ascites

Disorders of the heart and circulation:
    Congestive heart failure: left and right; pulmonary edema; multiple pulmonary emboli; mitral stenosis; aortic stenosis
    Congenital heart disease: tetralogy of Fallot; atrial or ventricular defects; patent ductus arteriosus
    Pericardial effusion
    Pulmonary hypertension

Miscellaneous:
    Psychogenic dyspnea (anxiety, neurosis); anemia; acidosis

Iatrogenic Causes of Dyspnea

Drug-induced pulmonary disease with dyspnea

Bleomycin	Hydrochlorothiazide	Narcotics overdose
Busulfan	Mecamylamine	Nitrofurantoin
Cyclophosphamide	Methotrexate	Oral contraceptives
Diphenylhydantoin	Methysergide	Penicillin
Hexamethonium	Mineral oil (nose	Pituitary snuff
Hydralazine	drops)	Sulfonamides

Drug-induced bronchoconstriction
Acetylsalicylic acid
Aerosolized drugs: cromoglycate disodium, isoproterenol; acetylcysteine
Propranolol

Drug-induced respiratory muscle paralysis

Colistin	Kanamycin	Polymyxin B
Gentamycin	Neomycin	Streptomycin

QUESTIONNAIRE

Possible *meaning of response*

1 Mode of onset

1.1 How long have you had shortness of breath?
    More than 5 months: (<u>COLD</u>); <u>left-heart failure</u>

1.2 Did the dyspnea appear
   • suddenly?

Pneumothorax; pulmonary embolism; pulmonary edema; bronchial asthma; pneumonia; **sudden occlusion of a major airway** (foreign body); **inhalation of noxious gases or fumes;** farmer's lung; hyperventilation

   • progressively?
      • over weeks or months?

Congestive cardiac failure; anemia; obesity; pregnancy; pleural effusion; tuberculosis; pericardial effusion; subacute occlusion of a major airway (tumor); Hamman-Rich syndrome

      • over months or years?

Chronic bronchitis and emphysema; pneumoconiosis; the pulmonary fibroses

1.2*a* If the onset was acute, what were you doing?

E.g., eating → foreign-body aspiration; straining at stool → pulmonary embolism

2 Character

2.1 Do you have any difficulty during
   • inspiration?
   • expiration?
   • inspiration and expiration?

Upper-airway obstruction
Lower-airway obstruction
Not specific

2.2 *Do you feel that you do not breathe in a sufficient quantity of air?*

Psychogenic dyspnea

2.3 Is the dyspnea
   • constant?

COLD; chronic static course of pneumoconiosis

   • variable?

Due to changes in bronchial secretions or the degree of bronchospasm: asthma; asthmatiform bronchitis

• continuous, with paroxysmal episodes?	Asthma; any chronic lung disease which is made worse by superimposed infection
• *paroxysmal, with asymptomatic intervals?*	<u>Bronchial asthma; psychogenic dyspnea</u>

2.3*a* What is the
  • frequency of the episodes?
  • duration of the episodes?

3 *Precipitating or aggravating factors*

3.1 Does the dyspnea occur

• *on exertion?*	Dyspnea only on exertion is strong evidence for organic disease: <u>early heart disease; COLD</u>; interstitial lung disease; anemia; obesity; pregnancy; pulmonary hypertension; <u>asthma</u>
• at rest?	**Pneumothorax;** bronchial **asthma; pulmonary edema; massive pulmonary embolism;** pneumonia; pleural effusion; **obstruction of airways;** <u>psychogenic dyspnea</u>
• *only at rest and not on exertion?*	Almost invariably psychogenic dyspnea (exception: spasmodic asthma)
• in erect position?	Platypnea: in severe COLD
• *when lying flat?*	Orthopnea: suggests the presence of organic disease: left-heart failure; may also occur in asthma and COLD (asthma may occur during the night)

3.2 Is the dyspnea aggravated by

• <u>atmospheric conditions?</u> smog? dusts? smoking?	All varieties of COLD

• cough? emotions? laughing?

Causing sudden variations in the level of pulmonary ventilation

3.3 In case of exertional dyspnea, are you short of breath when:

• running?

FEV_1: 45 to 60 percent

• walking up hills, climbing stairs, or walking fast on level ground?
• walking with people your own age on level ground?

FEV_1: 30 to 45 percent

Increasing severity of COLD or of left-heart failure or mitral valve disease

• walking more than 100 yd, on the level, at your own speed?

FEV_1: 20 to 30 percent

• washing or dressing?

FEV_1: <20 percent

4 *Relieving factors*

4.1 Is the dyspnea relieved by
• bronchodilators? corticosteroids?

Asthma

• digitalis? diuretics?

Left-heart failure

4.2 In case of orthopnea, is it relieved by
• *sitting up in bed?*
• *standing up?*

Left-heart failure

5 *Accompanying symptoms*

5.1 Is the dyspnea accompanied by
• wheezing?

Bronchial obstruction

• inspiratory?

Stridor: **upper-airway obstruction at larynx or above**

• inspiratory and/or expiratory?	Asthma; acute bronchitis
• fever?	Pneumonia; diffuse bronchiolitis; tuberculosis
• cough and/or expectorations?	COLD; acute infection; tuberculosis
• hemoptysis?	Tuberculosis; cancer; pulmonary infarction; pneumonia; acute bronchitis; bronchiectasis
• thoracic pain?	Could be **myocardial infarction** with congestive failure
• *increased when you take a deep breath?*	Pleuritic (or pericardial) involvement: pneumonia; pneumothorax; pulmonary infarction; lung tumor
• palpitations?	Cardiac arrhythmia with resultant congestive heart failure
• hoarseness?	Upper-airway obstruction; n. recurrens involvement in lung cancer
• *sighing?* anxiety? yawning? vertigo? tingling and/or numbness of the extremities or around the mouth?	Psychogenic dyspnea; hyperventilation
• swollen legs?	Congestive heart failure; deep-vein thrombosis
• blueness of your skin?	Cyanosis: COLD; venoarterial shunt
• difficulty swallowing?	Dysphagia: esophageal disease (e.g., scleroderma) with aspiration of foreign material
• pain in your joints?	Sarcoidosis; connective-tissue disorders; rheumatoid arthritis with "rheumatoid lung"; Caplan's syndrome
• diarrhea?	Carcinoid syndrome; parasitic disease of the lung; mucoviscidosis

6 *Iatrogenic factors*   see Etiology

7 *Environmental factors*

7.1 Do you <u>smoke</u>? Since when? How many cigarettes a day?

7.1*a* How long have you been smoking at your present rate?

Cigarette smoking is the most important predisposing factor to <u>chronic bronchitis</u> and is a major factor for squamous cell <u>tumors</u> of the lung

7.2 Have you ever
• worked in any mines?
• worked as a farmer?
• been exposed to asbestos? beryllium? sandblasting?

Inorganic and organic dust pneumoconioses

7.3 Do you have any pets? birds? pigeons?

Psittacosis; allergy to cat or dog dander

7.4 Have you ever lived in
• California? Arizona? Texas? Utah? New Mexico? Nevada?

Coccidioidomycosis

• Eastern and Midwestern US?

Histoplasmosis

7.5 Have you ever been exposed to someone with active tuberculosis?

8 *Personal antecedents pertaining to the complaint*

8.1 Have you ever had a chest x-ray? breathing tests? allergic skin tests? When? With what results?

8.2 Do you have any of the following conditions: emphysema? chronic bronchitis? asthma? allergy? tuberculosis? a past chest operation?

• a heart disease? hypertension?

Congestive heart failure

• repeated colds or bronchitis?

COLD; bronchiectasis; cystic fibrosis; immunologic deficiencies

- past radiation therapy to the chest?

  Pneumonitis and/or fibrosis in exposed area

- phlebitis?

  Pulmonary embolism

9   *Family medical history pertaining to the complaint*

9.1   Is there someone in your family with a pulmonary condition?

Tuberculosis; alpha-1-antitrypsin deficiency; mucoviscidosis

PHYSICAL SIGNS PERTINENT TO THE COMPLAINT

Finding	*Possible significance*
Stridor; retraction of the supra-clavicular fossae and intercostal spaces with inspiration	Acute upper-airway obstruction
Hypertension; abnormal heart sounds; heart murmurs; cardiomegaly; basilar moist rales	Cardiac origin of dyspnea: left ventricular failure
Distended jugular veins; hepatomegaly; edema; cardiomegaly; basilar moist rales; pleural effusion	Combined (right and left) congestive heart failure
Numerous bilateral moist rales; gallop rhythm; cardiomegaly	Acute left ventricular failure: pulmonary edema
Fever; tachypnea; localized dullness; increased tactile and vocal fremitus; bronchial breath sounds, rales, wheezes	Pulmonary signs of consolidation: bacterial pneumonia; lung abscess
Prolonged expiration; generalized wheezing and rhonchi	Obstruction of intrathoracic airways; asthma
Underweight patient; overinflated chest; prominent accessory muscles; hyperresonance; prolonged expiration; distant breath sounds; end-expiratory wheezes	Chronic obstructive lung disease, type A ("pink puffers"): emphysematous type

Plethoric patient; cyanosis at rest; prolonged expiration; well-heard breath sounds, rhonchi; right ventricular failure	COLD, type B ("blue bloater"): bronchitic type
Dullness to percussion; decreased fremitus; decreased to absent breath sounds; pleural friction rub in some cases	Pleural effusion
On affected side: **decreased chest movement; hyperresonance; decreased fremitus and breath sounds; tracheal deviation to the opposite side**	Pneumothorax
Deep-vein thrombosis; tachypnea; tachycardia; accentuation of the pulmonary second sound; gallop rhythm; rales; pleural friction rub	Pulmonary embolism and infarction (nonspecific signs)
On affected side: diminished chest movement; deviation of mediastinum toward the affected side; dullness to percussion; absent breath sounds	Atelectasis
Deformed chest; severe kyphoscoliosis; spondylitis; pectus excavatum	Thoracic cage abnormalities with hypoventilation
Neurologic or muscular disorder	Neuromuscular disease with weakness of respiratory muscles
Clubbing	Bronchial carcinoma; suppurative disease (pulmonary abscess; bronchiectasis); interstitial fibrosis; congenital heart disease
Nicotine stains on the fingertips	Prolonged excessive cigarette smoking

LABORATORY TESTS PERTAINING TO THE COMPLAINT

Procedure	Finding	Diagnostic possibilities
Blood		
Hematocrit	Increased ($>$ 50 percent)	Polycythemia secondary to chronic hypoxemia; e.g., COLD
WBCs	Increased	COLD with superimposed infection; bacterial pneumonia
	Eosinophilia	Asthma
Arterial oxygen tension (N: 80 to 100 mmHg)	Decreased ($<$ 75 mmHg)	Hypoxemia may be present in all pulmonary causes of chronic dyspnea
Arterial carbon dioxide tension (N: 35 to 45 mmHg)	Increased ($>$ 50 mmHg)	Hypercapnea: in COLD, predominant bronchitis
	Low to normal	Tachypnea in: COLD, predominant emphysema; interstitial lung disease
Alpha-1-globulin	Decreased	Alpha-1-antitrypsin deficiency
Sputum		
Gram's stain	Polymorphonuclear cells (PMNs)	Infection
Acid-fast stain	Positive	Tuberculosis
Wright's stain	Eosinophilia	Asthma
Culture	Positive	Bacterial, mycoplasmal, fungal infection
Cytology	Positive	Bronchogenic carcinoma

Pleural Fluid (PF)

$\dfrac{\text{PF protein}}{\text{Serum protein}}$ >0.5

Lactic dehydrog- >200 U
enase (LDH)

$\dfrac{\text{PF LDH}}{\text{Serum LDH}}$ >0.6

One or more of these three characteristics present: exudate: malignancy, tuberculosis, parapneumonic effusion, pulmonary infarction
None present: transudate: congestive heart failure, cirrhosis, nephrotic syndrome

Pulmonary function tests

Vital capacity (VC), liters†	Decreased	COLD; restrictive lung disease
Forced expiratory volume in 1 s (FEV₁), liters†	Markedly decreased	COLD
	Slightly decreased or N	Restrictive lung disease
FEV₁/VC (N: men: 66 to 77 percent; women: 74 to 82 percent)	Decreased	COLD
	N or high	Restrictive lung disease

† *Predicted normal values:*
Vital capacity (VC), liters:
 men: $(-0.020 \times \text{age, yr}) + (4.81 \times \text{height, m}) - 2.81$
 women: $(-0.022 \times \text{age, yr}) + (4.04 \times \text{height, m}) - 2.35$
Forced expiratory volume in 1 s (FEV₁), liters:
 men: $(-0.033 \times \text{age, yr}) + (3.44 \times \text{height, m}) - 1.00$
 women: $(-0.028 \times \text{age, yr}) + (2.67 \times \text{height, m}) - 0.54$

Procedure	*To detect*
Chest x-ray	Hyperinflation of the lungs, cor pulmonale: COLD
	Interstitial infiltrate: infiltrative lung disease
	Lobar consolidation: bacterial pneumonia
	Alveolar infiltrate, cardiomegaly: left ventricular failure
	Pneumothorax; pleural effusion; acute pulmonary embolism
ECG	Right axis deviation, P pulmonale, right ventricular strain pattern: chronic pulmonary

	disease; acute dyspnea in pulmonary embolism
Skin tests*	Tuberculosis; histoplasmosis; coccidioidomycosis; blastomycosis
Lung scan, ventilation/perfusion scan, pulmonary angiogram*	Pulmonary embolism; parenchymal lung disease
Fiberoptic bronchoscopy*	Tumors; granulomatous lesions
Bronchography*	Bronchiectasis; obstruction in distal bronchi; tracheobronchial distortion or malformation
Lung biopsy*	Type of diffuse infiltrative disease of the lungs

* If appropriate.

USEFUL REMINDERS AND DIAGNOSTIC CLUES

Misleading Factors

In patients with angina pectoris, shortness of breath may be closely linked to "tightness" in the chest; this combination of symptoms usually is associated with exertion and characteristically requires immediate complete cessation of activity, in contrast to dyspnea during exertion by patients with emphysema, which may allow continuance at a slower pace.

In Küssmaul respiration (metabolic acidosis: uremia, diabetes), the patient's minute ventilation may be greatly increased, yet the patient will be unaware of this augmentation.

Diagnostic Considerations

Chronic obstructive lung disease

Emphysematous type ("pink puffers")	*Bronchitic type ("blue bloaters")*
History of exertional dyspnea	History of cough and sputum production

Patient underweight	Patient overweight
Pink mucous membranes	Cyanosis at rest
Hematocrit less than 55 percent	Hematocrit greater than 55 percent
Chest x-ray: narrow cardiac shadow	Chest x-ray: cardiac enlargement
Pathology: panacinar emphysema prominent	Pathology: centriacinar emphysema prominent

In chronic bronchitis, dyspnea which develops during exertion almost invariably is preceded by a long history of cough and expectorations.

Early age of onset of emphysema suggests alpha-1-antitrypsin deficiency or mucoviscidosis.

Some patients with intrinsic asthma, nasal polyposis, and sinusitis are subject to violent attacks of asthma following the ingestion of aspirin.

Acute dyspnea with generalized wheezing does not necessarily imply asthma: it may be due to acute pulmonary embolism.

In interstitial lung disease, exertional dyspnea is present in the early stages and dyspnea may be present at rest in the advanced form of the disease.

Loss of consciousness or a swallowing disorder predisposes to aspiration pneumonia.

Functional dyspnea related to anxiety or tension is the most common cause of dyspnea and is said to occur in 10 percent of patients attending offices of internists.

In case of	*Suspect*
Persistent dyspnea in a digitalized patient in heart failure	Recurrent pulmonary embolism
Sudden onset of dyspnea in an ill patient or a postoperative patient	Pulmonary embolism

SELECTED BIBLIOGRAPHY

Burrows B, Hasan FM: *Abnormalities in Small Airways,* Disease-a-Month, Chicago, Year Book, July 1977

Ingram RH, Jr: Chronic bronchitis, emphysema, and chronic airway obstruction, in Thorn GW et al (eds), *Harrison's Principles of Internal Medicine,* 8th ed, pp 1355–1361, New York: McGraw-Hill, 1977

————, Braunwald E: Dyspnea and pulmonary edema, in ibid, pp 166–170

Rapaport E: Dyspnea: Pathophysiology and differential diagnosis. Progr Cardiovasc Dis 13:532–545, 1971

Williams MH, Jr (ed): Pulmonary disease. Med Clin North Am 61:1161–1408, 1977

4

Edema

DEFINITIONS AND PATHOPHYSIOLOGY

Edema swelling produced by an increase in the extravascular component of the extracellular fluid volume.

Ascites accumulation of fluid in the peritoneal cavity.

Anasarca gross generalized edema.

The movements of fluid between the plasma volume and the interstitial space are governed by (1) the gradient in hydrostatic pressure between the intravascular and interstitial spaces, and (2) the colloid oncotic pressure gradient resulting from the difference in protein concentration between plasma and interstitial fluid. At the arterial end of the microcirculation, hydrostatic pressure favors movement of fluid into the interstitial spaces against the osmotic pressures exerted by the plasma proteins. At the venous end of the capillary bed, fluid returns to the vascular compartment because the hydrostatic pressure falls below plasma oncotic pressure. (In addition, fluid is returned from the interstitial space into the vascular system by way of the lymphatic vessels.)

Localized edema Movement of plasma fluid into the interstitium may be caused by a localized increase in capillary permeability (due to chemical, bacterial, thermal, or mechanical agents) or by any localized increase in the capillary pressure (due to local obstruction in venous and lymphatic drainage).

Generalized edema In congestive heart failure, the increased venous pressure produces an elevated capillary hydrostatic pressure, promoting the formation of edema. The decreased cardiac output is associated with a decreased effective arterial blood volume and a decreased renal blood flow. Renin is released, angiotensin is produced, stimulating aldosterone release with resultant sodium retention. Vasopressin release is stimulated by diminished distention of volume receptors apparently located in the head and atria.

   In cirrhosis, effective arterial blood volume is diminished, probably as a consequence of splanchnic venous pooling, hypoalbuminemia, and diminished peripheral resistance. The increased portal venous pressure favors increased formation of intraperitoneal fluid (ascites). Hypoproteinemia causes a shift of plasma water into interstitial spaces, leading to generalized edema.

Hypoproteinemia resulting from protein loss (as in the nephrotic syndrome or in protein-losing enteropathy), or from nutritional deficiency, is associated with reduced oncotic pressure and increased fluid movement into the interstitium. This decreases plasma volume, and the kidney responds with salt and water retention.

Decreased glomerular filtration rate is usually not a major factor limiting sodium excretion until late in the disease. However, some causes of renal failure involve the renal vasculature and the glomeruli and impair sodium excretion early in their course.

ETIOLOGY

Generalized edema
Congestive heart failure; constrictive pericarditis
Nephrotic syndrome; acute glomerulonephritis; acute tubular necrosis
Cirrhosis
Hypoalbuminemia: malabsorption; protein-losing gastroenteropathies; malnutrition
Endocrine: myxedema; secondary hyperaldosteronism; Cushing's syndrome
Angioneurotic edema
Allergy; serum sickness
Toxemia of pregnancy
Idiopathic cyclic edema

Regional causes of edema of extremities
Acute cellulitis
Deep-vein thrombosis
Lymphatic obstruction: malignancy, resection of lymph nodes, irradiation
Lower extremities:
  Chronic venous insufficiency (postphlebitic syndrome)
  Gravitational: prolonged sitting or standing, pregnancy
  Pretibial myxedema
  Primary lymphedema; lipedema

Upper extremities: superior vena cava syndrome; thoracic outlet syndromes

Iatrogenic Causes of Edema of Lower Extremities

Antihypertensive drugs: guanethidine; hydralazine; reserpine; methyldopa; diazoxide
Anti-inflammatory drugs: phenylbutazone
Hormones: corticosteroids; estrogen; oral contraceptives; testosterone; aldosterone-like substances
Antidepressants, monoamine oxidase inhibitor type; carbenoxolone

QUESTIONNAIRE

Possible *meaning of response*

1 Location of edema

1.1 Where is the edema localized?	
• around the eyes? the face?	Nephrotic syndrome; acute glomerulonephritis; angioneurotic edema; hypoproteinemia; myxedema; trichinosis; constrictive pericarditis
• *the face, the neck, the upper arms?*	Superior vena cava syndrome (lung cancer)
• in an (upper or lower) extremity?	Venous thrombosis; lymphatic blockage (secondary lymphedema); cellulitis (may be uni- or bilateral)
• in the abdomen and legs?	Ascites: liver cirrhosis, congestive heart failure
• both legs?	Any cause of generalized edema; primary lymphedema (dorsum of feet)
• generalized edema?	Anasarca: nephrotic syndrome; congestive heart failure; cirrhosis; hypoproteinemia

2 Mode of onset and duration

2.1 In case of facial edema, has the edema appeared
- rapidly?

Angioneurotic edema; serum sickness; allergy

- gradually?

Nephrotic edema

2.2 In case of ascites and edema of the legs, has the ascites
- *appeared first?*

Cirrhosis; constrictive pericarditis

- *followed the edema of the legs?*

Cardiac or renal edema

2.3 In case of edema of lower limb(s), did the swelling occur
- suddenly?

Venous thrombosis; acute cellulitis; cyclic edema

- gradually?

Lymphedema; venous thrombosis; any cause of generalized edema

2.3a For how long has (have) your leg(s) been swollen?
- congenital?

Primary lymphedema (uni- or bilateral): Milroy's disease

- noticed in childhood?

Lipedema (bilateral; in girls)

- for years?

Repeated attacks of deep-vein thrombosis causing chronic edema; chronic lymphatic obstruction

3 Character of edema

3.1 In case of edema of both legs, is the edema
- symmetrical?

Systemic cause: cardiac, hypoproteinemia; lipedema

• asymmetrical?	Additional vascular or lymphatic factor; additional unilateral (pelvic) obstruction
• present or most pronounced in the evening?	Congestive heart failure; edema due to gravitation or dependency
• present all day?	Advanced stage of heart failure; hypoproteinemia; venous or lymphatic fibrosed edema

3.2 In case of generalized or localized edema, is the edema

• intermittent?	Angioneurotic edema; cyclic edema

4   Precipitating or aggravating factors

4.1 In case of generalized intermittent edema, does the edema occur

• after eating certain foods?	
• after an infection? an emotional stress?	Angioneurotic edema
• *with the menstrual periods?*	Idiopathic cyclic edema

4.2 In case of edema in the lower extremities, does the edema appear or worsen

• on prolonged standing?	Chronic venous insufficiency; cyclic edema; congestive heart failure
• at the end of the day?	Congestive heart failure; chronic venous insufficiency
• on prolonged sitting?	
• in hot weather?	Chronic venous insufficiency
• before or during the menstrual periods?	Cyclic edema

5 Relieving factors

5.1 In case of edema in the lower extremities, does the edema
- subside overnight?
- decrease by elevation of your legs?

Gravitational edema; chronic venous insufficiency; congestive heart failure

6 Accompanying symptoms

6.1 Has your weight increased?

Weight gain in excess of 1 kg/day almost invariably implies excess fluid retention

6.1a *Does your evening weight exceed your morning weight by more than 2 lb (1 kg)?*

Increased fluid retention; idiopathic cyclic edema

6.2 Do you have shortness of breath?

Congestive heart failure; **pulmonary edema;** pleural effusion; elevation of diaphragm due to ascites; **angioneurotic edema with laryngeal edema** (and stridor); **pulmonary embolism** secondary to deep-vein thrombosis

6.2a Has shortness of breath preceded the edema of the legs?

Edema due to poor function of left ventricle; mitral stenosis; cor pulmonale

6.3 Do you have
- a decrease in the volume of your urine?
- a smoky color of your urine?
- chronic diarrhea?

- abdominal pain?

Acute glomerulonephritis; congestive heart failure; cirrhosis
Acute glomerulonephritis

Malabsorption; protein-losing enteropathy with hypoproteinemia
Angioneurotic edema

6.4 In case of edema of lower extremities, do you have

• pain in your leg(s)?	Local cause of edema: acute cellulitis; lymphangitis; <u>acute thrombophlebitis</u>; ulcer (cardiac edema usually does not cause pain because the tissues stretch gradually)
• a red, warm, painful area on your leg?	Inflammation or hypersensitivity; acute <u>venous thrombosis</u>; lymphangitis
• leg ulcers? pigmentation, eczema, on the legs?	Past attacks of deep-vein thrombosis with <u>postphlebitic syndrome</u>; chronic venous insufficiency
• fever?	Acute lymphangitis; <u>venous thrombosis</u>

7 *Iatrogenic factors*   see Etiology

8 *Environmental factors*

8.1 What is your intake of beer? alcohol? wine?	Edema due to <u>cirrhosis</u>; alcoholic cardiomyopathy with heart failure; nutritional edema
8.2 Do you eat a particular kind of diet?	Possible nutritional deficiency with hypoalbuminemia and edema

9 *Personal antecedents pertaining to the edema*

9.1   Have you ever had liver, renal function tests? a chest x-ray? an ECG? When? With what results?

9.2   In case of edema of an extremtiy, have you ever had phlebitis? surgery to the extremity? irradiation of involved area or near the edematous area?

9.3   Do you have any of the following conditions: a cardiac condition? a high blood pressure? a kidney disease? a liver disease? allergy? varicose veins?

10 *Family medical history pertaining to the edema*

10.1 In case of edema of lower
extremities, does some-
one in your family have

• varicose veins? A positive family history is common

• "edema" of the legs? Lipedema

PHYSICAL SIGNS PERTINENT TO THE COMPLAINT

Finding	**Possible** *significance*
Generalized edema	
Cardiomegaly; gallop; basilar rales; distended jugular veins; hepatomegaly	Congestive heart failure
Jaundice; hepatomegaly; spider angiomas; palmar erythema; gynecomastia	Edema of hepatic origin; cirrhosis
Severe malnutrition	Edema of nutritional origin
Paradoxical pulse	Pericardial tamponade; occasionally in constrictive pericarditis; severe pulmonary disease with airway obstruction
Friction rub; distant heart sounds; pulsus paradoxus; distended jugular veins; hepatosplenomegaly; ascites, edema	Pericardial effusion; pericardial constriction (murmurs are usually absent)
Localized edema	
Facial edema	Constrictive pericarditis; allergic reaction; angioneurotic edema; nephrotic syndrome; myxedema; trichinosis
Edema and cyanosis of head, neck, upper extremities; dilated venous collaterals over upper portion of chest and abdomen	Superior vena caval obstruction: bronchogenic carcinoma; mediastinal lymphoma; aneurysm of the aorta

Edema of one leg; edema of one or both arms	Venous and/or lymphatic obstruction
Symmetrical edema in the lower extremities	Systemic cause: cardiac, hypoproteinemia; lipedema
Asymmetrical edema in the lower extremities	Additional vascular or lymphatic factor; unilateral pelvic obstruction
Ulceration, pigmentation of the skin on the legs	Past attacks of deep-vein thrombosis with postphlebitic syndrome; chronic venous insufficiency
Localized edema with red, warm, tender area; fever	Inflammation or hypersensitivity; acute venous thrombosis; cellulitis; lymphangitis
Swollen leg with local cyanosis	Venous obstruction

LABORATORY TESTS PERTAINING TO THE COMPLAINT

Procedure	*Finding*	*Diagnostic possibilities*
Urine Proteinuria	Absent	Liver disease; protein-losing enteropathy; malnutrition
	Slight to moderate	Congestive heart failure; renal disease
	Heavy (> 4 g/24 h)	Nephrotic syndrome
Sediment	RBCs, RBC casts, proteinuria	Acute glomerulonephritis
Blood BUN, creatinine	Elevated	Acute glomerulonephritis; congestive heart failure with renal hypoperfusion

Liver function tests	Abnormal	Cirrhosis of liver
Serum proteins	Hypoalbuminemia (< 2.5 g/100 mL)	Nephrotic syndrome; cirrhosis; severe malnutrition; protein-losing enteropathy
Cholesterol, other lipids	Elevated	Nephrotic syndrome
Thyroid function tests	Abnormal	Myxedema
Venous pressure (antecubital: N: 70 to 140 mmH$_2$O)	Normal	Cirrhosis
	Elevated	Congestive heart failure; chronic constrictive pericarditis; obstruction of superior vena cava

Procedure	*To detect*
Chest x-ray	Cardiomegaly, pulmonary edema: congestive heart failure; pericardial effusion Calcifications: constrictive pericarditis
ECG	Myocardial ischemia and/or arrhythmias with congestive heart failure; pericarditis; myocarditis; cardiomyopathies
Echocardiography	Pericardial effusion
Fecal excretion of ^{51}Cr*	Protein-losing enteropathy

* In case of hypoalbuminemia with normal liver function tests and normal urinalysis

USEFUL REMINDERS AND DIAGNOSTIC CLUES

Misleading Factor

Excess fluid retention may occur without a gain in weight, because of concomitant malnutrition or excessive kidney or bowel loss of protein.

General Considerations

In an adult of average size without increased capillary permeability or urinary loss of protein, the presence of generalized edema implies a weight gain of at least 5 kg.

Pitting edema is virtually never seen in the presence of pure water excess.

Edema is generally accompanied by secondary aldosteronism; it is absent in primary aldosteronism.

Diagnostic Considerations

Pitting edema of the arms and face occurs rarely and only late in the course of heart failure.

In the rare types of cardiac diseases, such as tricuspid stenosis and constrictive pericarditis, in which orthopnea may be absent and the patient may prefer the recumbent posture, the factor of gravity may be equalized and facial edema observed.

Absence of proteinuria is evidence against (but does not exclude) either cardiac or renal disease as a cause of edema.

Unilateral edema occasionally results from cerebral lesions affecting the vasomotor fibers on one side of the body; paralysis also reduces lymphatic and venous drainage on the affected side.

In case of	*Suspect*
Painless swelling of an extremity in an elderly male	Carcinoma of the prostate
Recurrent thrombophlebitis of either superficial cr deep vein	Visceral carcinoma (body or tail of pancreas, lung)
Ascites and edema of the legs without dyspnea and	
with distended neck veins	Constrictive pericarditis
without distended neck veins	Cirrhosis of liver

SELECTED BIBLIOGRAPHY

Braunwald E: Edema, in Thorn GW et al (eds): *Harrison's Principles of Internal Medicine*, 8th ed, pp 176–182, New York: McGraw-Hill, 1977

Cannon PJ: The kidney in heart failure. N Engl J Med 296:26–32, 1977

Johnson DH, Pflug J: *The Swollen Leg: Causes and Treatment*, London: Heinemann, 1975

5
Heart Murmurs

DEFINITIONS AND MECHANISMS OF PRODUCTION

Murmur   any prolonged sound produced by the heart and blood vessels.

Organic murmur   due to anatomic abnormalities within the heart or central circulation.

Physiologic murmur   related to altered function within an anatomically normal heart.

Normal blood flow is laminar and produces no audible murmur. Cardiac murmurs are attributed to vibrations arising in the heart or great vessels as a result of turbulent blood flow and/or the formation of eddies and bubbles. This occurs when the rate of blood flow is increased, when blood is propelled vigorously across a valvular or vascular constriction or into a dilated vessel, or when there is regurgitation, as in valvular insufficiency.

Systolic murmurs may be classified as (1) ejection murmurs (aortic and pulmonic stenosis), occurring predominantly in midsystole and related to a disproportion between blood flow and the size of the orifice which it traverses; and (2) regurgitant pansystolic murmurs (mitral and tricuspid insufficiency), involving two chambers which have widely different pressures throughout systole. Late systolic murmurs are attributed to papillary muscle dysfunction caused by infarction or ischemia of these muscles.

Early diastolic murmurs (aortic or pulmonic regurgitation) are due to a regurgitant flow of very high velocity. Middiastolic murmurs (mitral stenosis) usually arise from the auriculoventricular valves and are due to disproportion between valve orifice size and flow rate.

Continuous murmurs depend on a continuous blood flow from a chamber or vessel of higher pressure to one of lower pressure, such pressure difference persisting in diastole as well as systole (patent ductus arteriosus).

ETIOLOGY

Table 5-1   Systolic Murmurs

Apex and left lower sternal border	Right second interspace	Left second interspace
Mitral regurgitation (chronic rheumatic heart disease)	Aortic stenosis	Pulmonary stenosis
Ventricular septal defect	Aortic sclerosis	Atrial septal defect
Mitral valve prolapse	Hypertension	Idiopathic dilatation of pulmonary artery
Papillary muscle dysfunction	Bicuspid aortic valve	Partial anomalous pulmonary venous return
Idiopathic hypertrophic subaortic stenosis	Aortic dilatation	
Tricuspid regurgitation	Aortic aneurysm	Physiologic murmur
Aortic stenosis (transmitted)	Aortic regurgitation (severe)	
	Carotid bruit	
	Mitral regurgitation (transmitted)	

Table 5-2   Diastolic Murmurs

Apex	Base (right and left second interspace)
Mitral stenosis (chronic rheumatic heart disease)	Aortic regurgitation
Mitral regurgitation (diastolic flow murmur)	Pulmonary regurgitation
Aortic regurgitation (transmitted)	Diastolic component of continuous murmur (transmitted)
Aortic regurgitation with Austin Flint murmur	
Tricuspid stenosis	
Atrial septal defect ⎫ increased	
Ventricular septal defect ⎬ pulmonary	
Patent ductus arteriosus ⎭ blood flow	
Lutembacher's syndrome	
Atrial myxoma	

Table 5-3 Aortic and Mitral Regurgitation

Aortic	*Mitral*
Rheumatic aortic regurgitation	Rheumatic valvulitis
Syphilitic aortic regurgitation	Papillary muscle rupture or dysfunc-
Bacterial endocarditis	tion (ischemic heart disease)
Arteriosclerosis	Ruptured mitral chordae tendinosae
Aortic dilatation	Secondary to left ventricular
Ascending aortic aneurysm	dilatation
Severe systemic hypertension	Bacterial endocarditis
Cystic medial necrosis of aorta	Calcified mitral annulus fibrosis
(Marfan's syndrome, Hurler's	Idiopathic hypertrophic subaortic
syndrome)	stenosis
Congenital defects (bicuspid aortic	Floppy-valve syndrome
valve)	Congenital defects (endocardial
Aortic stenosis and regurgitation	cushion defect, Marfan's syn-
Ankylosing spondylitis, rheumatoid	drome, Ehlers-Danlos syn-
arthritis	drome)
Trauma	

QUESTIONNAIRE

Possible *meaning of response*

1 Mode of onset and evolution

1.1 How long have you known that you have a heart murmur?

From birth and childhood: congenital heart disease; congenital aortic regurgitation; idiopathic hypertrophic subaortic stenosis (IHSS)

1.2 How was it detected?
  • during a routine examination?
  • because of health complaints?

1.3 How long have you known that you have a heart murmur without having any complaint?	Patients with mitral regurgitation, aortic stenosis, and aortic regurgitation remain relatively asymptomatic for 10 to 20 years; in rheumatic mitral stenosis, symptoms usually become apparent in young adulthood; mitral regurgitation is the best tolerated of all valvular diseases
1.4 *Was the heart murmur detected during an acute episode of chest pain?*	Angina pectoris with mitral regurgitation occurring during transient periods of ischemia involving a papillary muscle

2 *Accompanying symptoms*

2.1 Do you have • shortness of breath?	Dyspnea is the earliest manifestation of mitral stenosis, mitral regurgitation, aortic stenosis
• at rest?	Severe heart failure; congenital cyanotic heart disease
• on exertion?	Mitral stenosis: increased cardiac output and tachycardia of exercise with elevation of left atrial pressure, pulmonary venous hypertension, and increased lung stiffness; aortic stenosis and regurgitation: elevation of the left ventricular end-diastolic, mean left atrial, and pulmonary capillary pressures
2.1a How long have you had shortness of breath on exertion?	Dyspnea beginning in early adulthood: mitral stenosis; in late adulthood (age 55 to 60): aortic stenosis or regurgitation

2.2   Do you have
   • chest pain?

May occur in severe mitral stenosis: may be due to pulmonary hypertension or myocardial ischemia; in aortic regurgitation: may be due to excessive cardiac pounding on the chest wall and/or myocardial ischemia

   • on exertion?

Angina pectoris: in one-third of patients with aortic stenosis; ischemic heart disease; pulmonary hypertension; aortic regurgitation

   • palpitations?

An early complaint in aortic regurgitation; atrial fibrillation in mitral stenosis

   • swollen legs?

Congestive heart failure: late symptom in mitral regurgitation

   • syncope
      • *on exertion?*

Occurs in 10 to 20 percent of patients with aortic stenosis: due to decline in arterial pressure caused by vasodilatation in the exercising muscles in the face of a fixed cardiac output or to transient arrhythmia; primary pulmonary hypertension; IHSS

      • *with alterations in position?*

Atrial ball-valve thrombus in mitral stenosis obstructing the stenotic mitral valve; left atrial myxoma

   • a dry cough?

Aortic aneurysm impinging on the trachea or bronchi

   • bloody expectorations?

Hemoptysis: in mitral stenosis: rupture of pulmonary-bronchial venous connections or atrial fibrillation with pulmonary infarction

   • hoarseness?

Compression of recurrent laryngeal nerve by an aneurysm of the aorta

• difficulty in swallowing?

Dysphagia: compression of the esophagus by a dilated left atrium of mitral stenosis, an aneurysm of the aorta

• pain in the back? the joints?

Aortic regurgitation may be associated with ankylosing spondylitis and rheumatoid arthritis; bacterial endocarditis with arthralgia; acute rheumatic carditis

• *episodes of facial flushes? diarrhea? wheezing?*

Carcinoid syndrome with tricuspid regurgitation or pulmonic stenosis

• *fever?* sweating? weight loss?

Subacute bacterial endocarditis superimposed on normal or abnormal valves; acute rheumatic carditis; atrial myxoma

• frequent episodes of bronchitis?

Pulmonary infections commonly complicate mitral stenosis

2.3 Do you feel tired?

Early symptom in mitral regurgitation (low cardiac output); severe heart failure; subacute bacterial endocarditis; anemia with functional murmur

3 Personal antecedents pertaining to the heart murmur

3.1 Have you ever had a chest x-ray? an ECG? a cardiac catheterization? When? Where? With what results?

3.2 Have you ever had
• rheumatic fever? "growing pains"?
• St Vitus' dance? (chorea)

Acute rheumatic fever producing chronic rheumatic heart disease; such a history is elicited in two-thirds of the patients with mitral stenosis

3.2a How long after the episode of rheumatic fever was the murmur heard?

The murmur of mitral regurgitation is commonly heard during or soon after the acute rheumatic episode, in contrast to the relatively late development of the murmur of mitral stenosis

3.3 Have you ever had
  • a trauma to the heart?   Traumatic aortic regurgitation
  • a myocardial infarction?   Functional mitral regurgitation; papillary muscle dysfunction

3.4 Have you recently had dental extractions? urologic manipulations?   Subacute bacterial endocarditis (SBE) may be superimposed on rheumatic heart disease; SBE is rare in pure mitral stenosis but is not uncommon in combined mitral stenosis and regurgitation

3.5 Do you have
  • arterial hypertension?   Functional mitral regurgitation; ischemic heart disease; aortic dilatation in the elderly

  • a venereal disease?   Syphilitic aortic regurgitation

4 Family medical history pertaining to the heart murmur

4.1 Does someone in your family have a cardiac disease?   Familial form of IHSS represents 50 percent of the disease

PHYSICAL SIGNS PERTINENT TO THE COMPLAINT

Intensity of Heart Murmurs
Grade 1   very faint, just audible
Grade 2   faint, soft
Grade 3   moderately loud
Grade 4   very loud
Grade 5   extremely loud
Grade 6   exceptionally loud, audible without a stethoscope

Finding	**Possible** *significance*
Murmur accentuated during inspiration	Murmur arising on the right side of the heart

Murmur changing with the body position	Atrial ball-valve thrombus; atrial myxoma
Crescendo middiastolic murmur at the apex, opening snap, loud first sound	Mitral stenosis
Blue-tinged facies; malar flush	Advanced cases of mitral stenosis
Holosystolic murmur maximum at apex, radiating to axilla, soft first sound	Mitral regurgitation
Crescendo-decrescendo aortic ejection systolic murmur ending before the second heart sound, faint or absent second aortic sound; slow-rising peripheral arterial pulse	Aortic stenosis
Decrescendo diastolic murmur at the base and along the left sternal border; elevated systolic pressure; depressed diastolic pressure; water-hammer pulse; capillary pulsations; to-and-fro murmur over compressed femoral arteries	Aortic regurgitation
	Duroziez's sign
Apical systolic click; mid- to late systolic murmur; slender body habitus	Mitral valve prolapse syndrome
Systolic murmur, left second interspace; wide split of second sound unaffected by inspiration	Atrial septal defect
Systolic murmur over the precordium, loudest along the left sternal border	Ventricular septal defect
Continuous murmur in interscapular region; hypertension; *blood pressure lower in the legs than in the arms*	Coarctation of the aorta

Continuous machinery murmur; wide pulse pressure	Patent ductus arteriosus
Hypertension	Causing cardiomegaly with functional mitral regurgitation; ischemic heart disease; aortic dilatation in the elderly
Cyanosis	Congenital cyanotic heart disease; congestive heart failure with peripheral cyanosis
Systolic hepatic pulsations	Tricuspid regurgitation
Fever	Subacute bacterial endocarditis; acute flare-up of the rheumatic process; atrial myxoma
Anemia	Subacute bacterial endocarditis; atrial myxoma
Fever; petechiae; splinter hemorrhages; Osler's nodes (pulp of the fingers); splenomegaly; systemic emboli; anemia	Subacute bacterial endocarditis (systemic emboli may occur in left atrial myxoma)

LABORATORY TESTS PERTAINING TO THE COMPLAINT

Procedure	*To detect*
Phonocardiogram	Precise timing of cardiac sounds and murmurs; configuration and frequency composition of cardiac murmurs
Chest x-ray	Straightening of left-heart border, left atrial enlargement, prominence of the pulmonary arteries, Kerley B lines, mitral valve calcifications: mitral stenosis
	Left atrial and left ventricular enlargement, pulmonary congestion: mitral regurgitation
	Left ventricular hypertrophy, calcified aortic valve, dilated ascending aorta: aortic stenosis

	Left ventricular enlargement, dilated aortic root: aortic regurgitation
	Increased pulmonary vascularity with right ventricular enlargement: atrial septal defect
	Increased pulmonary vascularity with left atrial and left ventricular enlargement: ventricular septal defect
	Decreased pulmonary vascularity: tetralogy of Fallot; primary pulmonary hypertension
ECG	Left atrial enlargement, right ventricular hypertrophy, right axis deviation: mitral stenosis
	Left ventricular hypertrophy, left atrial enlargement: mitral regurgitation
	Left ventricular hypertrophy: aortic stenosis; aortic regurgitation
	Atrial fibrillation: mitral stenosis; mitral regurgitation
Echocardiogram	Mitral stenosis; prolapsing mitral valve; idiopathic hypertrophic subaortic stenosis; atrial myxoma; congenital cardiac diseases; pericardial effusion
Cardiac catheterization* Angiocardiography*	Nature and severity of a mechanical valvular defect (in anticipation of surgery); type of congenital heart disease

* If appropriate.

USEFUL REMINDERS AND DIAGNOSTIC CLUES

General Consideration

Diastolic murmurs are rarely heard in the absence of organic heart disease.

Mitral Stenosis

Mitral stenosis is the most common single valvular lesion to follow acute rheumatic fever, accounting for over half the patients with chronic rheumatic heart disease.

About two-thirds of the patients with mitral stenosis are female.

Silent mitral stenosis should be suspected in every patient with signs and symptoms of pulmonary hypertension.

Mitral Regurgitation

Mitral regurgitation occurs more frequently in men than in women by a factor of 3:2.
The presence of aortic valve disease associated with mitral regurgitation favors a rheumatic cause.

Aortic Regurgitation

Approximately 70 percent of all patients with pure or predominant aortic regurgitation are males; females predominate among patients with aortic regurgitation who have associated mitral valve disease.
A hypertensive patient who suddenly develops free aortic regurgitation may have ruptured a cusp.

Aortic Stenosis

About 80 percent of adult patients with symptomatic valvular aortic stenosis are male.
During the first two decades, aortic stenosis is usually due to congenital abnormality of the cusps or of the outflow tract of the left ventricle. Between the ages of 30 and 50, the usual cause is rheumatic fever. In elderly persons, degenerative distortion of the valves predominates.

SELECTED BIBLIOGRAPHY

Barondess JA: Aortic regurgitation, in Barondess JA (ed), *Diagnostic Approaches to Presenting Syndromes*, pp. 24–78, Baltimore: Williams & Wilkins, 1971

Fortuin NJ, Kelly DT, and Ross RS: Cardiac murmurs and other manifestations of valvular and cyanotic congenital heart disease, in Harvey AM et al (eds): *The Principles and Practices of Medicine*, 19th ed, pp 272–297. New York: Appleton-Century-Crofts, 1976

O'Rourke RA and Braunwald E: Physical examination of the heart, in Thorn GW et al (eds), *Harrison's Principles of Internal Medicine*, 8th ed, pp. 1131–1138, New York: McGraw-Hill, 1977

Roberts WC, Perloff JK: Mitral valvular disease. Ann Intern Med 77:939–975, 1972

6
Hemoptysis

DEFINITION AND GENERAL CONSIDERATIONS

Hemoptysis expectoration of sputum either streaked or grossly contaminated with blood.

Bleeding from the lungs and bronchi is influenced by the degree of aeration and the presence of mucus and pus. Hemoptysis in tuberculosis may be due to ulceration of the bronchial mucosa or slough of a caseous lesion; it is usually minor in degree, but massive hemorrhage occasionally occurs when a vessel is eroded. In severe pulmonary edema caused by acute left ventricular failure, the frothy fluid that pours from the bronchial tree is often blood-tinged, owing to the escape of red cells into the alveoli from the congested vessels of the lungs. In mitral stenosis, hemoptysis is caused by rupture of dilated endobronchial vessels which appear to form collateral channels between the pulmonary and bronchial venous systems; it tends to occur most frequently in patients who have elevated left atrial pressure without marked elevation of the pulmonary vascular resistance. Hemoptysis in pulmonary thromboembolism is present only when infarction, with necrosis and hemorrhage into the alveoli, has occurred. In lung carcinoma, hemoptysis of bright red blood or "rusty" sputum may be due to vascular invasion or to pneumonia developing behind the tumor. In bronchiectasis, bleeding from the lungs may result from necrosis of the mucosa or rupture of pulmonary-bronchial venous connections.

ETIOLOGY

Infections: tuberculosis; bronchiectasis; lung abscess; pneumonia; acute bronchitis; fungus infections (aspergillosis); psittacosis
Neoplasms: bronchogenic carcinoma; bronchial adenoma; miscellaneous rare tumors
Cardiovascular lesions: pulmonary infarction; left ventricular failure;

mitral stenosis; primary pulmonary hypertension; arteriovenous malformations; hereditary telangiectasia; polyarteritis nodosa; Goodpasture's syndrome; Wegener's granulomatosis; pulmonary hemosiderosis; intrabronchial leakage of an aortic aneurysm

Miscellaneous: hemorrhagic diseases (purpura, leukemia, hemophilia); anticoagulant therapy; broncholith; foreign body; congenital cystic disease; lung contusion; hydatid cyst

**Table 6-1   Incidence of Hemoptysis
(combined medical-surgical series)**

	Percentage
Bronchiectasis	30
Carcinoma	20
Bronchitis	15
Tuberculosis and other infections	10–20
Others	10
Undiagnosed	5–15

Iatrogenic Causes of Hemoptysis

Oral anticoagulants, heparin
Immunosuppressive drugs (with thrombocytopenic purpura)
Contraceptive pills (deep-vein thrombosis with pulmonary infarction)

QUESTIONNAIRE

Possible *meaning of response*

1   Duration

1.1   How long have you noticed the presence of blood in your sputum?

Recent onset in a male smoker over 40: <u>bronchogenic carcinoma</u>; chronic process: <u>bronchiectasis, chronic bronchitis</u>; chronic recurrent in a young (otherwise normal) female: bronchial adenoma

2 *Amount of blood coughed up*

2.1 Can you give an estimate of the amount of blood?

Most patients tend to exaggerate the amount of blood coughed up

2.2 Do you have
- slight, persistent bleeding?

Of recent onset: <u>bronchogenic carcinoma</u>

- recurrent episodes of minor bleeding?

<u>Bronchiectasis</u>; endobronchial <u>tuberculosis; mitral stenosis</u> (bleeding from the deep respiratory tract usually recurs over a period of several hours or days)

- large amounts of blood coughed up?

<u>Pulmonary infarction</u>; bleeding within a tuberculous cavity; upper lobe bronchiectasis; Goodpasture's syndrome

3 *Character of hemoptysis*

3.1 Is the sputum
- streaked with blood?

Chronic bronchitis; bronchogenic carcinoma

- intimately mixed with blood?

Bronchogenic carcinoma; lung abscess

- "rusty"?

Pneumococcal pneumonia (due to degradation products of hemoglobin)

- blood mixed with pus?

Pneumonia; bronchiectasis; lung abscess

- frankly bloody? (without mucus or pus)

Pulmonary thromboembolism; mitral stenosis; bronchiectasis (upper lobes); tuberculosis (usually bright red)

- *bright red and frothy?*

Blood from the lung (vomiting of blood excluded); pulmonary edema

- at first red and becoming progressively darker for 24 to 48 h?

Prolongation of hemoptysis; common in <u>pulmonary infarction</u>

• brown? • mixed with food particles?	Vomiting of blood from the stomach rather than hemoptysis from the lung

4 Precipitating or aggravating factors

4.1 Has hemoptysis occurred after

• nausea? vomiting? retching?	Suggests hematemesis rather than hemoptysis
• coughing?	Hemoptysis from the trachea, the bronchi, or the lung occurs typically after cough; violent coughing could cause hemoptysis

5 Accompanying symptoms

5.1 Do you

• cough? • expectorate?	The blood is usually mixed to some extent with sputum
• clear? gray sputum?	Chronic obstructive lung disease
• yellowish-green sputum?	Purulent: lung infection; lung abscess
• for days to weeks?	Acute bronchitis; pneumonia; tuberculosis; bronchogenic carcinoma
• for months to years?	Chronic productive cough: bronchiectasis; chronic bronchitis

5.2 Do you have

• chest pain? • of sudden onset? • *worse by inspiration?*	Pleural involvement: pulmonary infarction, bronchogenic carcinoma; pneumonia
• fever? (chills?)	Pulmonary infection: pneumonia; lung abscess; tuberculosis
• night sweats?	Tuberculosis
• shortness of breath?	Mitral stenosis; chronic bronchitis; pulmonary infarction; bronchogenic carcinoma

• palpitations?	Pulmonary infarction, pneumonia, with tachycardia
• irregular heartbeat?	Atrial fibrillation with pulmonary thromboembolism
• hoarseness?	Bronchogenic carcinoma; tuberculous laryngitis
• a loss of weight?	Bronchogenic carcinoma; tuberculosis; lung abscess
• a swollen, painful leg?	Deep-vein thrombosis with pulmonary thromboembolism

6 *Iatrogenic factors* see Etiology

7 *Environmental factors*

7.1 Do you smoke?	The heavy smoker is liable to chronic obstructive lung disease, bronchogenic carcinoma
7.2 Have you recently been exposed to a person with tuberculosis?	
7.3 Have you ever worked in a coal mine?	Pneumoconiosis
7.4 Do you have any birds? pigeons?	Psittacosis
7.5 Have you ever lived in	
• the Southern United States? California? Arizona? Texas?	Coccidioidomycosis (hemoptysis infrequent)
• Eastern and Midwestern United States? Mississippi Valley?	Histoplasmosis (blastomycosis: anywhere in the United States)

8 *Personal antecedents pertaining to the hemoptysis*

8.1 Do you have	
• frequent episodes of bronchitis? pneumonia?	Bronchiectasis; chronic bronchitis; mitral stenosis
• a chronic sinusitis?	Frequently present in bronchiectasis

• a heart condition?	Congestive heart failure with deep-vein thrombosis and pulmonary infarction; left-heart failure with pulmonary edema; mitral stenosis
• a bleeding tendency?	Telangiectasia of the lung (hemoptysis is rare in other bleeding tendencies)

8.2 Have you ever had
  • tuberculosis?
  • a recent operation?   Deep-vein thrombosis with pulmonary thromboembolism

9   *Family medical history pertaining to the hemoptysis*

9.1 Is there a history of blood sputum in your family?	Tuberculosis; hereditary hemorrhagic telangiectasia with pulmonary arteriovenous malformations

PHYSICAL SIGNS PERTINENT TO THE COMPLAINT

Finding	**Possible** *significance*
Prolonged expiration; diffuse rhonchi and wheezes	Bronchitis; bronchiectasis with airway obstruction
Coarse rales altered by coughing	Chronic bronchitis; bronchiectasis
Increased tactile and vocal fremitus; bronchial breath sounds; fine rales	Pulmonary signs of consolidation: bacterial pneumonia, lung abscess, lung tumor, pulmonary infarction
Localized wheeze	Bronchial obstruction: bronchogenic carcinoma, foreign body
Pleural friction rub	Pleurally based lesion: pulmonary embolism with infarction, lung abscess
Heart murmur	Mitral stenosis; congenital heart disease with pulmonary hypertension

Deep-vein thrombosis Atrial fibrillation }	Pulmonary embolism with infarction
Fever; weight loss; posttussive crepitant rales; apical rales	Tuberculosis
Clubbing	Bronchogenic carcinoma; lung abscess; bronchiectasis
Foul breath (halitosis)	Bronchiectasis; lung abscess
Telangiectases on skin and mucosae; continuous murmur over the lung fields	Hereditary hemorrhagic telangiectasia with pulmonary arteriovenous malformation

LABORATORY TESTS PERTAINING TO THE COMPLAINT

Procedure	*To detect*
Chest x-ray	Ring shadows, "tram lines," cyst formation: bronchiectasis
	Mass lesion: pulmonary neoplasm; pulmonary arteriovenous malformation
	Primary complex, apical infiltration, cavitary lesion: tuberculosis
	Cavitary lesion, air-fluid level: lung abscess
	Lobar consolidation: bacterial pneumonia
	Segmental consolidation: pulmonary infarction
	A mass within a cavity: aspergilloma
	Characteristic cardiac silhouette, Kerley B lines: mitral stenosis
Blood Hematocrit	Iron-deficiency anemia: in Goodpasture's syndrome, idiopathic pulmonary hemosiderosis
BUN, creatinine	Uremia: in Goodpasture's syndrome, Wegener's granulomatosis
Hemostasis studies	Bleeding tendency

Serologic studies	*Aspergillus* precipitins
Sputum examination	Tubercle bacilli; fungi; bronchogenic carcinoma; hemosiderin-laden macrophages: Goodpasture's syndrome
Urinalysis	Protein, RBCs, casts: Goodpasture's syndrome; Wegener's granulomatosis
Fiberoptic bronchoscopy	Abnormalities (tumor, granulomas, etc.) of the tracheobronchial tree; precise site of bleeding
ECG	Right axis deviation, P pulmonale, right ventricular hypertrophy: pulmonary hypertension
Bronchography	Localized or diffuse bronchiectasis
Pulmonary angiography*	Pulmonary thromboembolism; congenital or acquired lesions of the pulmonary vessels
Lung biopsy*	Idiopathic pulmonary hemosiderosis; Goodpasture's syndrome

* If appropriate.

USEFUL REMINDERS AND DIAGNOSTIC CLUES

Misleading Factors

Hemoptysis should be distinguished from blood coming from the gastrointestinal tract or the nasopharynx with secondary aspiration of blood.

Ascribing recurrent episodes of hemoptysis to a previously established diagnosis, such as chronic bronchitis or bronchiectasis, may result in missing a serious, potentially treatable lesion.

Occurrence of hemoptysis during the course of a viral or bacterial pneumonia should raise the question of a more serious underlying process.

Diagnostic Considerations

It is estimated that at least one-fourth of all patients with chronic bronchitis have hemoptysis at some time during their illness.

True hemoptysis in mitral stenosis must be distinguished from the bloody sputum that occurs with pulmonary edema, pulmonary infarction, and bronchitis, three conditions frequently noted in mitral stenosis.

The commonest cause of hemoptysis in patients past the age of 45 is primary bronchogenic carcinoma.

Hemoptysis is rare in metastatic carcinoma to the lung.

Hemoptysis occurs in 25 to 50 percent of patients with bronchogenic carcinoma, in 50 percent of patients with bronchiectasis.

In case of	*Suspect*
Profuse and persistent hemoptysis associated with severe nephritis	Goodpasture's syndrome
Hemoptysis associated with purulent rhinorrhea and renal disease	Wegener's granulomatosis

SELECTED BIBLIOGRAPHY

Pierce J: Hemoptysis, in Mac Bryde CM, Blacklow RS (eds), *Signs and Symptoms*, 5th ed, chap 18, pp 337–340, Philadelphia: Lippincott, 1970

7
Hypertension

DEFINITION AND GENERAL CONSIDERATIONS

Hypertension arterial pressure above 150/90 mmHg in a resting adult.

The blood pressure is determined by the product of cardiac output and peripheral resistance. These factors are in turn modified by blood volume, stroke volume, pulse rate, blood viscosity, elasticity of blood vessels, and neurogenic and humoral stimuli. Various physiologic and pathologic influences may produce hypertension. Excessive intake or administration of salt and water, administration or excessive secretion of mineralocorticoids can expand blood volume. Systemic vascular resistance can be increased by adrenergic stimuli, circulating catecholamines (pheochromocytoma) and angiotensin, and stiffness of the arteriolar walls (secondary to an increased sodium content?).

Most renal diseases are associated with hypertension. Reduced perfusion of renal tissue activates the renin-angiotensin system. Angiotensin is a potent vasoconstrictor and also causes the liberation of aldosterone, which acts at the renal tubule to facilitate sodium reabsorption and expansion of intravascular volume. Hypertension in renal parenchymal disease has also been attributed to failure by the kidney to destroy an extrarenal pressor substance, failure to produce a vasodilator substance, production of an unidentified vasopressor substance, and retention of sodium.

If a defined cause of hypertension is found, the patient has secondary hypertension. In essential hypertension (90 percent of cases), no cause can be identified. Increased peripheral resistance (presumably related to increased neurogenic tone, "waterlogging" of small resistance vessels, or arteriolar hypertrophy) is the hallmark of essential hypertension.

Systolic hypertension with a normal or decreased diastolic pressure is usually secondary to another pathologic process (decreased compliance of the aortic wall, increased stroke volume).

ETIOLOGY

Combined systolic and diastolic hypertension

Renal causes: chronic pyelonephritis; acute and chronic glomerulo-nephritis; diabetic nephropathy; polycystic renal disease; partial occlusion of renal artery; renal infarction; arteriolar nephrosclerosis; polyarteritis nodosa; systemic lupus erythematosus; renin-producing tumor

Endocrine causes: adrenal cortical hyperfunction (Cushing's syndrome, primary hyperaldosteronism, adrenogenital syndromes); pheochromocytoma; acromegaly; hyperparathyroidism

Miscellaneous: coarctation of the aorta; increased intravascular volume (overhydration, polycythemia); hypercalcemia; acute porphyria; acute lead poisoning; increased intracranial pressure; familial dysautonomia; toxemia of pregnancy

Unknown etiology: essential hypertension

Systolic hypertension

Decreased compliance of aorta: arteriosclerosis

Increased stroke volume or cardiac output: arteriovenous fistula; aortic valvular insufficiency; thyrotoxicosis; fever; hyperkinetic heart syndrome; patent ductus arteriosus; psychogenic factors

Iatrogenic Causes of Hypertension

Amphetamines; carbenoxolone; contraceptive pills; corticosteroids; epinephrine, norepinephrine; licorice; concomitant administration of monoamine oxidase inhibitors and sympathomimetic amines

QUESTIONNAIRE

1 Mode of onset and evolution

Possible *meaning of response*

1.1 At what time was high blood pressure first observed?

Before age 35: secondary hypertension; acute glomerulonephritis; between the ages of 35 and 55: essential hypertension; after age 55: secondary hypertension; renovascular cause

1.2 How was your high blood pressure detected?	Many patients with hypertension are identified in the course of routine examination and have no symptoms referable to the high blood pressure
1.3 Is your blood pressure • variable?	Most patients with labile hypertension eventually develop sustained hypertension
• constantly elevated?	
1.3*a* What was the highest level of your blood pressure?	Important in determining the approach to treatment
1.4 Has your blood pressure recently increased over previous high levels?	**Accelerated or malignant hypertension**

2 *Precipitating or aggravating factors*

2.1 For female patients: Are you pregnant?	Toxemia of pregnancy (usually pregnant 24 weeks or more)
2.1*a* Do you take contraceptive pills?	Hypertension due to contraceptive pills is reversible within 3 months after use of the pills is discontinued

3 *Accompanying symptoms*

Reflect complications of the hypertensive state

3.1 Do you have
• headaches?

Episodic: pheochromocytoma

• *occipital?*
• *upon awakening in the morning?*
• wearing off during the day?

Typical in hypertension; uncommon at diastolic pressures less than 120 mmHg

• giddiness?

Transient cerebral ischemia

• syncope? dizziness?

• upon standing?	Cerebrovascular insufficiency; diabetic neuropathy; postural hypotension in pheochromocytoma
• shortness of breath?	Left ventricular failure complicating hypertension: rise in left atrial and pulmonary venous pressure
• foot or ankle swelling?	<u>Congestive heart failure</u>
• chest pain on exertion?	<u>Angina pectoris</u> due to accelerated coronary artery sclerosis
• pain in the calves when walking?	Arteriosclerotic involvement of the blood vessels of the legs with intermittent claudication
• pain on urination? ⎫ • blood in your urine? ⎭	Renal cause of hypertension
• an increased amount of urine passed? increased thirst?	Polyuria and polydipsia suggest renal or endocrine disease; polyuria is observed in potassium deficiency (primary hyperaldosteronism)
• frequent micturition during the night?	Nocturnal frequency may be an early manifestation of hypertension, usually occurring when diastolic pressure is 120 mmHg or more
• blurred or dimmed vision? ⎫ • a decrease in visual acuity? ⎬ ⎭	Hypertensive retinopathy: retinal papilledema or hemorrhage
• a recent weight gain?	Cushing's syndrome
• a recent weight loss?	Pheochromocytoma
3.2 Do you have spells of sweating? palpitations? nervousness?	Pheochromocytoma

4 *Iatrogenic factors* **see Etiology**

5 *Personal antecedents pertaining to the hypertension*

5.1 Have you ever had a chest x-ray? an ECG? a urinalysis? an IV pyelogram? an eye examination? When? With what results?

5.2 Do you have any of the following conditions:

• a heart disease? a heart murmur?	Coarctation of the aorta; aorta regurgitation
• a kidney disease? repeated urinary infections?	Renal cause of hypertension
• diabetes?	Frequently associated with hypertension

5.3 Do you smoke? — Cigarette smoking is a risk factor for the development of arteriosclerotic cardiovascular disease

6 *Family medical history pertaining to the hypertension*

6.1 Is there someone in your family who has

• hypertension?	Essential hypertension; inherited and environmental factors may lead to similar arterial pressures in members of certain families; a positive family history does not exclude the possibility of secondary causes
• a renal disease?	Polycystic disease
• a myocardial infarction? cerebrovascular disease? diabetes?	A family history of early deaths due to cardiovascular disease may justify a more aggressive treatment of the patient

PHYSICAL SIGNS PERTINENT TO THE COMPLAINT

Finding	**Possible** *significance*
Response of diastolic blood pressure to standing:	
orthostatic drop	Pheochromocytoma; antihypertensive medications

orthostatic rise	Essential hypertension
Cardiomegaly; left ventricular lift; accentuated aortic second sound; presystolic (atrial) gallop rhythm	Hypertensive heart disease with left ventricular hypertrophy: severe and/or long-standing hypertension
Bilateral basilar rales	Left-heart failure with pulmonary congestion
Peripheral edema; hepatomegaly; distended jugular veins	Right-heart failure
Bruit over carotid arteries	Atherosclerotic involvement of carotid arteries; stenosis of a carotid artery (may be associated with a renal arterial lesion)
Systolic murmur over the base of the heart; palpable collateral circulation on chest; decreased and/or delayed femoral pulses; *blood pressure in legs 20 to 30 mmHg lower than in arms*	Coarctation of the aorta
Bruits in the epigastrium or in the flanks	Renal artery stenosis
Enlarged kidneys	Polycystic renal disease
Renal mass	Renal carcinoma; polycystic renal disease
Round plethoric facies; truncal obesity; purple striae; hirsutism	Cushing's syndrome
Abnormal neurologic examination	Previous cerebrovascular accident; intracranial pathologic change
Café-au-lait spots	Neurofibromatosis with associated pheochromocytoma
Funduscopic examination: diminution in size of the arterioles: A-V ratio: ½; localized constriction of the vessels	Grade I hypertensive retinopathy

A-V ratio: ⅓; "copper" wiring; arteriovenous nicking	Grade II: associated arteriolar sclerosis (thickening of arterioles suggests that hypertension has been present for at least 10 to 15 yr)
A-V ratio: ¼; hemorrhages, exudates	Grade III: progression or acceleration of hypertension
Papilledema, hemorrhages, exudates; arterioles threadlike or invisible	Grade IV: malignant hypertension; often associated with arteriolar nephronecrosis and a poor prognosis

LABORATORY TESTS PERTAINING TO THE COMPLAINT

Procedure	*To detect*
Urine Urinalysis	Proteinuria: malignant phase of hypertension; congestive heart failure; primary renal disease
	Glycosuria: diabetes mellitus; pheochromocytoma with associated hyperglycemia
	Proteinuria and glycosuria: Kimmelstiel-Wilson syndrome
	Alkaline pH (in the presence of potassium deficiency): hyperaldosteronism
Sediment	RBCs, RBC casts: acute glomerulonephritis; polyarteritis nodosa; malignant phase of hypertension
	Pus cells, bacteria: chronic pyelonephritis
Vanillyl mandelic acid (N: < 8 mg/24 h)	Pheochromocytoma
Catecholamines (N: < 100 μg/24 h)	Pheochromocytoma

Blood

BUN, creatinine	Impairment of renal function
Electrolytes	Hypokalemia: previous diuretic therapy; primary aldosteronism; Cushing's syndrome; heavy licorice ingestion
	Base line prior to treatment with diuretics
Fasting glucose Glucose tolerance test	Diabetes mellitus associated with renal vascular disease or diabetic nephropathy; primary aldosteronism; Cushing's syndrome; pheochromocytoma associated with hyperglycemia
	Base line prior to treatment with diuretics
Uric acid	Gout; gouty nephropathy; base line prior to treatment with diuretics
Calcium	Hypercalcemic states with hypertension
Cholesterol Triglycerides	Hyperlipemia predisposing to arteriosclerosis
Plasma cortisol*	Cushing's syndrome
ECG	Left ventricular hypertrophy
Chest x-ray	Cardiomegaly; pulmonary venous congestion
	Aortic dilatation or elongation, rib notching: coarctation of aorta
Rapid-sequence IV pyelogram	Renal arterial obstruction; renal parenchymal lesion; polycystic disease; chronic pyelonephritis; etc.
Renal arteriography* Isotope renogram*	Renovascular hypertension
Renal vein plasma renin activity*	Renovascular hypertension

* If appropriate

Plasma aldosterone*	High: primary or secondary aldosteronism
Plasma renin activity*	High (with elevated plasma aldosterone level): secondary aldosteronism low (with elevated plasma aldosterone level): primary aldosteronism

* If appropriate.

USEFUL REMINDERS AND DIAGNOSTIC CLUES

Misleading Factor

Falsely high blood pressure readings may be obtained if the bladder inside a blood pressure cuff does not cover 75 percent of the arm circumference.

Diagnostic Considerations

Chronic renal disease is the most common cause of secondary hypertension.

The incidence of renal artery stenosis is less than 1 percent of the hypertensive population.

Pheochromocytoma is a rare cause of hypertension (1 in 1000 hypertensive patients).

Primary hyperaldosteronism represents approximately 1 percent of the hypertensive population in a referral hospital clinic. On the other hand, secondary hyperaldosteronism is common in patients with malignant hypertension.

Hydronephrosis, however impressive otherwise, rarely causes hypertension, unless pyelonephritis is also present.

Those patients with chronic pyelonephritis or polycystic renal disease who are salt wasters do not develop hypertension.

A difference in blood pressure greater than 15 mmHg between the right and left arms suggests: an aberrant radial artery; pulseless disease; aneurysm of the thoracic aorta; subclavian steal syndrome; thoracic outlet syndrome; coarctation of the aorta; arterial thrombosis.

In case of hypertension	*Suspect*
Of sudden onset within the preceding 6 months	Renal artery stenosis; acute renal parenchymal disease
Triggered by abdominal palpation	Pheochromocytoma

SELECTED BIBLIOGRAPHY

Jagger PI, Braunwald E: Hypertensive vascular disease, in Thorn GW et al (eds), *Harrison's Principles of Internal Medicine*, 8th ed, pp 1307–1318, New York: McGraw-Hill, 1977

Maronde RF: The hypertensive patient: An algorithm for diagnostic work-up. JAMA 233:997–1000, 1975

Strong CG, Northcutt RC, Sheps SG: Clinical examination and investigation of the hypertensive patient, chap 15, pp 640–660, in Genest J, Koiw E, Kuchel O (eds), *Hypertension: Physiopathology and Treatment,* New York: McGraw-Hill, 1977

8
Palpitations

DEFINITIONS AND GENERAL CONSIDERATIONS

Palpitation   unpleasant awareness of the heart's action, whether slow or fast, regular or irregular.

Sinus tachycardia   a sinus rate in excess of 100 beats per minute (for adults).

Premature beats (extrasystoles)   cardiac contractions of ectopic origin which occur earlier than expected in the dominant or usual rhythm.

Arrhythmia   generation of an impulse at any site in the heart other than the sinoatrial node, whether the resultant ventricular rate is slow, normal, or rapid.

The healthy subject of average temperament is unaware of the beating of the heart under ordinary circumstances. Palpitation is a normal sensation when the force of the heartbeat and its rate are considerably elevated, as in strenuous physical effort or emotional stress. Certain pathologic conditions (anemia, high fever, thyrotoxicosis) may be associated with increased contractility and tachycardia, and may give rise to palpitation.

Common causes of palpitations are ectopic tachycardias (ventricular tachycardia rarely is manifested as palpitation, probably because of asynchrony and impaired force of ventricular contraction) and unusual movements of the heart (ectopic beats, compensatory pause following extrasystoles). Heavy and regular palpitation is usually due to an augmented stroke volume (aortic or mitral regurgitation, ventricular septal defect). The onset of bradycardia (sudden development of heart block) may also give rise to palpitation.

In anxious patients the threshold of consciousness of the heart's beating may be so lowered that palpitation may occur with normal rhythm and rate.

ETIOLOGY

Disorders of the mechanism of the heartbeat (with arrhythmias):
Extrasystoles: atrial, ventricular

Sick-sinus syndrome (bradycardia-tachycardia syndrome)
Ectopic tachycardias: paroxysmal atrial tachycardia; atrial fibrillation; atrial flutter; ventricular tachycardia; Wolff-Parkinson-White syndrome
Disorders of auriculoventricular conduction
Disturbances originating outside the circulatory system (without arrhythmia)
Sinus tachycardia: anemia; fever; circulatory collapse; congestive heart failure; thyrotoxicosis; hypoglycemia; pheochromocytoma; arteriovenous fistula; alcohol; tobacco; coffee; tea; drugs
Miscellaneous: aortic aneurysm; marked cardiomegaly (aortic valvular disease, hypertensive cardiovascular disease)
Anxiety state; neurocirculatory asthenia

Table 8-1   Causes of Some Common Arrhythmias

Paroxysmal atrial tachycardia:
Atrial septal defect; mitral valve disease; Wolff-Parkinson-White syndrome; chronic obstructive lung disease; digitalis toxicity; emotional upset; fatigue; indigestion; alcohol ingestion
Atrial fibrillation:
Paroxysmal: acute infections (pneumonia); acute myocardial infarction; anesthesia; chest surgery; potassium deficiency; digitalis intoxication; thyrotoxicosis; mitral stenosis; ischemic heart disease
Permanent: mitral stenosis; ischemic heart disease; thyrotoxicosis; constrictive pericarditis; myocardial disease; hypertension
Ventricular tachycardia:
Ischemic heart disease; following a myocardial infarction; digitalis or quinidine intoxication; during cardiac catheterization and angiography; following dc shock; during syncope in patients with Stokes-Adams syndrome; in myxedema coma; during proper function or malfunction of pacemaker; ventricular aneurysm; anesthetic agents; spontaneously in otherwise healthy subjects

Iatrogenic Causes of Palpitation

Sinus tachycardia: sympathomimetic amines; aminophylline; atropine; thyroid hormone; nitrites, nitrates; monoamine oxidase inhibitor drugs concurrently with sympathomimetic drugs

Ventricular tachycardia: toxic doses of digitalis, epinephrine, quinidine, procainamide
Ventricular extrasystoles: sympathomimetic drugs
Any arrhythmia: digitalis intoxication

QUESTIONNAIRE

Possible *meaning of response*

1 Duration of palpitations

1.1 How long have you had palpitations?

1.2 *Do you have recurrent attacks of palpitations?*

Paroxysmal atrial or ventricular tachycardia; paroxysmal atrial fibrillation or flutter; Wolff-Parkinson-White syndrome; pheochromocytoma

1.2*a* How frequently do these episodes occur?

1.2*b* How long do these attacks last?
- an instant? about a minute?
- a few minutes? an hour or more?

Extrasystoles
(Paroxysmal) ectopic tachycardia

2 Character

2.1 Do you feel
- heart fluttering? beating rapidly?

Tachycardia

- skipped beats? "flopping"?

Extrasystoles; atrioventricular (AV) block with dropped beats

- slow beating?

Heart block

- chest "pounding"?

First ventricular contraction succeeding a compensatory pause

- as if your heart stopped beating?

Pause following the premature contraction

2.2 Are onset and cessation of
the attacks
- *abrupt?*   Paroxysmal ectopic tachycardia
- gradual?   Sinus tachycardia; anxiety state

2.3 Is the rapid heart action
- regular?   Anxiety state; sinus tachycardia;
                                  paroxysmal ectopic tachycardias
- irregular?   Atrial fibrillation; fibrillo-flutter

2.4 How fast is your pulse rate
during the palpitations?
- less than 140 beats per   Sinus tachycardia; anxiety state;
  minute?   digitalis-induced atrial tachy-
                                  cardia with AV block
- *about 150 beats per minute?*   Atrial flutter
- more than 170 beats per   Ectopic tachycardia
  minute?
- too fast to be counted?   Atrial fibrillation; ectopic tachy-
                                  cardia

3 *Precipitating or aggravating factors*

3.1 Do you have palpitations
- after strenuous physical ac-   Normal awareness of an over-
  tivity?   active heart; paroxysmal atrial
                                  tachycardia
- on exertion? when   Mild anemia; heart failure
  walking?
- on standing?   Postural hypotension
- at rest? independently of   Atrial fibrillation; atrial flutter;
  exercise or excitement?   thyrotoxicosis; febrile states;
                                  hypoglycemia; severe anemia,
                                  anxiety states
- when lying on your left   Occasionally in healthy subjects:
  side?   better transmission of the heart
                                  sounds to the ear
- after a meal? after drinking   Precipitating factors in any ar-
  coffee? tea? alcohol?   rhythmia; extrasystoles; sinus
                                  tachycardia

• when tired? anxious? upset?

Anxiety state; an emotional upset may precipitate paroxysmal
ectopic tachycardia

4 Relieving factors

4.1 Are your palpitations relieved by
• lying down?
• *massaging the neck?*
stooping? *inducing gagging,*
vomiting?

• belching?

• medications? which ones?

Paroxysmal ectopic tachycardia
Vagal stimulation (carotid sinus
pressure, Valsalva maneuver)
bringing to an end paroxysmal
atrial tachycardia

Aerophagia; associated anxiety
state

5 Accompanying symptoms

5.1 Are your palpitations accompanied by
• syncope?

May occur during a supraventricular or ventricular tachyarrhythmia; total cardiac asystole
or extreme bradycardia following
the termination of a tachyarrhythmia; Stokes-Adams attack
in AV block; hypoglycemia

• anxiety? giddiness? tingling in hands, around the
mouth?
• a blurring of vision? buzzing in the ears?

Anxiety states with hyperventilation

Decrease in cerebral circulation
secondary to the tachycardia;
hypoglycemia

• sweating?

Anxiety states; thyrotoxicosis;
hypoglycemia; pheochromocytoma

• a sensation of hunger?
• trembling? weakness?

Hypoglycemia

∘ headaches?	Pheochromocytoma; hypoglycemia; anxiety state
• breathing trouble?	Anxiety state with hyperventilation; dyspnea in anemia, congestive heart failure
• chest pain?	Angina pectoris may develop during tachyarrhythmias in patients with ischemic heart disease; anxiety states
• fever?	Acute infections; incipient tuberculosis; subacute bacterial endocarditis; acute rheumatic fever with carditis; thyrotoxicosis
• intolerance to heat?	Thyrotoxicosis
• a lump in your throat?	<u>Anxiety state</u>

5.1*a* Do you urinate more than usual after your episodes of palpitations?

Polyuria following paroxysmal supraventricular tachycardia

6 *Iatrogenic factors*   see Etiology

7 *Personal antecedents pertaining to the palpitations*

7.1 Have you ever had an ECG? a thyroid examination? When? With what results?

7.2 Do you have any of the following conditions: a cardiac condition? high blood pressure? anemia? a thyroid condition? emotional problems? diabetes?

PHYSICAL SIGNS PERTINENT TO THE COMPLAINT

Finding	**Possible** *significance*
Palpitation with normal heart rate and regular rhythm	Anxiety state
Irregular rhythm with normal heart rate	Frequent premature beats; atrial fibrillation with ventricular rate slowed by digitalis; sinus arrhythmia; partial heart block with dropped beats

Regular tachycardia (> 100 beats per minute) with	
< 140 beats per minute	Sinus tachycardia; anxiety state; ectopic tachycardia with AV block
150 beats per minute	Atrial flutter
≥ 170 beats per minute	Ectopic tachycardia
Tachycardia with regular rhythm	Sinus tachycardia; paroxysmal atrial tachycardia; ventricular tachycardia; atrial flutter with 1:1 response or with unchanging degree of block
Tachycardia with irregular rhythm	Atrial fibrillation; atrial flutter with varying block; paroxysmal atrial tachycardia with block; sinus tachycardia with numerous premature beats; bradycardia-tachycardia syndrome
Irregular tachycardia with a predictable basic cadence	"Regular irregularity": frequent premature beats
Entirely unpredictable cadence	"Irregular irregularity": atrial fibrillation
Regular bradycardia (< 60 beats per minute)	Sinus bradycardia; sick-sinus syndrome; nodal rhythm; severe partial heart block with constant degree of block
with ≤ 45 beats per minute	Complete AV block
Irregular bradycardia	Sinoatrial bradycardia with marked sinus arrhythmia or frequent premature beats; partial block with frequent dropped beats or changing degrees of block
Constant intensity of first heart sound and amplitude of peripheral pulse	Sinus, paroxysmal atrial, junctional tachycardia

Variable intensity of first heart sound and amplitude of peripheral pulse	Complete AV heart block; ventricular tachycardia; atrial flutter
Inspection of jugular venous pulse:	
"cannon wave"	Right atrium contracting against a closed tricuspid valve during ventricular systole: complete AV block; nodal or ventricular tachycardia
A waves at 250 to 350 beats per minute	Atrial flutter
Effect of exercise on an irregular rhythm:	
disappearance of irregularity	Extrasystoles
increase of irregularity	Atrial fibrillation
Effect of carotid sinus massage on tachycardia:	This maneuver (performed with caution) elicits vagal efferent impulses influencing automaticity and conduction
no change in rate	Ventricular tachycardia; may also occur in atrial tachycardia
abrupt termination persisting after discontinuation of massage	Atrial tachycardia
temporary slowing lasting only during massage	Atrial flutter; sinus tachycardia
with gradual return to previous rate	Sinus tachycardia
with abrupt return to previous rate	Atrial flutter
Enlarged thyroid; tremor; warm, moist skin	Thyrotoxicosis

LABORATORY TESTS PERTAINING TO THE COMPLAINT

Procedure	Finding	Diagnostic possibilities
Blood Hematocrit	Low	Anemia causing palpitations
Glucose	Low	Hypoglycemic episodes with palpitation
	Elevated	Diabetes mellitus; pheochromocytoma with episodes of palpitation
Thyroid function tests	Abnormal	Hyperthyroidism

Procedure	To detect	
ECG		
Long-term electrocardiographic monitoring	Cardiac arrhythmias	
His bundle electrogram*		
Chest x-ray	Cardiac disease	

* If appropriate.

USEFUL REMINDERS AND DIAGNOSTIC CLUES

The pulse rate in general rises about 9 beats per minute for each degree Fahrenheit of temperature elevation.

Chronic atrial fibrillation may be the only feature suggesting the possibility of thyroid disease.

In atrial fibrillation, failure of ventricular rate to slow after full doses of digitalis suggests the presence of fever, thyrotoxicosis, a recent myocardial infarction, multiple pulmonary infarcts, acute rheumatic carditis, constrictive pericarditis, cardiomyopathy, anemia, hypokalemia, unrecognized digitalis toxicity, severe lung disease with chronic cor pulmonale, the Wolff-Parkinson-White syndrome. Palpitation is particularly prominent when the precipitating cause for increased heart rate or contractility or arrhythmia is recent, transient, and episodic.

Recurrent episodes of supraventricular tachycardia in otherwise normal individuals occur in the Wolff-Parkinson-White syndrome.

SELECTED BIBLIOGRAPHY

Braunwald E: Palpitation, in Thorn GW et al (eds), *Harrison's Principles of Internal Medicine*, 8th ed, pp 182–185, New York: McGraw-Hill, 1977

Massie E: Palpitation and tachycardia, in Mac Bryde CM, Blacklow RS (eds), *Signs and Symptoms*, 5th ed, chap 16, pp 304–323, Philadelphia: Lippincott, 1970

Resnekov L (ed): Symposium on cardiac rhythm disturbances. Med Clin North Am 60:1–386, 1976

9
Thoracic Pain

GENERAL CONSIDERATIONS

Thoracic pain may have its origin in the various tissues of the chest wall, the intrathoracic structures, the neck, or areas below the diaphragm.

Cardiac pain The myocardium gives rise to pain when the oxygen supply to the heart is deficient in relation to the oxygen needs; this occurs when coronary blood flow is inadequate (e.g., coronary atherosclerosis). Pain from myocardial disease is felt to arise within the first to fourth or fifth thoracic segments. These spinal segments also receive sensory fibers from other structures: the esophagus, mediastinal contents, osseous and muscular structures; diseases of these structures may cause pain that is difficult to distinguish from cardiac pain. The pain of myocardial ischemia may be felt along the inner aspect of the left arm, owing to the common innervation of the heart and the affected area of the skin by the eighth cervical and first thoracic segments. However, almost any disorder involving the deep afferent fibers of the left upper thoracic region may produce pain in the chest, the left arm, or both areas. Pain associated with *pericarditis* is believed to be due to inflammation of the adjacent parietal pleura; the visceral surface of the pericardium is ordinarily insensitive to pain.

Pleuritic pain The parietal pleura is supplied by pain nerve endings whose impulses are transmitted by the intercostal and phrenic nerves. The parenchyma of lung and its visceral pleura are insensitive to pain.

Pain arising in the chest wall The pain-sensory innervation of the integuments and the muscles of the chest wall is conveyed to the dorsal roots through the cutaneous and the intercostal nerves. Generally pain arising from the thoracic integuments and other superficial tissues is sharply localized.

ETIOLOGY

Pain originating in the heart
Myocardial ischemia
  Due to coronary artery disease: angina pectoris; coronary insufficiency; preinfarction angina; variant angina pectoris; myocardial infarction due to coronary thrombosis or embolism
  Due to relative ischemia: extreme exertion; thyrotoxicosis; low diastolic pressure (aortic insufficiency); severe anemia
  Aortic stenosis (endocardial and valvular disease)
Myocarditis
Pericarditis: viral; tuberculosis; uremia; trauma; neoplasm; connective-tissue disease; postinfarction (Dressler's syndrome)
Right ventricular hypertension
Fabry's disease; carcinoid syndrome
Systolic click–systolic murmur syndrome
Post-cardiac-injury syndrome

Pain originating in noncardiac intrathoracic structures
Aorta: dissecting aneurysm (hypertension; pregnancy; coarctation; blunt trauma; Marfan's syndrome); syphilitic aneurysm
Pulmonary artery: pulmonary embolism
Bronchopulmonary tree and pleura: pneumonia; pleuritis; emphysema; tracheobronchitis; tumors of bronchi, lungs, or pleura; pneumothorax; hemothorax
Mediastinum: mediastinal (interstitial) emphysema; tumors or suppurative infections of lymph nodes and other mediastinal structures
Esophagus: hiatus hernia; esophagitis; Mallory-Weiss syndrome; tumors; ulcerations; diverticuli; dilatation due to cardiospasm
Diaphragm: hiatus hernia

Pain originating in the tissues of the neck or chest wall
Skin: herpetic neuralgia; radiculitis; thoracic outlet syndrome (cervical rib syndrome)
Muscles: precordial catch syndrome; Bornholm's disease; intercostal cramp
Skeletal (cervicodorsal spine): Tietze's syndrome; osteoarthritis; herniated intervertebral disk; fractures; tumors; bursitis
Mammary glands
Spinal cord and sensory nerves

Pain referred from subdiaphragmatic structures
Peptic ulcer; pancreatitis; gallbladder (cholecystitis, biliary colic); splenic flexure syndrome; spleen; kidneys; peritoneum

Pain of functional origin
Anxiety neurosis; factitious (malingerer); addict

Iatrogenic Causes of Thoracic Pain

Contraceptives, withdrawal from propranolol (myocardial infarction)
Hydralazine (pericarditis with systemic lupus erythematosus)
Antihypertensive drugs, ergot, methysergide, oxytocin, vasopressin (ischemic heart disease)

QUESTIONNAIRE

Possible *meaning of response*

1 Location and radiation of the pain

1.1   Where do you have pain? | Pain arising in the skin or superficial structures is usually accurately localized by the patient: chest-wall pain; Tietze's syndrome (if costochondral area)

1.1*a Can you point to the pain?* | If so: excludes anginal pain

1.1*b* Is the pain diffuse? difficult to localize? | Pain arising in deeper structures

1.2   Is the pain localized
• *in the middle of your chest?* | Substernal: <u>coronary artery disease</u>, pericarditis, esophageal origin, **pulmonary embolism**

• under the left nipple? | Precordial: usually a <u>noncardiac condition</u>: anxiety state, osteoarthritis, splenic flexure syndrome, gaseous distention of the stomach

• in the anterior part of the chest? | **Myocardial infarction; dissecting aneurysm of aorta** (proximal dissection, above the aortic valve)

• between the shoulder blades?	Myocardial infarction; hiatus hernia; dissecting aortic aneurysm (distal dissection, beyond the left subclavian artery)
• in an upper costochondral junction?	Anterior chest-wall (Tietze's) syndrome

1.3 Is the pain

• superficial?	Chest-wall conditions; herpes zoster; pain of <u>pleural origin</u>
• deep?	Visceral pain

1.4 Does the pain radiate to the

• *left arm? left shoulder?*	**Coronary artery disease; pericarditis;** disorders of the <u>cervical spine</u>
• right arm? right shoulder?	Occasionally observed in angina pectoris; disorders of the <u>cervical spine</u>
• both arms?	Occasionally in myocardial infarction; dissecting aortic aneurysm
• neck? jaw?	Angina; myocardial infarction; pericarditis
• back?	Coronary artery disease; dissecting aortic aneurysm (rupture distal to the left subclavian artery)
• abdomen?	Dissecting aortic aneurysm

2 Mode of onset and evolution

2.1 How long have you had pain in your chest?	To be kept in mind when interpreting blood enzyme changes; pain persisting for 20 min or longer: myocardial infarction, dissecting aneurysm, pulmonary embolism, acute pericarditis, gallbladder colic, acute pancreatitis; anginal pain is of brief duration, usually lasting from 2 to 10 min

2.2 Do you have recurrent episodes of chest pain?

Angina pectoris; cervical radiculitis; anterior chest-wall conditions; functional GI disorders; anxiety

2.2*a* How long have you had attacks of chest pain?

2.2*b* What is the duration of the episodes?

Less than 30 s: anginal pain may be excluded; 2 to 10 min: anginal pain; longer duration: musculoskeletal pain; hiatus hernia; psychogenic pain; variable duration; musculoskeletal condition; anxiety states

2.2*c* What is the frequency of the episodes per day? per week?

If angina pectoris is present: reflects the intensity of the process

2.2*d* Are the frequency, the intensity, the duration, of the attacks
• increasing?

Recent coronary thrombosis; may presage an impending myocardial infarction

• decreasing?

May be due to limited activity

3 Intensity of the thoracic pain

3.1 Is the pain
• mild? moderately severe?

Pericarditis; angina pectoris (the discomfort of angina is usually moderate in intensity, although any degree of intensity may occur)

• severe? unbearable?

Myocardial infarction; massive pulmonary embolism; dissecting aortic aneurysm

4 Character of the pain

4.1 Is the pain
• *squeezing? constricting?*

Coronary artery disease; spasm of esophagus; hiatus hernia

• pressing? boring? gripping?	Angina pectoris
• crushing?	Myocardial infarction
• dull? aching?	Musculoskeletal pain; lesion of bone (also angina pectoris, pericarditis)
• sticking? jabbing?	Musculoskeletal pain (excludes anginal pain)
• throbbing?	Chest-wall pain; lesion of bone
• sharp? knifelike? fleeting?	Not typical of angina; lesion of the spinal cord and nerve roots; anxiety states
4.1a *Do you feel as though a weight is on your chest?*	Coronary artery disease

5 *Precipitating or aggravating factors*

5.1 (Acute episode): Did the pain appear	
• at rest?	Myocardial infarction; pneumothorax; pleural disorder
• *on exertion?*	Angina: pneumothorax; myocardial infarction (may appear without relation to effort)
• after protracted vomiting?	Mallory-Weiss syndrome: tear in the lower portion of the esophagus
5.2 (Recurrent chest pain): Does the pain appear	
• at rest?	Anxiety states; radicular pain; Prinzmetal variant of angina
• while bending over?	Radicular pain; disk pain; osteoarthritis with involvement of the nerve roots of the cervical and upper thoracic spine; esophageal pain
• when moving your neck?	Herniated cervical intervertebral disk
• while eating?	Spasm of the esophagus; hiatus hernia

• after a heavy meal?	Hiatus hernia; angina pectoris
• when under emotional strain?	Angina pectoris; psychogenic pain
• when exhausted?	Psychogenic pain
• at night?	Angina decubitus; esophageal pain
• when lying down?	
• *on exertion? (moving the body as a whole)*	
• *while walking against the wind? walking rapidly in the cold?*	Angina pectoris
• *during sexual intercourse?*	

5.3 Is the pain made worse by

• swallowing?	Acute pericarditis; esophageal pain
• lying flat?	Myocardial infarction; hiatus hernia; reflux esophagitis; acute pericarditis
• inspiration?	Pleural disorder; pericarditis; pneumothorax
• coughing?	Pericarditis; pleural disorder; radicular pain; herniated cervical disk
• sneezing? straining at stool?	Radicular pain
• movements of the neck? chest? arm? head?	Lesion of the cervicodorsal spine

6 *Relieving factors*

6.1 Is the pain relieved by

• *remaining immobile?*	Angina pectoris (the pain of myocardial infarction is not relieved by rest)
• walking around?	The pain of myocardial infarction causes the patient to move about in an attempt to find a comfortable position

• belching? passing gas?	Gaseous distention of the stomach or splenic flexure; angina pectoris
• sitting up? standing erect?	Reflux esophagitis; acute pericarditis; angina decubitus
• lying down?	Angina pectoris
• *leaning forward?*	Pericardial pain
• an alcoholic drink?	Anginal pain
• food?	Peptic ulcer
• holding the breath in deep expiration?	Pleural lesion
• antacid therapy?	Reflux esophagitis; peptic ulcer
• *nitroglycerin?*	Angina pectoris (the pain of myocardial infarction is not relieved by coronary dilator drugs); the pain of esophagitis may be relieved by nitroglycerin

6.1*a* How quickly is the pain relieved by?

• nitroglycerin? ⎫	2 to 3 min: angina pectoris
• rest? ⎭	10 min or more: evidence against the diagnosis of angina pectoris

7 *Accompanying symptoms*

7.1 Do you have

• nausea? vomiting?	Myocardial infarction
• belching?	The need to belch during an anginal attack is common
• shortness of breath?	Congestive heart failure; pulmonary edema secondary to myocardial infarction; pneumothorax; pulmonary embolism
• palpitations?	Arrhythmias accompanying a myocardial infarction

• *a sensation of imminent death?*	Myocardial infarction
• coughing?	Pulmonary or pleural origin of pain: pneumonia; lung tumor
• leg pain or swollen leg?	Deep-vein thrombosis with pulmonary embolism
• bloody expectorations?	Pulmonary infarction; lung tumor
• fever?	Pneumonia; viral pericarditis; low-grade fever frequently appears on the second or third day after myocardial infarction
• *frequent sighing?* anxiety? depression?	Psychogenic pain
• abdominal pain?	Thoracic pain referred from subdiaphragmatic structure

8   *Iatrogenic factors*   see Etiology

9   *Environmental factors*

9.1 Do you smoke? How many cigarettes a day?	Smoking is a major risk factor for myocardial infarction
9.2 What is your daily physical activity?	Many patients with angina pectoris learn to modify their daily activity to avoid pain

10   *Personal antecedents pertaining to the thoracic pain*

10.1   Have you ever had an ECG? a chest x-ray? past cardiac catheterization? When? With what results?

10.2   Have you recently had

• an operation?	Deep-vein thrombosis with pulmonary embolism
• an upper respiratory infection?	May precede viral pericarditis

10.3   Do you have any of the following conditions:

• high blood pressure?

Proneness to coronary artery disease; dissecting aneurysm

• a cardiac disease?

Aortic stenosis, hypertrophic subaortic stenosis, aortic regurgitation, mitral stenosis, right ventricular hypertension: may be associated with anginal pain

• emphysema? chronic bronchitis?

Proneness to pneumothorax

• diabetes? obesity?

• elevated serum cholesterol level?

Hypercholesterolemia, cigarette smoking, and hypertension are the three major risk factors for myocardial infarction

11   Family medical history pertaining to the thoracic pain

11.1   Does someone in your family have high cholesterol? diabetes? hypertension? (premature death?)

PHYSICAL SIGNS PERTINENT TO THE COMPLAINT

Finding

Possible *significance*

At the time of an acute episode of pain:

Tachycardia; rise in blood pressure; fourth heart sound; abnormal parasternal heave

Coronary ischemia with left ventricular dysfunction and localized noncontracting myocardium

Systolic murmur at apex

Angina pectoris with papillary muscle dysfunction secondary to localized ischemia

Restless patient; cool skin; sweating; fourth heart sound; thready pulse; reduced blood pressure; basilar rales; friction rub; arrhythmias

Acute myocardial infarction

Precordial friction rub

Acute pericarditis

Pleural friction rub	Pleurally based lesion; pulmonary thromboembolism, pneumonia, tumor; pneumothorax
Hypertension; unequal peripheral pulses; aortic insufficiency murmur; neurologic abnormalities	Dissecting aortic aneurysm
Tachycardia; tachypnea; accentuation of P2; S3 or S4 gallop; rales; friction rub	Pulmonary embolism and infarction
Deep-vein thrombosis	Pulmonary thromboembolism
On affected side: **hyperresonance; diminished breath sounds**	Pneumothorax
Fever	Infectious cause of pain: bacterial or viral pneumonia; viral pericarditis
Heart murmur	Aortic and subaortic stenosis; aortic insufficiency; mitral stenosis or septal defects associated with pulmonary hypertension may produce chest pain resembling that of coronary ischemia
Rapid heart rate	Ectopic tachycardia may provoke chest pain, particularly if there is associated coronary artery disease
Local tenderness or swelling	Local musculoskeletal disease; fractured rib
of upper costochondral cartilages	Tietze's syndrome
Crepitus in the neck; crushing noise synchronous with the heartbeat	Mediastinal emphysema

LABORATORY TESTS PERTAINING TO THE COMPLAINT

Procedure	Finding	Diagnostic possibilities
Blood Enzymes and iso-enzymes: Creatinine phosphokinase (CPK)	Elevated	Myocardial infarction; intramuscular injection; electrical cardioversion; stroke; cardiac catheterization; myopathy associated with chronic alcoholism; clofibrate therapy
Serum glutamic oxaloacetic transaminase (SGOT)	Elevated	Myocardial infarction; right ventricular failure with hepatic congestion; primary muscle disease; hemolytic crisis; cardiac operations; acute pancreatitis; infarction of spleen, kidney, intestine; extensive CNS lesion; opiates
Lactic dehydrogenase (LDH)	Elevated	Myocardial infarction; right ventricular failure with hepatic congestion; pulmonary embolism; pancreatitis; opiates

Procedure	To detect
ECG: at rest	Ischemic heart disease; pulmonary embolism; pericarditis
after exercise	Plateau-type ST segment depression of at least 0.1 mV lasting more than 0.08 s: myocardial ischemia
Chest x-ray	Pericarditis; pneumothorax; pleural effusion; pneumomediastinum; pulmonary thromboembolism; widening of aortic shadow: dissecting aortic aneurysm; calcification in a coronary artery: ischemic heart disease
Cervical and thoracic spine x-ray	Skeletal disease pain; cervical rib: thoracic outlet syndrome
X-ray of sternum and ribs	Traumatic injury
Acid-barium swallow*	Esophageal origin of thoracic pain
Esophageal motility*	Reflux esophagitis; hiatus hernia
Lung scan* Pulmonary angiography*	Pulmonary thromboembolism
Coronary arteriography*	Arterial narrowing: obstructive coronary artery disease
Echocardiography* Cardiac blood pool scan*	Acute pericarditis with pericardial effusion

* If appropriate.

USEFUL REMINDERS AND DIAGNOSTIC CLUES

Misleading Factors

Long-standing skeletal pain in the chest wall or shoulder girdles is frequent in persons with angina pectoris. This coexistence of two different types of chest pain in the same patient is a frequent cause of a confusing history.

The presence of spinal arthritis or an upper abdominal disorder (hiatus hernia, disease of the gallbladder, pancreatitis, peptic ulcer) may affect the radiation of the pain of angina pectoris.

Nitroglycerin deteriorates with age; one must be sure that the patient has used a potent preparation before ascribing failure of nitroglycerin to a nonanginal pain.

There is little correlation between the severity of chest pain and the gravity of its cause, or between the geography of the chest pain and its source.

Diagnostic Considerations

Coronary artery disease

Angina pectoris is rarely found in patients with complete heart block (bradycardia).

Pain or a burning sensation in the tongue or hard palate induced by effort or emotional tension and relieved by rest or nitroglycerin has been noted in angina pectoris.

When asked about the attack, the patient with angina pectoris may clench his fist and hold it over the sternum, illustrating the constrictive nature of the discomfort (Levine's sign).

Angina pectoris induced by exertion is usually mild at the onset and becomes progressively more severe until the patient is forced to rest.

If the pain subsides while the exercise continues at the same rate, the diagnosis of angina pectoris should be questioned.

Right ventricular hypertension occasionally produces exertional pain which is indistinguishable from that of angina pectoris.

Miscellaneous

Rib fracture as a cause of chest-wall pain must be carefully looked for in alcoholics; these patients frequently do not recall a history of trauma.

In over 90 percent of the cases, significant chest pain is due to coronary disease, spinal root compression, or psychogenic disturbances.

In case of	*Suspect*
Severe chest pain with normal ECG neurologic signs	Dissecting aortic aneurysm
Chest pain with sighing respiration	An anxiety state

SELECTED BIBLIOGRAPHY

Braunwald E, Harrison TR: Pain in the chest, in Thorn GW et al (eds), *Harrison's Principles of Internal Medicine,* 8th ed, pp 28–33, New York: McGraw-Hill, 1977

Hurst JW, King III SB: The problem of chest "pain." JAMA 236:2100–2103, 1976

Kleiger RE: Chest pain in patients seen in emergency clinics. JAMA 236: 595–597, 1976

Digestive System

10

Abdominal Distention

DEFINITIONS AND GENERAL CONSIDERATIONS

Tympanites gaseous distention of the bowel.
Ascites accumulation of fluid in the peritoneal cavity.

In normal subjects, volumes of gas present in the intestine at any one time range from 30 to 200 mL. Gases are produced within the colon from bacterial fermentation of unabsorbed nutrients (especially dietary carbohydrates) or organic substances secreted into the lumen. Stomach gas has the composition of swallowed air. Increased amounts of gas in the intestinal tract may be due to aerophagia (excessive swallowing of air) or to increased intestinal gas production following the ingestion of certain foods containing nonabsorbable carbohydrates or in conditions associated with abnormal bacterial colonization of the small intestine.

Subjective abdominal distention is usually transient and often related to a functional gastrointestinal disorder when it is not accompanied by objective physical findings of increased abdominal girth or local swelling.

Ascites may result from increased permeability of the peritoneal capillaries (inflammatory and neoplastic diseases of the peritoneum), decreased plasma colloid osmotic pressure (severe hypoalbuminemia), or elevation of the hydrostatic pressure within the hepatic sinusoids (cirrhosis, congestive heart failure, constrictive peri-carditis, hepatic vein or inferior vena cava obstruction). Ascites formation may be aggravated by increased renal retention of sodium and water.

ETIOLOGY

Abdominal Distention without Ascites (increased amounts of gas in the gastrointestinal tract)

Irritable colon
Aerophagia
Malabsorption
Chronic pancreatic insufficiency

Partial bowel obstruction
Acute bowel obstruction
Following surgical procedures

Ascites

Transudative
Cirrhosis
Congestive heart failure; constrictive pericarditis
Nephrotic syndrome
Hepatic vein obstruction (Budd-Chiari syndrome)
Inferior vena cava obstruction; portal vein obstruction
Protein-losing gastroenteropathy

Exudative
Peritonitis: ruptured viscus: peptic ulcer, appendicitis, diverticulitis, cholecystitis
Tuberculous peritonitis; bacterial peritonitis
Pancreatitis; bile peritonitis
Tumors: metastatic to the liver; lymphoma, leukemia; primary hepatoma and cholangiocarcinoma

Chylous (lymphatic obstruction)
Abdominal neoplasm, lymphoma; mediastinal tumors
Trauma to the thoracic duct in the chest
Filariasis
Occasionally: tuberculosis; cirrhosis

Miscellaneous   Meigs' syndrome: ovarian fibroma; myxedema

Causes of Ascites According to Frequency

Common cirrhosis; congestive heart failure; nephrotic syndrome; disseminated carcinomatosis

Less common constrictive pericarditis; hepatic vein obstruction; ovarian fibroma; pancreatitis; pyogenic peritonitis; tuberculous peritonitis

Iatrogenic Causes of Obstruction or Ileus

Aluminum hydroxide; enteric-coated potassium chloride or potassium
Chloride-thiazides; ganglionic blockers; narcotic analgesics

QUESTIONNAIRE

Possible *meaning of response*

1 Mode of onset and duration

1.1 How long have you had a distended abdomen?

1.2 Did you notice it because of
- a sensation of pressure or fullness in the abdomen?

  Not specific; <u>irritable colon</u> or ascites
- *a progressive increase in your belt or clothing size?*

  Organic abdominal swelling; ascites
- the development of a localized swelling?

  Neoplastic peritoneal involvement; metastatic liver

2 Character

2.1 Is the abdominal distention
- intermittent?

  Increased amounts of gas in the gastrointestinal tract; <u>irritable colon</u>

- permanent?

  Ascites; intraabdominal mass(es)

2.2 If the abdominal distention is permanent, has it appeared

• rapidly? (days)

Rapid accumulation of ascites; rapidly expanding mass; intestinal obstruction

• gradually? (weeks)

Ascites formation may be insidious

3   Precipitating and relieving factors

3.1   If the abdominal distention is intermittent, does it occur after eating?

3.1*a*   It is relieved by the passing of gas? belching? defecation?

Gaseous distention of the GI tract

4   Accompanying symptoms

4.1   Has your weight
• decreased?

Neoplastic intraabdominal process; cirrhosis of the liver; carcinomatosis with peritoneal involvement; tuberculous peritonitis; hepatoma

• *increased?*

Ascites

• remained unchanged?

Increased amounts of gas in the GI tract

4.2   Do you have pain in the abdomen?

Pain is uncommon in cirrhosis with ascites

• localized?

Involvement of an abdominal organ, e.g., passively congestive liver, large spleen, colonic tumor

• diffuse?

Peritonitis; pancreatitis; **intestinal obstruction**

4.2*a*   Have you recently had an episode of acute abdominal pain?

Pancreatitis with formation of a pseudocyst

4.3 Are your legs swollen?

Ascites with generalized edema

4.3*a* Were the legs swollen
- *before the appearance of the abdominal distention?*

Dependent edema appears prior to ascites in right-sided congestive heart failure

- after the appearance of the abdominal distention?

Ascites usually occurs early, prior to dependent edema, in cirrhosis, constrictive pericarditis

4.4 Do you have
- vomiting?

Intestinal obstruction; vomiting occurs earlier and is more severe, the higher the intestinal obstruction

- recent severe constipation?

Intestinal obstruction

- shortness of breath?

Combined congestive heart disease; elevation of the diaphragm due to ascites or abdominal tumor; coexistent pleural effusion

- puffiness of your face?

Generalized edema; nephrotic syndrome

- a change in the volume of your urine?

Commonly decreased in ascites

  - bloody urine?

Acute glomerulonephritis

  - brown urine?

Hepatic disease with bilirubinuria

- a loss of appetite?

Cirrhosis; peritoneal carcinomatosis; hepatoma

  - with fever?

Tuberculous peritonitis

- a change in your bowel habits?

Colonic tumor with peritoneal seeding

- chronic diarrhea?

Malabsorption with abdominal distention

5 *Iatrogenic factors* see Etiology

6   *Environmental factors*

6.1   What is your alcohol intake?

Cirrhosis with ascites

6.2   What is your occupation?

Bartenders, brewery workers:
liable to alcoholism with cirrhosis and ascites

6.3   What is your usual diet?

May reveal malnutrition with
hypoalbuminemia and edema

7   *Personal antecedents pertaining to the abdominal distention*

7.1   Have you ever had liver or renal tests? When? With what results?

7.2   Do you have a liver condition? alcoholism? a cardiac disease?
a renal disease?
  • a hernia?

**May become incarcerated and
give mechanical obstruction**
with abdominal distention

  • a past abdominal operation?

**Postoperative adhesions may
give intestinal obstruction**

PHYSICAL SIGNS PERTINENT TO THE COMPLAINT

Finding	**Possible** *significance*
Abdominal percussion:	
Increased tympany	Gaseous distention
Central dullness with resonance in the flanks	Large ovarian cyst
Everted umbilicus; bulging flanks; shifting dullness; fluid wave	Ascites
Ascites with palmar erythema, spider angiomas, jaundice, hepatomegaly	Liver cirrhosis (with portal hypertension)

Prominent abdominal venous pattern with	
Blood flow away from the umbilicus	Caput medusae (rare): portal hypertension
Flow upward toward the umbilicus	Inferior vena cava obstruction
Flow downward toward the umbilicus	Superior vena cava obstruction
Venous hum at the umbilicus	Portal hypertension; increased collateral blood flow around the liver
Portal hypertension with	
A soft liver	Extrahepatic obstruction to portal flow
A firm liver	Cirrhosis
A very hard or nodular liver	Tumor with neoplastic ascites
Friction rub over the liver	Hepatoma
Ascites; distended jugular veins; hepatomegaly; peripheral edema	Congestive heart failure
Ascites; distended jugular veins; pulsus paradoxus; tender hepatomegaly; minimal peripheral edema	Constrictive pericarditis
Fever; ascites; diffuse abdominal tenderness	(Tuberculous) peritonitis
Ascites with pulsatile liver	Tricuspid insufficiency
Localized abdominal swelling	Neoplastic peritoneal involvement; metastatic liver
Tympanites with high-pitched rushing bowel sounds; visible hyperperistalsis	Early intestinal obstruction
Tympanites with absent bowel sounds	Paralytic ileus
Rectal and pelvic examination	May reveal otherwise undetected masses due to tumor or infection

LABORATORY TESTS PERTAINING TO THE COMPLAINT

Procedure	Finding	Diagnostic possibilities
Paracentesis Ascitic fluid: protein, g/100 mL	<2.5	Transudate: cirrhosis, nephrosis, congestive heart failure
	>2.5	Exudate: neoplasm, tuberculous peritonitis, pyogenic peritonitis (occasionally congestive heart failure)
WBC per cubic millimeter	<250	Transudate: cirrhosis, nephrosis
	<1000 (predominantly mesothelial)	Congestive heart failure
	>1000 (variable cell type)	Neoplasm
	>1000 (predominantly lymphocytes)	Tuberculous peritonitis
	>1000 (predominantly PMNs)	Pyogenic peritonitis
Glucose, mg/100 mL	<60	Neoplastic ascites
Triglycerides	In excess of plasma concentration	Chylous ascites
Amylase	Elevated (>500 U)	Pancreatic ascites
Cytology study	Abnormal	Intraabdominal malignancy
Gram's and acid-fast stains, and culture	Positive	Infection of peritoneum

Procedure	*To detect*
Blood	
Liver function tests	Liver cirrhosis
Amylase	Pancreatitis
RBCs	Anemia in malignancy; macrocytic anemia: liver cirrhosis, malabsorption
Plain abdominal films	Intestinal obstruction; ascites; size of liver and spleen
Barium studies of the GI tract*	Esophageal and/or gastric varices: cirrhosis; malabsorption pattern; colonic obstruction
Liver scan	Intrahepatic space-occupying lesions
Ultrasonic scan Computerized tomography	Intraabdominal or retroperitoneal lesions
Laparoscopy and liver biopsy	Cirrhosis; hepatoma; intraabdominal neoplasm

* Upper GI series: contraindicated in complete intestinal obstruction. Barium enema: contraindicated in suspected perforation.

USEFUL REMINDERS AND DIAGNOSTIC CLUES

Misleading Factors

Conditions that may mimic ascites: pregnancy; ovarian cyst; pancreatic cyst; mesenteric cyst.

Considerable abdominal enlargement may go unnoticed for weeks or months either because of coexistent obesity or because of ascites formation that has been insidious without pain or localizing symptoms.

Diagnostic Considerations

Ascites is usually demonstrable clinically when 500 mL or more of fluid has accumulated in the peritoneal cavity.

A finding of more than 250 white blood cells per cubic millimeter in

a transudative ascitic fluid is atypical for cirrhosis, nephrosis, or congestive heart failure, and suggests tumor or infection.
Pleural effusion (usually right-sided) occurs in some 5 percent of patients with ascites.

In case of	*Suspect*
Pain in a cirrhotic patient with ascites	Hepatoma; pancreatitis; peritonitis
Worsening of ascites in a cirrhotic patient	Hepatoma; portal vein thrombosis; tuberculous peritonitis; spontaneous bacterial peritonitis

SELECTED BIBLIOGRAPHY

Glickman RM, Isselbacher KJ: Abdominal swelling and ascites, in Thorn GW et al (eds), *Harrison's Principles of Internal Medicine,* 8th ed, pp 223–226, New York: McGraw-Hill, 1977

Hyman S, Villa F, and Steigmann F: Mimetic aspects of ascites. JAMA 183: 651–655, 1963.

11

Acute Abdominal Pain

DEFINITIONS AND GENERAL CONSIDERATIONS

Visceral pain   initiated by a stimulus acting upon sensory nerve endings in an abdominal viscus. True visceral abdominal pain is mediated over afferent visceral fibers accompanying the sympathetic trunks. The location of the pain corresponds generally to the segmental level of the affected organ. However, the pain originating in deep visceral structures cannot be localized closer than two to three sensory segments. The pain usually results from distention or exaggerated muscular contraction of a hollow viscus; the threshold to such stimuli may be lowered by inflammation. Acute stretching of the capsules of solid organs (liver, spleen, kidney, ovary) and tension on the mesentery also produce pain, presumably by acting on stretch receptors similar to those in muscle. Ischemia causes abdominal pain by increasing the concentration of tissue metabolites in the region of the sensory nerves.

Parietal (somatic) pain   pain sensations which arise from noxious stimulation of the parietal peritoneum. Parietal pain is transmitted by cerebrospinal afferent nerves supplying the peritoneum and is located directly over the inflamed area.

Referred pain   pain not localized by the patient in the diseased viscus, but in remote areas supplied by the same neurosegment as the diseased organ, because of shared central pathways by afferent neurons from different sites.

ETIOLOGY

Intraabdominal sources
Peritoneal inflammation:
    Local: acute appendicitis; acute cholecystitis; acute pancreatitis; acute diverticulitis; salpingitis; ruptured ovarian follicle (Mittelschmerz); mesenteric lymphadenitis

Perforation of a hollow viscus: lower esophagus, stomach, duodenum, small bowel, gallbladder, urinary bladder
Tuberculous peritonitis
Intraperitoneal hemorrhage: rupture of spleen; ectopic pregnancy; dissecting aortic aneurysm
Retroperitoneal hemorrhage: laceration of kidney; fracture of spine; coagulation abnormality

Obstruction of a hollow viscus:
Obstruction of the small or large intestine
Obstruction of the biliary tree: gallstones
Obstruction of the ureter: calculi, blood clots

Vascular occlusion:
Mesenteric embolism or thrombosis
Torsional occlusion: ovarian cyst or tumor; undescended testes
Portal vein thrombosis
Sickle cell anemia

Abdominal wall:
Rectus sheath hematoma; trauma or infection of muscles

Acute stretching of visceral surfaces:
Hepatic, splenic, or renal capsules

Infectious diseases:
Enteric infections; hepatitis; acute pyelonephritis

Referred pain from extraabdominal sources
Thoracic: diaphragmatic pleuritis: pneumonia, pulmonary infarction; acute myocardial infarction; pericarditis
Neurologic: nerve root compression; tabes; spinal cord tumor or abscess
Genitalia: torsion of the testicle

Metabolic and systemic disorders
Diabetic ketoacidosis; uremia; Addisonian crisis; hyperlipemia; hypercalcemia; hyperparathyroidism; acute porphyria; hereditary angioneurotic edema; familial Mediterranean fever; connective-tissue diseases: systemic lupus erythematosus, polyarteritis nodosa, Henoch-Schönlein purpura; rheumatic fever

Poisons and Toxins
Heavy metals (lead, arsenic, mercury); mushrooms; arachnoidism

Iatrogenic Causes of Abdominal Pain

Barbiturates in patients with porphyria
Enteric-coated potassium chloride tablets: mucosal ulceration
Anticoagulants: hemorrhage
Aspirin, indomethacin, phenylbutazone, corticosteroids: peptic ulceration
Aluminum hydroxide, ganglionic blockers, narcotics, analgesics: obstruction
Atropine-like drugs in prostatism: acute urinary retention
Corticosteroids, thiazides: pancreatitis
Narcotic withdrawal

QUESTIONNAIRE

Possible *meaning of response*

1   Location and radiation of pain

1.1   Where do you have pain?

1.1*a   Can you point to it?*

Epigastric pain of peptic ulcer

1.2   Is the pain
  • *diffuse? difficult to localize?*

Visceral pain: inflammation; biliary colic; colonic pain; acute hepatitis; **obstruction of small intestine;** vascular pain; diaphragmatic irritation

  • *well localized?*

Parietal peritoneal inflammation; appendicitis; pain due to nerve root stimulation: spinal cord tumor, herpes zoster

1.2*a*   Has the pain changed in its location?

The shifting of pain to a localized site suggests a local inflammation of the parietal peritoneum with a circumscribed inflammatory process: appendicitis; cholecystitis

1.2*b* In case of diffuse pain: At the onset, where was the maximum intensity of the pain localized?	Chronologic sequence of events may be more important than emphasis on the location of pain
• upper part of the abdomen?	**Perforated duodenal ulcer**
• lower part of the abdomen?	**Ruptured ectopic pregnancy**
1.3 Is the pain felt as being deep to the surface?	Visceral pain; deep musculoskeletal pain; referred pain
1.4 Do you have pain in the	
• midline?	Unpaired structures
• (mid)epigastrium?	Structures innervated by T6 to T8: stomach, duodenum, pancreas, liver, biliary tree; associated parietal peritoneum
• periumbilical region?	Structures innervated by T9 to T10: small intestine, appendix (early stages), upper ureters, testes, ovaries
• hypogastrium?	Structures innervated by T11 to T12: colon, bladder, lower ureters, uterus
• right upper quadrant (RUQ)?	Liver: stretching of liver capsule in acute congestive heart failure; infectious hepatitis; gallbladder; bile tract; duodenum; hepatic flexure; pancreas (head); diaphragmatic pleuritis
• left upper quadrant (LUQ)?	Pancreas (body and tail); spleen, perisplenitis; transverse colon; upper descending colon; splenic flexure; diaphragmatic pleuritis
• left lower quadrant (LLQ)?	Pelvic colon and rectosigmoid (functional and organic lesion); diverticulitis; left urinary tract; left adnexa

- right lower quadrant (RLQ)?

Appendix; terminal ileum; cecum; right urinary tract; right adnexa; subnephritic collection

- suprapubic region?

Obstruction of urinary bladder; rectosigmoid distention

- widespread over the abdomen?

Perforated peptic ulcer; peritonitis; diabetic acidosis; lead colic

- *the entire abdomen, immediately or shortly after onset?*

Flooding of the peritoneal cavity with an irritating fluid: **perforated ulcer, ruptured ectopic pregnancy, ruptured pyosalpynx, ruptured aneurysm**

- the upper part of the abdomen?

Acute pancreatitis; intrathoracic disease

1.5 Does the pain radiate
  - from the epigastrium to the
    - tip of right shoulder?

Acute cholecystitis

    - upper part of the lumbar region?

Distention of the common bile duct

    - shoulder tips?

Perforated peptic ulcer; involvement of undersurface of the diaphragm by acute peritonitis

    - midline of the back?

Penetrating peptic ulcer; gallbladder disease; dissecting aneurysm; pancreatitis; tumor of pancreas; hiatus hernia

    - jaws and/or down the arms?

Hiatus hernia

  - from the RUQ to the
    - *right shoulder?*
    - *tip of right scapula?*

Biliary colic, acute cholecystitis (acute distention of the gallbladder)

  - from the LUQ to the left shoulder?

Splenic disorder; splenic flexure syndrome

  - from flank to hypochondrium? down to the groin? into the genitalia?

Ureteral stone, renal colic

• from suprapubic area to the lumbosacral region?	Uterine pain

2   Mode of onset and duration

2.1 How long have you had pain in your abdomen?	Acute abdominal pain which has persisted for more than 6 h usually indicates a surgical problem; acute appendicitis evolves steadily over 12 h without remission
2.1a *Do you have recurrent episodes of abdominal pain?*	Medical diagnosis: peptic ulcer; pancreatic lesion; gallbladder disease; porphyria; regional enteritis; ulcerative colitis; irritable colon (see Chap. 14)
2.2 Did the pain appear • suddenly?	**Perforation of a viscus:** perforated peptic ulcer; **ruptured ectopic pregnancy; occlusion of the blood supply to an organ; strangulation** of a loop of intestine; mesenteric thrombosis; torsion of the pedicle of an ovarian cyst; occasionally acute pancreatitis; biliary colic
• gradually?	Inflammatory lesion: appendicitis; cholecystitis; salpingitis; intestinal obstruction

3   Character and intensity of the pain

3.1 Is the pain • severe? intense?	Biliary colic; renal colic; perforated peptic ulcer; acute pancreatitis; dissecting aortic aneurysm; mesenteric occlusion; ruptured ectopic pregnancy
• mild or moderate?	Peptic ulcer; small intestinal pain; appendicular pain; colonic pain

3.2 Is the pain
- dull?   Epigastric: pain of peptic ulcer
- burning?   Epigastric: psychogenic; duo-
                                         denal ulcer
- crushing?   Dissecting aortic aneurysm; pep-
                                         tic ulcer; hiatus hernia
- sticking in nature?   Regional enteritis; functional GI
                                         disorder
- aching?   Visceral pain: peptic ulcer;
                                         cholecystitis; tumor
- cramping?   Colic: colonic, renal; mesenteric
                                         vascular occlusion (crampy pain
                                         in early stage)

3.3 Is the pain
- steady? continuous?   Inflammatory process in an ab-
                                         dominal organ; parietal perito-
                                         neal inflammation; ischemia from
                                         strangulation obstruction (later
                                         stage); occlusion of the superior
                                         mesenteric artery; pain arising
                                         from the abdominal wall
- crampy at the onset,   Strangulation obstruction
  becoming continuous
  later?
- persistent and mild or   Peptic ulcer; appendicular pain
  moderate?
- persistent and severe?   Gallstone colic (sudden disten-
                                         tion of the biliary tree)
- fluctuant and severe?   Ureteral colic
- intermittent? colicky?   Pain of obstruction of a hollow
                                         abdominal viscus: intestinal and
                                         colonic pain
- pulsatile?   Abdominal aneurysm of the
                                         aorta

3.4 Does the pain
- *recur for several seconds*   Proximal obstruction; intestinal
  about three times a minute,   colic
  with pain-free intervals of
  4 to 5 min?

• *last 1 to 5 min with pain-free intervals of 10 to 20 or 30 min?*	Distal obstruction; colonic pain

4 Precipitating or aggravating factors

4.1 Is the pain worsened by

• coughing? sneezing?	Peritoneal inflammation; pain arising from abdominal wall (hematoma of rectus sheath); referred pain from the spine (prolapsed intervertebral disk)
• *recumbency?*	Pancreatic pain: distention of pancreatic ducts
• bending over?	Hiatus hernia; reflux esophagitis
• deep inspiration?	Involvement of diaphragm; acute cholecystitis, when the movement of the diaphragm brings the inflamed organ against the peritoneum

5 Relieving factors

5.1 Is the pain relieved by

• *leaning forward?* sitting up?	Pancreatic pain
• *lying still? avoiding motion?*	Peritoneal inflammation; perforation of peptic ulcer
• *changing your position? moving about frequently?*	Obstructed hollow organ: <u>ureteral</u> or biliary colic
• vomiting?	Gastric outlet obstruction; pain due to an inflammatory lesion (appendicitis) is not relieved by vomiting

5.2 Have you received any drugs for your pain?   Analgesics may modify the clinical picture

6 Accompanying symptoms

6.1 Is the pain associated with

- sweating? nausea? vomiting?

Severe abdominal pain: appendicitis; perforated ulcer; obstructive lesion; pancreatitis; cholecystitis; biliary colic; volvulus; intraperitoneal hemorrhage

- severe constipation? (last bowel movement more than 24 h ago)

Intestinal obstruction; appendicitis; cholecystitis; **volvulus**

- black, tarry stools?

Intussusception; mesenteric vascular occlusion; obstructing neoplastic or inflammatory lesion

- diarrhea?

Acute enteritis; unusual position of appendix

- bloody diarrhea?

Mesenteric arterial occlusion

- abdominal distention?

Intestinal obstruction

- decreased appetite?

Anorexia is the rule in acute intraabdominal disease

- fever? chills?

Cholecystitis; acute pyelonephritis

- jaundice?

Gallstone colic

- burning on urination?
- bloody urine?

Renal colic

- dark urine?

Gallstone colic (bilirubinuria); porphyria

- purulent urine?

Urinary infection

6.2 For the female patient: What date did your last menstrual period begin?

Last menstrual period more than 6 weeks previous: ectopic pregnancy

6.2a *Have you noticed any vaginal hemorrhage?*

7 *Iatrogenic factors*   see Etiology

8 *Environmental factors*

8.1 What is
- your occupation?

Professional hazards (lead)

- your alcohol intake?

Pancreatitis; acute peptic ulcer

8.2 Are there any other peo-   Food poisoning
ple in your immediate
surroundings who also
have abdominal pain?

9 *Personal antecedents pertaining to the abdominal pain*

9.1 Have you ever had an x-ray of your stomach? gallbladder?
intestine? kidneys? When? With what results?

9.2 Have you recently had a   Rupture of the spleen may occur
trauma to your abdomen?   after a minor injury

9.3 Do you have any of the following conditions:
  • peptic ulcer?   Pain due to perforated ulcer
  • gallstone disease?   Biliary colic; pancreatitis
  • kidney stones?
  • any prior abdominal sur- Postoperative adhesions; pa-
    gery?   tients with porphyria frequently
                             have abdominal operations

  • a heart disease?   Acute congestive heart failure
                             with stretching of liver capsule
                             and pain in RUQ; embolic mes-
                             enteric arterial occlusion in atrial
                             fibrillation or recent myocardial
                             infarction
  • diabetes?   Pain of impending diabetic coma

10 *Family medical history pertaining to the abdominal pain*

10.1 Is there a family history   Medical diagnosis: familial Medi-
of similar attacks?   terranean fever; acute intermit-
                            tent porphyria

PHYSICAL SIGNS PERTINENT TO THE COMPLAINT

Finding   **Possible** *significance*
Patient lying immobile in bed, Diffuse peritonitis
resisting movement and change
in position

Restless patient, changing posi-   Obstruction of ureter, bile ducts,
tion frequently   or small bowel early in its course

Hypotension; rapid, weak pulse; cold, moist skin; restlessness	Shock: peritonitis; bowel infarction; intestinal obstruction; rupture of an abdominal aortic aneurysm
Fever	Infectious process: peritonitis, appendicitis, diverticulitis, tissue necrosis (the temperature is usually normal early with most causes of "surgical" abdomen)
Temperature over 102°F	Acute urinary tract or pulmonary infection more likely than an acute surgical condition of the abdomen
Tenderness on abdominal palpation; **generalized rebound tenderness**	Diffuse peritonitis
Involuntary guarding	Reflex muscle spasm due to underlying peritoneal irritation; perforated intraabdominal viscus
Localized direct and rebound tenderness	Surgical condition; localized peritonitis; vascular necrosis of an ischemic organ
Tenderness on palpation in RLQ	Acute appendicitis
Abdominal mass	Tumor; abscess; ruptured aortic aneurysm; distended loop of bowel; distended gallbladder
Auscultation of the abdomen: Absent bowel sounds	Later stage of mechanical obstruction; paralytic ileus; generalized peritonitis; ischemia and strangulation of the bowel
Hyperactive high-pitched bowel sounds	Early stage of mechanical obstruction of the bowel
Vascular bruit	Dissecting arterial aneurysm
Abdominal distention; absent bowel sounds; absence of liver dullness	Free intraperitoneal air: perforated viscus

Inspection of umbilicus and groin	May reveal an incarcerated hernia, a common cause of small-bowel obstruction; metastasizing intraabdominal malignancy at the umbilicus
Scars of previous surgery	Obstruction caused by adhesions; porphyria
Rectal examination: Tenderness	Pelvic inflammation; appendicitis; etc.
Mass	Abscess; tumor; etc.
Abnormal pelvic examination	Masses of uterus or adnexae; pelvic inflammatory disease; twisted ovarian cyst; peritonitis; etc.

LABORATORY TESTS PERTAINING TO THE COMPLAINT

Procedure	Finding	Diagnostic possibilities
Urine		
Urinalysis	RBCs	Renal stone; tumor of the genitourinary (GU) tract
	RBC casts	Glomerulitis
	Glycosuria	Diabetic acidosis
	Pyuria	Urinary tract infection
Porphobilinogen	Positive	Porphyria
Blood		
RBCs	Anemia	Intraabdominal hemorrhage; dissecting aneurysm

	Increased	Hemoconcentration; hypovolemia
	Sickling	Sickle cell crisis
WBCs	Leukocytosis	Perforation of a viscus; appendicitis; acute cholecystitis; pancreatitis; intestinal infarction; pelvic inflammatory disease (a normal WBC count does not exclude perforation of abdominal viscera)
Electrolytes	Abnormal	Dehydration; vomiting; imbalances needing correction prior to eventual surgery
Calcium	Low	Acute pancreatitis
BUN, creatinine	Elevated	Renal disease; dehydration secondary to vomiting and deficient fluid intake
Glucose	Elevated	Diabetes mellitus
Amylase (N: 60 to 180 Somogyi U/100 mL)	Elevated	Pancreatitis; perforated ulcer; strangulating intestinal obstruction; acute cholecystitis; acute common duct obstruction
Bilirubin	Elevated	Biliary tract or pancreas disorder
Amylase/creatinine clearance ratio	>5 percent	Acute pancreatitis

Procedure	*To detect*
Flat and upright films of the abdomen	Free air in the peritoneal cavity: perforation of a hollow viscus; acute small-bowel obstruction; calculus in biliary or urinary tract; soft-tissue masses; pancreatic calcifications; "sentinel loops": acute pancreatitis; absent psoas shadow: retroperitoneal mass or bleeding; displaced stomach or bowel shadows
Chest x-ray	Extraabdominal condition mimicking acute abdominal situation; pneumonia; free air under the diaphragm
IV cholangiogram	Biliary tract obstruction or inflammation
IV pyelogram	Ureteral obstruction; hydronephrosis
Barium enema	Site and nature of colonic obstruction
ECG	Extraabdominal condition: myocardial infarction; acute pericarditis

USEFUL REMINDERS AND DIAGNOSTIC CLUES

Misleading Factors

Sudden distention of the biliary tree produces a steady rather than a colicky type of pain: the term "biliary colic" is misleading.

The possibility of intrathoracic disease must be considered in every patient with abdominal pain, especially if the pain is in the upper part of the abdomen.

Embolism or thrombosis of the superior mesenteric artery may be associated, at the onset, with a mild, continuous, diffuse type of pain.

Diagnostic Considerations

Disorders which may simulate perforated ulcer: coronary thrombosis; dissecting aneurysm; severe biliary or renal colic; pneumonia involving diaphragmatic segments; acute pancreatitis; acute duodenal ulcer; acute perforation of appendix; mesenteric thrombosis; ruptured ectopic pregnancy.

Gallstones may cause abdominal pain, but they are present in 10 to 20 percent of the adult population and do not usually cause symptoms.

Vomiting appearing at about the same time as the abdominal pain is seen in patients with peritonitis, acute obstruction of choledochus or ureter, and high intestinal obstruction. Vomiting appearing some hours after the onset of the pain is seen in low intestinal obstruction and appendicitis.

In case of	*Suspect*
Severe distress with minimal abdominal findings	A medical condition
Abdominal pain of obscure origin	A metabolic cause

SELECTED BIBLIOGRAPHY

Jones RS: An approach to the acute abdomen and intestinal obstruction, in Sleisenger MH, Fordtran JS (eds), *Gastrointestinal Disease: Pathophysiology, Diagnosis, Management,* pp 338–351, Philadelphia: Saunders, 1973
Steinheber FU: Medical conditions mimicking the acute surgical abdomen. Med Clin North Am 57:1559–1567, 1973

12
Constipation

DEFINITIONS AND GENERAL CONSIDERATIONS

Constipation   delay in the evacuation of feces, with passage of unduly hard and dry fecal material; stools of insufficient size (less than 50 g/day).

Obstipation   a condition in which constipation is so severe that the patient has no movement without an enema.

Obstruction   a condition in which there is interference with the passage of intestinal contents (gas, fluid, and solid) onward through the bowel lumen.

Chyme passes through the small intestine rapidly, so that 5 or 6 h after a meal, the greater proportion is in the cecum. In the large bowel, the fecal mass progresses more slowly, about 12 h being required for a part of it to pass from the cecum to the sigmoid and descending colon. An additional 6 or 8 h usually elapses before evacuation of the residue of ingesta occurs. Normally the fecal mass does not pass beyond the sigmoid into the rectum until the act of defecation is about to occur. The mass peristaltic movement which propels the fecal matter into the rectum is usually initiated by the ingestion of food at breakfast time. The desire to defecate is initiated by distention of the rectum by the fecal mass as a result of the mass peristaltic movement.

Repeatedly ignoring the desire to defecate results in blunting of the "defecation sense of the rectum" and constitutes a frequent cause of constipation (rectal constipation or dyschezia). In rectal constipation, rectal examination discloses a rectum filled with feces. Patients with spastic constipation have a motility abnormality of the sigmoid and descending colon; transfer of feces into the rectum is delayed, and the rectum is relatively empty. Stools are small and excessively hard, owing to increased absorption of fluid as a result of prolonged contact of the luminal contents with the colonic mucosa consequent to delayed transit. Inadequate propulsion of feces may also result from mechanical obstruction (e.g., carcinoma of the sigmoid colon) or from diminished contraction of the proximal intestine (e.g., paralytic ileus).

ETIOLOGY

Table 12-1   Acute Constipation

Mechanical intestinal obstruction
   Narrowing of the lumen
      Strictures:
         Congenital
         Acquired: neoplastic, traumatic, vascular, inflammatory
      Obturation: gallstones, fecaliths, foreign bodies, worms
      Compression from without
   Obstruction from adhesions or bands: congenital, inflammatory, traumatic, neoplastic
   Hernia: external, internal
   Volvulus
   Intussusception

Adynamic ileus: inhibition of bowel motility
   Intraabdominal causes:
      Peritoneal irritation: traumatic, bacterial, chemical
      Vascular changes: strangulation, mesenteric thrombosis
      Extraperitoneal irritation: hemorrhage, infection, renal colic
   Extraabdominal:
      Toxic: pneumonia, empyema, uremia, systemic infection
      Neurogenic: injuries of the spinal cord, fractures of the lower ribs, irritation of the splanchnic nerves, cerebrovascular accident

Table 12-2   Recent Progressive Constipation

Partial bowel obstruction: malignant and benign tumors of colon or rectum; fecal impaction, fecaliths; partial intussusception; volvulus; neoplastic or inflammatory stricture; adhesions
Pressure on the bowel from without: uterine fibroids, ovarian cysts, pregnancy; any large abdominal tumors; ascites
Carcinoma of stomach, gallbladder, pancreas (initial symptom)
Hypothyroidism; hyperparathyroidism
Tuberculosis; urinary tract disease; congestive heart failure
Neurologic disorder: multiple sclerosis; parkinsonism; spinal cord lesion
Severe psychoses; profound depression
Myasthenia gravis
Drugs; plumbism
Porphyria; systemic lupus erythematosus
Anal painful lesions: fissures, hemorrhoids, anusitis

Table 12-3   Chronic Constipation

Social improprieties: dietary factors; lack of roughage; laxative abuse; improper training; poor bowel habits; improper posture at defecation; lack of toilet facilities; lack of exercise

Diminished expulsive power: weakness of diaphragm (chronic obstructive lung disease, emphysema); weakness of abdominal wall muscles (frequent pregnancies, obesity); weakness of pelvic floor (frequent pregnancies)

Loss of rectal defecation reflex: repeated neglect of the normal desire to move the bowels; laxative abuse

Irritable colon

Megacolon: idiopathic; acquired

Spasm of anal sphincter (painful anal lesions): anusitis, fissures, ulcer, hemorrhoids

Iatrogenic Causes of Constipation

Antacids: aluminum hydroxide, calcium carbonate

Anticholinergics; ganglionic-blocking agents

Large amounts of sedatives (any sedatives may augment a tendency toward constipation); opiates: morphine, codeine

The bland nonresidue diet often prescribed to patients with gastric disorders

QUESTIONNAIRE

Acute Onset of Severe Obstipation

Possible *meaning of response*

1   When did you have your last bowel movement?

1.1   Do you still pass gas?   Failure to pass gas suggests complete intestinal obstruction

2   Do you have

• abdominal pain? cramps?   **Mechanical intestinal obstruction** (see Chap. 11)

• abdominal distention?   Adynamic ileus; distention may be quite marked late in any form of obstruction

• nausea? *vomiting?*   **Intestinal obstruction**

3	Do you hear bowel sounds? abdominal rumbling?	Borborygmi: bowel sounds are active at the onset of mechanical ileus
4	What were your bowel habits before this episode?	
	• abnormal?	Chronic intestinal disorder progressing to complete obstruction
	• constipation alternating with bouts of diarrhea?	Carcinoma of colon; irritable colon; diabetic autonomic neuropathy; fecal impaction
5	Have you taken any laxatives? enemas?	In high obstruction, the lower bowel may function well for a time, e.g., expelling an enema readily
6	Have you ever had an operation on the abdomen?	Postoperative adhesions or strictures interfering with the onward movement of the intestinal contents

Chronic Constipation

1   Mode of onset and duration

1.1	How long have you been constipated?	A long history suggests: <u>irritable colon, simple rectal constipation</u>; megacolon
1.2	How many stools do you have per day? or week?	
1.3	According to you, how many times a day should you have a movement?	Some patients are concerned because their bowel movements do not measure up to their expectations
1.3*a*	What do you regard as a normal defecatory pattern?	Defecatory habits are very varied among normal subjects

1.4   How many times a day, a week, do you feel the urge to defecate?

1.4a   Do you still feel a desire to defecate?

A decreasing desire is often due to repeated neglect to empty the colon when the desire to defecate occurs

2   Character of the stools

2.1   Are the stools
  • excessively hard?

Chronic constipation

  • like hard small pellets?

Spastic constipation; <u>irritable colon</u> (rare in simple constipation due to neglect of the bowels)

  • like ribbons (thin and narrow)?

Rectal cancer; functional bowel disorders, irritable colon

  • watery?

In an elderly, debilitated patient: <u>fecal impaction</u> (liquid stool above the fecal mass passing around the impaction)

  • of variable consistency?

Malignant lesion of the colon; <u>irritable colon</u>

2.2   What is the color of the stools?
  • streaked with blood?

Anal disease (fissures, ulcers, <u>hemorrhoids</u>)

  • mixed with blood?

Neoplasm of the large bowel

  • mixed with mucus?

Irritable colon

  • black, tarry?

Gastrointestinal bleeding

2.3   *Do you have periods of constipation alternating with bouts of diarrhea?*

Neoplasm of large bowel; <u>irritable colon</u>

2.4   Have you recently noticed
  • *a change in your bowel habits?*

Partial bowel obstruction (tumor)

  • a decrease in the size of the stools?

Neoplasm of rectum; proctitis; irritable colon

3 Accompanying symptoms

3.1 Do you have
- abdominal pain? distress?

  Obstructive process: carcinoma of colon; <u>irritable colon</u>

  - *relieved by defecation? passage of flatus?*

    Colonic disease; irritable colon
  - pain with defecation?

    Fissures; <u>hemorrhoids</u>; may reinforce the inhibitory impulses to defecation
  - pain at the anus?

    Thrombosis of external <u>hemorrhoids</u>

3.2 Do you
- often pass gas?
- frequently hear rumbling from your abdomen? bowel sounds?

  <u>Irritable colon; habitual constipation</u>

3.3 Do you experience a sensation of fullness or pressure in the rectum?

Constipation of rectal type: fecal accumulation in the rectum

3.4 Do you feel, after a bowel movement, that defecation was insufficient?

<u>Rectal constipation</u>; colon carcinoma

3.5 Do you have a loss of appetite? bloating? belching? headaches?

Symptoms generally related to the anxiety aroused by the constipation and the attendant disturbance of intestinal motility

3.6 Has your weight
- remained the same?

  Habitual constipation; irritable colon
- increased?

  Hypothyroidism
- decreased?

  Carcinoma of the colon

3.7 Have you recently noticed the appearance of
- frequent urination?

  Carcinoma of pelvic colon or rectum invading, or pressing against, the lower urinary tract

   • urinary retention?   Lesion in the cauda equina impairing the function of the parasympathetic innervation of the colon

4 *Iatrogenic factors*   see Etiology

4.1   Do you take laxatives? enemas? Since when? which ones? every day?   Constipation is complicated by the use or abuse of laxatives in almost all patients with this disorder; abuse of laxatives induces a loss of the sensitivity of the rectal defecatory reflexes

5 *Environmental factors*

5.1   What do you habitually eat?   Lack of roughage may induce constipation

5.1*a*   Did you recently modify your usual diet?   A marked change in dietary regime, particularly in combination with sedative drugs, may produce constipation

5.1*b*   Do you skip breakfast?   Absence of stimulation of bowel peristalsis

5.2   What is your occupation?   A sedentary occupation may produce constipation by blunting the defecatory reflex and diminishing expulsive power

6 *Personal antecedents pertaining to the constipation*

6.1   Has an examination of your stool ever been performed? When? With what results?

6.2   Have you ever had an x-ray examination of your intestine? a rectoscopy? When? With what results?

6.3   Have you ever had any of the following conditions: colitis? a thyroid condition?

   • an abdominal operation?   Postoperative adhesions or strictures

• hemorrhoids? anal ulcers? fissure?	Often a result of the constipation; these lesions may also induce a failure of relaxation of the anal sphincter
6.3*a* Have you recently been bedridden for a prolonged period? why? for how long?	May induce blunting of defecatory reflexes and diminished expulsive power
6.4 For the female patient: How many pregnancies have you had?	Multiple pregnancies may produce lax abdominal muscles and weaken the pelvic floor, resulting in rectal constipation

PHYSICAL SIGNS PERTINENT TO THE COMPLAINT

Finding	**Possible** *significance*
Hyperactive bowel sounds; visible peristalsis; abdominal mass	Mechanical ileus; intestinal obstructing lesion
Absent bowel sounds; distended abdomen	Adynamic ileus
Dry skin; delayed relaxation phase of the deep tendon reflexes	Myxedema
Rectal examination:	
Absence of stools	Primary disorder of defecation unlikely; point of obstruction at the rectosigmoid or above; irritable colon
Rectum packed with feces	Chronic habitual constipation
Fecal impaction	May be accompanied at first by constipation
Thrombosed hemorrhoids; anal ulcers	Disorders preventing the relaxation of the internal anal sphincter
Rectal mass	Carcinoma (up to 50 percent of all colonic cancers are within the reach of the index finger)

LABORATORY TESTS PERTAINING TO THE COMPLAINT

Procedure	Finding	Diagnostic possibilities
Blood Thyroid function tests*	Abnormal	Hypothyroidism
Calcium*	Elevated	Hyperparathyroidism with constipation
Electrolytes*	Hypokalemia	Inhibits intestinal peristalsis
Stool Occult blood tests	Positive	GI malignancy; anal disease

Procedure	To detect
Flat abdominal film	Megacolon
Proctosigmoidoscopy Barium enema	Carcinoma of the rectum or descending colon (indicated in constipation of recent onset)
Upper GI x-rays	Tumor of GI tract (in constipation of recent onset)

* If appropriate.

USEFUL REMINDERS AND DIAGNOSTIC CLUES

Some healthy persons go to stool on the average of three times daily and others evacuate the bowel once in 2 or 3 days: marked departures from the average normal passage rate of feces through the colon are commensurate with good health.

Constipation of the irritable colon may be differentiated from simple constipation by its intermittency. Not infrequently, in "irritable-colon" patients, normal bowel habit may be present for long periods of time between attacks of colonic dysfunction.

In high intestinal obstruction, the lower bowel may function quite well for a time, whereas in low intestinal obstruction and colon obstruction, obstipation occurs early.

Intermittent intestinal obstruction may be due to: neoplasm, adhesions, internal hernia, chronic inflammatory disease of the small bowel, intussusception, or volvulus.

Malignancy

Colorectal cancer is the most common cancer in the United States after skin cancer.

It has been found that the physician was responsible for delay in diagnosis in 28 percent of malignant disease of the colon.

A history of changed bowel habit, most frequently constipation, can be elicited from 60 percent of patients with carcinoma of the descending colon.

SELECTED BIBLIOGRAPHY

Almy TP: Constipation, in Sleisenger MH, Fordtran JS (eds): *Gastrointestinal Disease: Pathophysiology, Diagnosis, Management,* chap 23, pp 320–325, Philadelphia: Saunders, 1973

Peterson ML: Constipation and diarrhea, in Mac Bryde CM, Blacklow RS (eds), *Signs and Symptoms,* 5th ed, chap 22, pp 381–398, Philadelphia: Lippincott, 1970

13
Diarrhea

DEFINITION AND PATHOPHYSIOLOGY

Diarrhea   frequent passage of unformed stools.

The absorptive surfaces of the intestinal tract are normally presented with 10 L of liquid (dietary and secretions) per day. In the healthy subject, all but 1000 to 1500 mL is absorbed by the time the cecum is reached. Only 100 to 150 mL of that fluid volume remains unabsorbed and appears in the feces. Since the colon has a limited absorptive capacity (about 2.5 L per day), diarrhea appears if a larger volume is presented to the colon by the small intestine. This occurs if there is (1) an impaired intestinal absorption of water and solutes (osmotic diarrhea), due to inadequate functional absorptive surface, intestinal vascular insufficiency, ingestion of poorly absorbed solutes (some laxatives), maldigestion of ingested food, diffuse mucosal disease, lactase deficiency; or (2) increased fluid secretion (secretory diarrhea), e.g., toxin-induced (viral and bacterial enteritis), fatty acid–induced, peptide hormone–producing tumors.

Disordered colonic function may be the cause of diarrhea if there is (1) decreased colonic reabsorption of water and electrolytes because of diffuse mucosal disease (ulcerative colitis, shigellosis), or (2) increased colonic secretion induced by unabsorbed bile salts or fatty acids entering the colon, or caused by a fluid-secreting tumor such as villous adenoma.

Abnormalities of intestinal motility mediated by neurohumoral factors (serotonin, acetylcholine, prostaglandins) may also lead to diarrhea.

ETIOLOGY

Table 13-1   Acute Diarrhea

Infection: *Salmonella, Shigella,* enteropathogenic *Escherichia coli, Staphylococcus, Vibrio cholerae, Clostridium perfringens, Proteus,* viral pathogens, helminths, protozoa (*Entamoeba, Giardia*)

Table 13-1 (continued)

Toxic: chemical poisons: arsenic, lead, cadmium, mercury; mushrooms; drugs
Dietary: irritating foods
Acute episode in a patient with chronic disease process: ulcerative colitis; regional enteritis; diverticulitis
Ischemic colitis
Partial intestinal obstruction
Psychologic stress
Miscellaneous: pericolic and perirectal abscess; retroiliac appendicitis; pellagra; gastrointestinal allergy; acute radiation sickness

Table 13-2 Chronic Diarrhea (persisting for at least 3 weeks)

Diseases of the small intestine
Inflammatory: regional enteritis; systemic lupus erythematosus; polyarteritis nodosa; radiation enteritis
Absorption defects: malabsorption: see Table 13-3.

Diseases of the large intestine
Ulcerative colitis; irritable-bowel syndrome; diverticulitis; amebic colitis; uremic colitis; Crohn's disease of colon; radiation therapy; ischemic colitis; multiple polyposis; carcinoma of right colon; villous adenoma

Diseases of the stomach
Gastric carcinoma; pyloric stenosis; giant hypertrophic gastritis

Miscellaneous
Metabolic: hyperthyroidism; Addison's disease; hypervitaminosis D; diabetes mellitus; Cushing's syndrome; amyloidosis; hypoparathyroidism
Neoplastic (humorally mediated): carcinoid syndrome; sympathomimetic secreting tumors; Zollinger-Ellison syndrome; non-beta cell tumor of the pancreas with vasoactive intestinal peptide; medullary carcinoma of the thyroid
Hematologic: pellagra; pernicious anemia
Postoperative: vagotomy; gastrectomy; enteric fistula formation; blind-loop syndrome; inadvertent gastroileostomy
Allergy: eosinophilic gastroenteritis
Fecal impaction; drugs

Table 13-3   Causes of Malabsorption*

Inadequate digestion
Pancreatic insufficiency: chronic pancreatitis, carcinoma of pancreas, pancreatic resection
Inactivation of pancreatic enzymes by gastric secretion: Zollinger-Ellison syndrome
Postgastrectomy steatorrhea

Reduced bile salts (with inadequate micelle formation)
Hepatocellular disease; bile duct obstruction
Bacterial overgrowth (bile salt deconjugation): diabetic visceral neuropathy, scleroderma, multiple small-bowel diverticula, fistulas, strictures, blind loops
Ileal resection

Inadequate absorptive surface
Intestinal resection, gastrocolic fistula, gastroileostomy

Mucosal absorptive defects
Biochemical defects: sprue (gluten-induced enteropathy); disaccharidase deficiency; monosaccharide malabsorption; hypogammaglobulinemia; abetalipoproteinemia; cystinuria; Hartnup disease
Infiltration or inflammation of intestinal wall: amyloidosis; scleroderma; lymphoma; regional enteritis; Whipple's disease; tropical sprue

Lymphatic obstruction
Intestinal lymphangiectasia; Whipple's disease; lymphoma; tuberculosis

Altered blood supply
Mesenteric vascular insufficiency; constrictive pericarditis

Endocrine and metabolic
Diabetes mellitus; carcinoid syndrome; hyperthyroidism; hypoadrenocorticism

---

* Multiple defects may be responsible.

Iatrogenic Causes of Diarrhea (partial list)

Antibiotics: tetracycline; lincomycin, clindamycin (pseudomembranous enterocolitis); neomycin (malabsorption)

Antimetabolites
Arsenicals, gold, mercury
Cathartic habit
Cholestyramine
Cholinergic drugs
Colchicine
Digitalis

Ganglionic-blocking agents
Lactulose
Magnesium-containing antacids
Paraaminosalicylic acid
Phenformin
Quinine, quinidine
Thyroid extracts

QUESTIONNAIRE

Possible *meaning of response*

Acute Diarrhea

1 Mode of onset

1.1 How long have you had diarrhea?

1.2 How many stools a day do you have?

1.3 Did the diarrhea appear
  • abruptly?

Active <u>infection</u>: bacterial diarrhea, viral gastroenteritis; toxins; poisons; drugs

  • gradually?

Usual mode of onset of amebic colitis

1.4 Has the diarrhea appeared after a meal?
  • *almost immediately after ingestion?*

Chemical food poisoning: cadmium, sodium fluoride

  • *1 to 3 h after?*

<u>Staphylococcal food poisoning</u>

  • within 12 to 24 h of eating?

Preformed toxin ingested; viral gastroenteritis

  • without relation to a meal?

Viral gastroenteritis

1.4*a* What did you eat at this meal?
  • milk? cream? prepared foods?

Not properly refrigerated; staphylococcal food poisoning

  • egg products?

(Of infected fowl): *Salmonella*

• meat?	Of infected animals: *C. perfringens*
• fat? oil? unripe fruit? alcohol?	Dietary causes of acute diarrhea

2 Character of the stools

2.1 Are the stools

• watery?	Inflammatory disease of small intestine; viral gastroenteritis; giardiasis
• greenish?	Salmonellosis; giardiasis

2.2 Do the stools contain

• mucus and/or blood?	Shigellosis; diverticulitis; *Salmonella* enteritis; amebic colitis
• mucus without blood?	Irritable colon
• pus?	Acute enteritis; shigellosis
• none of the above?	<u>Functional disorder</u>

2.3 What is the odor of the stools?

• malodorous?	Salmonellosis; giardiasis
• lack of odor?	Shigellosis

3 Accompanying symptoms

3.1 Do you have

• loss of appetite? nausea? vomiting?	Inflammatory disease of small bowel: bacterial toxins, staphylococcal, *Clostridia*; viral
• abdominal cramps? pain?	Staphylococcal, shigellosis; viral gastroenteritis
• epigastric or periumbilical?	Inflammatory disease of small intestine
• *rectal urgency? a painful tension in the rectum with a frequent desire to move the bowels?* (tenesmus)	Colonic infection: diverticulitis, amebic dysentery (not in inflammatory disease of small intestine)
• fever?	Infectious origin: salmonellosis; shigellosis

• no fever?	Bacterial toxins (staphylococcal, *C. perfringens*); viral gastroenteritis; psychogenic diarrhea
• pain in your muscles? malaise?	Myalgia may occur in acute infectious diarrhea

4 *Iatrogenic factors*   see Etiology

5 *Environmental factors*

5.1 *Are there other people in your family, at your job, at school, who became ill with diarrhea?*	Viral gastroenteritis; infectious diarrhea
5.1*a* Did they eat the same food as you?	
5.2 Have you recently traveled to a tropical or an underdeveloped country?	Traveler's diarrhea (turista); amebic colitis; giardiasis (also in the United States) Cholera: Africa, Asia, Middle East Schistosomiasis: • *Schistosoma mansoni:* Africa, Arabian peninsula, Brazil, Puerto Rico • *S. japonicum:* Japan, Taiwan, the Philippines • *S. haematobium:* Nile Valley, Africa

Chronic Diarrhea (lasting more than 3 weeks)

1 *Mode of onset, frequency, duration*

1.1 How long have you had diarrhea?	Since infancy: celiac disease; disaccharidase deficiency
1.2 Is the diarrhea • continuous?	Regional enteritis; ulcerative colitis; fistulas; hyperthyroidism; gastric disorders; laxative abuse

• intermittent?	Allergy; diverticulitis; malabsorption; <u>irritable colon</u> (emotional disorders)
1.3 *Do you have bouts of diarrhea alternating with periods of constipation?*	<u>Carcinoma</u> of the colon; <u>diverticulitis; irritable colon</u>; partial intestinal obstruction; diabetic autonomic neuropathy; fecal impaction; diarrhea of chronic constipation and laxative habit

2 *Qualitative aspects of the diarrhea*

2.1 Are the stools

• loose?	Diseases of the left colon
• pasty?	Sigmoid hypomotility with poor water absorption
• watery?	Protein-losing enteropathy; villous adenoma; Zollinger-Ellison syndrome; cathartics; diabetic visceral neuropathy; "pancreatic cholera"; medullary carcinoma of the thyroid; internal fistulas; fecal impaction; emotional disturbances; severe inflammatory diseases of the bowel
• foamy? liquid?	Small intestine: lactase or sucrase deficiency; monosaccharide malabsorption
• *oily? floating?*	Small intestine: malabsorption syndrome; steatorrhea

2.2 Do your stools contain

• mucus?	<u>Ulcerative colitis; irritable colon</u>; amebiasis; cathartics
• without pus? blood?	Functional bowel disorder
• blood?	Chronic inflammatory process of small bowel or colon or both; amebic or bacillary dysentery; ulcerative colitis; diverticulitis; carcinoma; polyps; associated proctitis or anusitis

- pus? | Abscess; inflammatory bowel disease; ulcerating neoplasm

- undigested food? | Small intestine or colon; gastro-colic or gastroileal fistula

2.3 What is the color of your stools?
- pale? light in color? | Small intestine; steatorrhea
- black? | GI bleeding
- greenish? | Excessive amounts of bile: infection, laxative abuse

2.4 Do your stools have a foul odor? | Small intestine: malabsorption

2.5 At what time in the day do you have diarrhea?
- *in the early morning?* | Irritable colon
- only during the day? | Functional or organic
- *also during the night?* | Favors organic disease over irritable colon (but this is not always specific); ulcerative colitis; hyperthyroidism; diabetic visceral neuropathy; severe inflammatory disease

3 *Quantitative aspects of the diarrhea*

3.1 How many bowel movements per day do you have?
- *few? about six times (or less) daily?* (without urgency) | Small intestine, right colon: malabsorption
- *many? exceeding six times per day?* (with urgency) | Left colon, rectum: ulcerative colitis, amebiasis

3.2 What is the *volume* of your stools?
- *large, bulky?* | More than 300 g/day: small intestine, right colon: malabsorption; Crohn's disease

• *small?*

Less than 200 g/day: distal colon, rectum: ulcerative colitis, diverticulitis, cancer, irritable colon

4 Precipitating or aggravating factors

4.1 Do you have diarrhea
• after meals?

Osmotic diarrhea; irritable colon; regional enteritis; ulcerative colitis

• after eating cheese, ice cream, yogurt, milk?

Lactase deficiency

• without any relation to meals?

Secretory diarrhea; infectious disease; hyperthyroidism

• after emotional stress? anxiety?

Functional GI disorder

5 Relieving factors

5.1 Does the diarrhea
• *stop when you fast?*

Osmotic diarrhea: disaccharidase deficiency; monosaccharide malabsorption

• *persist during fasting?*

Secretory diarrhea: Zollinger-Ellison syndrome; pancreatic cholera; medullary carcinoma of the thyroid

6 Accompanying symptoms

6.1 Do you have
• abdominal pain?

Carcinoma of colon; Zollinger-Ellison syndrome

• in periumbilical region? RLQ?

Motor disorder in the small intestine, ileum, or right colon; regional enteritis; ischemic colitis

• in LUQ?

Irritable colon

• in LLQ?	Diverticulitis; disturbance in the rectosigmoid segment
• relieved by defecation?	Colonic disease
• not relieved by defecation?	Disease of small bowel
• *no cramps?*	Irritable colon; small-intestine disorder; hyperthyroidism; diabetes mellitus
• abdominal distention?	Malabsorption; chronic partial intestinal obstruction (due to adhesions or neoplasm)
• *urgency? a frequent desire to move the bowels?* (tenesmus)	Left colon, rectum: ulcerative colitis; amebiasis; carcinoma of rectum
• *no urgency?*	Small intestine, right colon: malabsorption; Crohn's disease
• pain with defecation?	Anus, rectum, colon; anal fissure; ulcerative colitis
• nausea? vomiting?	Partial intestinal obstruction (e.g., due to adhesions); uremia; diabetic autonomic neuropathy

6.2 Has your appetite

• remained the same?	Hyperthyroidism; malabsorption; allergy
• decreased?	Uremia; carcinoma

6.3 Has your weight

• remained the same?	<u>Functional bowel disease</u>; allergy; lactase deficiency
• increased?	Edema due to malabsorption with hypoproteinemia
• decreased?	In malabsorptive disorders: loss of calories; cancer of pancreas; regional enteritis

6.3a Did the weight loss

• precede the onset of diarrhea?	Malignancy; carcinoma of pancreas; hyperthyroidism; diabetes mellitus; malabsorption
• appear late after the onset of diarrhea?	Carcinoma of the colon

6.4   Do you have
- fatigue?

Anemia (in malabsorption: impaired absorption of iron, vitamin B_{12}, and folic acid); hypokalemia

- fever?

Chronic inflammatory bowel disease; regional enteritis; tuberculosis; lymphoma; hyperthyroidism

- no fever?

Absorptive defect of small intestine; chronic pancreatitis

- pain, weakness in your limbs?

Peripheral neuritis in malabsorptive disorders: deficiency of vitamin B_{12}

- pain in your joints?

Regional enteritis; ulcerative colitis; Whipple's disease; polyarteritis; colchicine treatment of gout

- bone pain?

In malabsorptive disorders: protein depletion with osteoporosis; calcium malabsorption with osteomalacia

- back pain?

Osteoporosis; osteomalacia; cancer of pancreas

- easy bruising?

Vitamin K malabsorption with hypoprothrombinemia

7   *Iatrogenic factors*   see Etiology

8   *Environmental factors*

8.1   What do you usually eat each day?

May disclose an avitaminosis or other dietary cause of diarrhea, such as eating uncooked or poorly cooked pork products (trichinosis)

8.2   Have you ever lived in, or traveled to, tropical or underdeveloped countries?

Amebiasis; schistosomiasis; strongyloidosis; capillariasis (Philippines); trichuriasis; tropical sprue (India, Far East, China, Central America)

9   *Personal antecedents pertaining to the diarrhea*

9.1   Have you ever had an examination of your stools? an x-ray of your abdomen? of your intestines? a rectoscopy? When? With what results?

9.2   Have you ever been treated for your diarrhea? Did it respond to

• corticosteroids?	Ulcerative colitis; regional enteritis; Whipple's disease; sprue
• *a gluten-free diet?*	Sprue
• antibiotics?	Blind-loop syndrome; Whipple's disease; tropical sprue

9.3   Do you have any of the following conditions: pancreatitis? ulcerative colitis? regional enteritis? diverticulosis?

• diabetes?	Visceral neuropathy; exocrine pancreatic insufficiency; abnormal bacterial proliferation in proximal small bowel; coexistent sprue
• a renal disease?	Uremia; avitaminosis
• asthma?	Carcinoid syndrome; polyarteritis nodosa
• chronic cough? shortness of breath?	Fibrocystic disease of pancreas; scleroderma
• a liver disease?	Ulcerative colitis; Crohn's disease; bowel disease with metastasis to the liver
• anemia?	Malabsorption with vitamin B_{12} or folic acid deficiency or iron-deficient anemia
• emotional problems?	Irritable colon

9.4 Have you ever had GI surgery?	Postgastrectomy diarrhea; blind-loop syndrome; gastrocolic fistula

PHYSICAL SIGNS PERTINENT TO THE COMPLAINT

Finding	**Possible** *significance*
Acute diarrhea	
Shock; thready radial pulse; poor skin turgor; cold extremities; flat neck veins	Acute loss of 8 to 12 percent of body weight
Fever; diffuse abdominal tenderness; active bowel sounds	Acute infectious diarrhea
Chronic diarrhea	
Fever	Inflammatory bowel disease; amebiasis; lymphoma
Edema; ascites	Protein-losing enteropathy with hypoalbuminemia; malabsorption of amino acids with hypoproteinemia; nephrotic syndrome with amyloidosis
Skin manifestations:	
Hyperpigmentation	
• generalized	Addison's disease
• sparing the mucosae	Whipple's disease
• of oral mucosae	Peutz-Jeghers syndrome
Flushing	Carcinoid syndrome
Erythema nodosum	Ulcerative colitis; regional enteritis
Petechiae, ecchymoses	Henoch-Schönlein purpura; vitamin K malabsorption with hypoprothrombinemia
Dermatitis	Pellagra
Clubbing	Regional enteritis; primary biliary cirrhosis
Edema of one limb	Lymphedema: in intestinal lymphangiectasia
Thrombophlebitis migrans	Carcinoma of pancreas
Lymphadenopathy	Whipple's disease; lymphoma

Glossitis; cheilosis	Malabsorption syndromes with deficiency of iron, vitamin B_{12}, folate, other vitamins
Macroglossia	Amyloidosis
Enlarged thyroid; tremor; tachycardia	Thyrotoxicosis
Heart murmur; attacks of wheezing; loud bowel sounds; flushing; hepatomegaly	Carcinoid syndrome
Chronic lung disease	Cystic fibrosis (may be observed in adults)
Left pleural effusion	Chronic pancreatitis
Right pleural effusion	Amebiasis with liver abscess
Abdominal mass, tenderness in RLQ	Carcinoma; regional enteritis
Abdominal mass, tenderness in LLQ	Carcinoma; diverticulitis
Perianal fistula or abscess	Crohn's disease; tuberculosis
Liver disease	Ulcerative colitis; Crohn's disease; bowel malignancy with hepatic metastases
Arthritis	Ulcerative colitis; Crohn's disease; Whipple's disease
Peripheral neuropathy	Diabetes with autonomic neuropathy; amyloidosis; malabsorption syndromes with deficiency of vitamin B_{12}
Postural hypotension	Diabetic diarrhea; Addison's disease
Stroke; atherosclerotic disease of large vessels	Ischemic injury to the gut: mesenteric arterial insufficiency
Abnormal rectal examination Fecal impaction	Malignancy, etc. Usually associated with liquid feces

LABORATORY TESTS PERTAINING TO THE COMPLAINT

Procedure	*Finding*	*Diagnostic possibilities*
Stool Examination for ova, parasites / Culture	Positive	Salmonellosis; bacillary dysentery; amebiasis; schistosomiasis; giardiasis; trichuriasis; etc.
Occult blood tests	Positive	GI tumor; amebic or bacillary dysentery; ulcerative colitis; regional enteritis
Fat (N:<6 g/24 h)	Increased	Steatorrhea: malabsorption, maldigestion (pancreatic insufficiency)
D-Xylose absorption (25 g orally; N: 5-h urinary excretion > 4.5 g)	Normal	Maldigestion: pancreatic insufficiency
	Decreased	Malabsorption
Blood Carotene (N: 50 to 300 μg/100 mL)	Decreased	Steatorrhea: malabsorption; maldigestion
Prothrombin time (N: 11 to 14 s)	Prolonged	Vitamin K deficiency: malabsorption; maldigestion
Iron (N: 75 to 175 μg/100 mL)	Normal	Maldigestion: pancreatic insufficiency
	Decreased	Chronic blood loss; impaired absorption
Calcium (N: 9 to 11 mg/100 mL)	Normal	Pancreatic insufficiency
	Low	Calcium malabsorption

Serum albumin (N: 3.5 to 5.5 g/100 mL)	Decreased	Protein depletion; protein-losing enteropathy
Cholesterol (N: 180 to 240 mg/100 mL)	Decreased	Steatorrhea: malabsorption; pancreatic insufficiency
BUN	Elevated	Dehydration; renal disease
Electrolytes	Abnormal	Electrolyte depletion; dehydration
RBCs	Anemia	Chronic blood loss; malabsorption; folic acid deficiency; pernicious anemia
WBCs	Leukocytosis	Infectious diarrhea
	Eosinophilia	Parasitic disease; allergy
Vitamin B_{12} absorption (N:>7 percent urinary excretion per 24 h)	Normal	Maldigestion: pancreatic insufficiency
	Decreased	Malabsorption: resection of the terminal ileum; terminal ileal disease; bacterial overgrowth; pernicious anemia; total gastrectomy
Secretin test	Normal	Malabsorption
	Abnormal	Maldigestion: pancreatic insufficiency
^{14}C bile acid breath test	Elevated	Bacterial overgrowth in the small bowel; ileal dysfunction

| *Procedure* | *To detect* |
| Plain abdominal films | Pancreatic calcifications: chronic pancreatitis |

	Calcified lymph nodes: tuberculosis Calcified adrenal glands: Addison's disease Colonic dilation: ulcerative colitis
Upper GI series	Peptic ulcer disease: Zollinger-Ellison syndrome; malabsorption pattern; inflammatory bowel disease; GI tumor; gastroileostomy Normal small-bowel pattern: pancreatic insufficiency
Barium enema	Ulcerative colitis; tumor; intestinal fistulas
Proctosigmoidoscopy	Rectal or colonic neoplasm; inflammatory disease; parasitic disease; melanosis coli: chronic usage of anthraquinone laxatives (indicated in acute bloody diarrhea or acute diarrhea persisting for more than 5 days)
Fiberoptic colonoscopy	Inflammatory vs. neoplastic lesions; nature of localized lesions
Small-bowel biopsy	Sprue; Whipple's disease; amyloidosis; etc.

USEFUL REMINDERS AND DIAGNOSTIC CLUES
Acute Diarrhea

	Incubation period, h	Duration of diarrhea, days	Source of infection
Salmonellosis	8–48	1–7	Poultry products
Shigellosis	24–48	c. 10	Food; water
Staphylococcal food poisoning	1–6	1–2	Poorly refrigerated foods (creamed foods, pies, salad, filling, mayonnaise)

Foods containing staphylococcal enterotoxin have normal appearance, odor, and taste.

Chronic Diarrhea

Chronic diarrhea and weight loss occur in: cancer of pancreas; partial intestinal obstruction with postprandial pain and a resultant decrease in food intake, as in regional enteritis; malabsorption;

uremia (due to anorexia); generalized disease affecting the intestinal tract (hyperthyroidism, Addison's disease, diabetes with autonomic neuropathy, lymphoma, leukemia, systemic lupus erythematosus, polyarteritis, scleroderma, carcinoid syndrome, tuberculosis).

Psychogenic factors are the most important cause of chronic diarrhea.

A common symptom of fecal impaction of the rectum is the frequent passage of small watery stools, forcefully passed around the impaction.

In case of chronic diarrhea	*Suspect*
With urinary complaints	Diverticulitis; regional enteritis with fistula of the bladder
Of undetermined origin	Habitual cathartic abuse

SELECTED BIBLIOGRAPHY

Almy TP: Chronic and recurrent diarrhea, in Barondess JA (ed), *Diagnostic Approaches to Presenting Syndromes*, pp 167–196, Baltimore: Williams & Wilkins, 1971

Greenberger NJ, Isselbacher KJ: Disorders of absorption, in Thorn GW et al (eds), *Harrison's Principles of Internal Medicine*, 8th ed, pp 1518–1537, New York: McGraw-Hill, 1977

Matseshe JW, Phillips SF: Chronic diarrhea: A practical approach. Med Clin North Am 62:141–154, 1978

Sleisenger MH: Diseases of malabsorption, in Beeson PB and McDermott W, *Textbook of Medicine*, 14th ed, Part XIV, Sec 3, pp 1217–1243, Philadelphia: Saunders, 1975

14
Dyspepsia (Chronic Abdominal Discomfort, Indigestion)

DEFINITIONS AND GENERAL CONSIDERATIONS

Dyspepsia abdominal distress associated with the intake of food. Dyspepsia may result from disease of the GI tract or may be associated with pathologic conditions in other organ systems.

Visceral abdominal pain of dyspepsia generally results from distention or exaggerated muscular contraction of a viscus. The pain of peptic ulcer is believed to be produced either directly by acid irritating exposed nerve endings in the ulcer or by alteration of the motor activity of the gastroduodenal segment that the patient appreciates as ulcer pain. Some patients with dyspepsia describe a sensation of abdominal distention and various complaints, some of which appear to be related to increased quantities of gas in the intestinal tract.

Aerophagia excessive swallowing of air. Aerophagia is generally a compulsive habit and a manifestation of emotional tension.

Belching forceful regurgitation of air from the esophagus or stomach.

Patients with dyspepsia may also complain of:

Heartburn a burning sensation located substernally or high in the epigastrium. Heartburn is generally attributed to an incompetent lower esophageal sphincter and the reflux of gastric juice into the esophagus.

Regurgitation effortless appearance of esophageal or gastric contents in the mouth. It may be due to an incompetent lower esophageal sphincter.

The symptoms of functional dyspepsia, with no demonstrable pathologic function, are ascribed to psychogenic causes.

ETIOLOGY

Functional: irritable colon; aerophagia; anxiety and/or depression
Peptic ulcer; carcinoma of stomach; hypertrophic gastritis
Esophageal reflux; reflux esophagitis; hiatal hernia

Chronic cholecystitis and cholelithiasis
Chronic relapsing pancreatitis; carcinoma of the pancreas
Episodes of diverticulitis; lactase deficiency; sprue; ulcerative colitis; chronic peritonitis (tuberculous infection)
Intermittent or chronic intestinal obstruction: postoperative adhesions; regional enteritis; neoplastic lesions (cancer of colon, left side); lymphoma of small bowel; intermittent incomplete volvulus; intestinal polyps (Peutz-Jeghers syndrome); small intestinal carcinoid; vascular: ischemic disease of the intestine, intestinal angina
Systemic diseases and intoxications: polyarteritis nodosa; systemic lupus erythematosus; lead poisoning; hypercalcemia; hyperparathyroidism; porphyria; hyperlipemia; uremia; congestive heart failure; pulmonary tuberculosis; neoplastic diseases; anemia

Iatrogenic Causes of Chronic Abdominal Discomfort

Aspirin	Indomethacin	Potassium chloride
Corticosteroids	Phenylbutazone	*Rauwolfia* alkaloids
Ferrous salts		

QUESTIONNAIRE

Possible *meaning of response*

1   Location of abdominal distress

1.1   Where do you have discomfort? distress? pain?

• in the epigastrium?

Peptic ulcer; carcinoma of stomach; peptic esophagitis; hiatus hernia stricture; carcinoma of esophagus; cholelithiasis, cholecystitis; pancreatitis; pancreatic carcinoma

• substernal?

Disease of esophagus or cardia of stomach; heart disease

• RUQ?

Cholelithiasis; cholecystitis; passive congestion of liver; hepatitis; cirrhosis; hepatic flexure syndrome; irritable colon; lesion of head of pancreas

• periumbilical?	Small-bowel disease; regional enteritis
• below the umbilicus?	Appendiceal, colonic (ulcerative colitis, carcinoma of colon, partial obstruction) or pelvic origin of pain
• LUQ?	Splenic flexure syndrome; <u>Irritable colon</u>; tail of pancreas
• LLQ? hypogastrium?	<u>Irritable colon</u>; diverticulitis

1.2 Is the pain (or discomfort)

• diffuse?	Visceral pain
• localized?	Somatic pain; referred pain; if epigastric: large or penetrating peptic ulcer

1.3 Does the pain

• remain in the same place?	Gastric ulcer pain: usually no radiation in the absence of posterior penetration of the ulcer

• radiate

• from epigastrium

• up into the middle of the chest?	Reflux of acid gastric juice into esophagus
• *through to the back?*	Posterior penetration of an ulcer; pancreatic lesion
• to RUQ?	Involvement of gallbladder or biliary ducts; carcinoma of head of pancreas
• to the left?	Carcinoma of body and tail of pancreas
• from LUQ to the left side of the chest? left shoulder?	Splenic flexure syndrome

2   *Mode of onset and chronology*

2.1   How long have you had pain in the abdomen?

For years: duodenal ulcer; functional dyspepsia

2.1*a*   Was it precipitated by a stressful event?

Functional dyspepsia

2.2   Is the pain (or discomfort)
  • constant?
  • intermittent?

Gastric carcinoma
May be associated with the use of certain drugs; chronic relapsing pancreatitis

2.3   If the pain is intermittent: what is the frequency, duration of the attacks?

2.4   *Does the pain occur in episodes of 2 to 10 weeks separated by pain-free periods lasting several months?*

Peptic ulcer

2.5   *Is the pain seasonal?*

Peptic ulcer: prominent in spring and autumn

3   *Character of the discomfort*

3.1   Do you have abdominal: pain? distress? discomfort? fullness?

Most patients have difficulty in accurately describing chronic abdominal pain

3.2   Do you have
  • a dull and aching distress?

Visceral pain; peptic ulcer (if epigastric)

  • epigastric hunger pain? gnawing, burning pain?

Peptic ulcer

  • vague, cramping pain or discomfort in the periumbilical area?

Intermittent intestinal obstruction; regional enteritis

  • colicky (wavelike) pain?

Forceful peristaltic contractions attempting to overcome an obstruction: in small intestine, colon, biliary tract

3.3 In case of epigastric pain:

- Does the pain gradually increase in intensity? does it remain steady for ½ to 2 h before gradually subsiding?

  Pain of peptic ulcer

- Does the pain reach a peak intensity within 15 to 45 min, subsiding over several hours?

  Biliary "colic" (sudden distention of the biliary tree produces a steady type of pain)

4 Precipitating or aggravating factors

4.1 Is the distress related to food?

4.1*a* Does it occur or worsen

- during, or minutes after, eating?

  Esophageal disease; pyloric obstruction; gastritis

- *1 to 3 or more hours after eating?*

  Peptic ulcer (epigastric); biliary tract lesion; intestinal angina; carcinoma of stomach; pyloric stenosis; gastric atony; pancreatic insufficiency; regional enteritis

- *after drinking milk?*

  Lactase deficiency, congenital or acquired (sprue, ulcerative colitis, regional enteritis)

- after eating
  - fatty foods?

    Pancreatic or biliary tract disease (not specific for gallbladder dysfunction); functional GI disease more likely

  - gluten-containing foods? (wheat, barley, rye)

    Nontropical sprue

  - vegetables?

    Fermentative action of bacteria on nonabsorbable sugars contained in vegetables, with increased gas production

• fried foods?	Chronic cholecystitis; gallstones; nonulcer dyspepsia
• large intake of alcohol?	Chronic relapsing pancreatitis; peptic ulcer
• others?	May initiate allergic reactions
• before breakfast?	Functional: infrequent in peptic ulcer; may occur in carcinoma of stomach

4.2 Is the distress caused or worsened by

• certain drugs?	Porphyria, following use of barbiturates
• stress?	Functional dyspepsia
• when lying flat?	Carcinoma of pancreas
• *1 to 2 h after retiring?*	Organic disease; duodenal ulcer (pain that occurs during the night should never be called "functional")

4.3 For the female patient:
Is the pain related to your menstruations?   Intestinal endometriosis

5 *Relieving factors*

5.1 Is the distress relieved by

• *eating? drinking milk?* antacids?	<u>Peptic ulcer</u> (especially duodenal) (biliary pain is not relieved by food or antacids)
• vomiting?	Peptic ulcer; gastritis; gastric carcinoma (if not relieved: pancreatic or biliary tract disease)
• defecation? passing gas?	Functional or organic lesion likely in colon or distal ileum; irritable colon; ulcerative colitis; splenic flexure syndrome
• belching?	Aerophagia
• standing? *leaning forward?* sitting upright?	Pancreatic pain: tumor, pancreatitis

6 *Accompanying symptoms*

6.1   Do you have heartburn?

Reflux of gastric juice into esophagus; peptic ulcer; may be psychogenic

6.1*a*   Is your heartburn evoked or worsened by
• a large meal? when lying down, bending over?

Gastroesophageal reflux, with or without esophagitis

6.1*b*   Is the heartburn relieved
• by standing up? drinking liquids, antacids?

Esophageal reflux

6.2   Do you have
• sour regurgitations?

Severe esophageal reflux; peptic ulcer

• difficulty swallowing?

Esophageal disease (see Chap. 15)

6.3   Do you have diffuse abdominal distention?

Nonulcer dyspepsia; increased amounts of gas in the GI tract; irritable colon; chronic pancreatic insufficiency; regional enteritis; biliary tract disease

• especially after eating a fatty meal?

Fats delay gastric emptying and hence the passage of swallowed air

• relieved by passing gas?

Increased amounts of gas in the GI tract

• with an increase in weight? swollen feet?

Ascites: cirrhosis; chronic peritonitis (tuberculosis)

6.4   Do you have
• frequent belching?

Not specific; aerophagia: poor eating habits, bad habit, chronic anxiety (also: actual intestinal disease)

• frequent bowel sounds? gas?

Aerophagia; diet containing large quantities of carbohydrates or vegetables; regional enteritis

• especially after eating vegetables?	Increased gas production due to fermentative action of bacteria on nonabsorbable sugars
6.5 Do you have	
• nausea? vomiting?	Peptic or nonulcer dyspepsia; biliary tract disease
• a loss of appetite? of weight?	Serious underlying disease; carcinoma of stomach; regional enteritis; malabsorption
• fever?	Chronic cholecystitis; regional enteritis; diverticulitis
• jaundice?	Biliary tract disease; carcinoma of pancreas
• *a change in your bowel habits?*	Significant
• constipation?	Obstructing lesion in the colon
• *alternating diarrhea and constipation?*	Carcinoma of left colon; irritable colon; intermittent obstructive symptoms; regional enteritis
• hard and small stools?	Irritable colon
• soft and poorly formed stools?	Regional enteritis
• containing mucus? blood?	Ulcerative colitis; rare in regional enteritis
• greasy stools?	Malabsorption
• black, tarry stools?	GI bleeding

7 *Iatrogenic factors*   see Etiology

8 *Environmental factors*

8.1 Do you smoke?	Smoking probably interferes with the healing of gastric ulcer and thus maintains its chronicity
8.2 Do you drink	
• alcohol? beer? wine?	Alcoholism with chronic pancreatitis; alcohol stimulates gastric secretion

• coffee? tea?

Caffeine and theophylline cause an increase in gastric acid secretion

9 *Personal antecedents pertaining to the dyspepsia*

9.1 Have you ever had an x-ray of the stomach? Intestine? gallbladder? When? With what results?

9.2 Do you have any of the following conditions: a peptic ulcer? alcoholism? hiatus hernia? colitis? diverticulosis? a liver disease (cirrhosis)? anxiety? depression?

9.3 Have you ever had
   • a biliary colic?
   • an operation on your abdomen?

Postoperative adhesions: dubious cause of dyspepsia

PHYSICAL SIGNS PERTINENT TO THE COMPLAINT

Finding	**Possible** *significance*
Abdominal distention; increased tympany	Increased amounts of intestinal gas; irritable-colon syndrome
Abdominal dullness	Ascites: cirrhosis; tuberculous peritonitis
Visible or palpable distended loops of bowel; visible peristalsis; hyperactive bowel sounds	Obstructive intestinal lesion; Crohn's disease; left carcinoma of colon
Abdominal masses	Neoplastic disease; inflammatory disease
Epigastric mass	Tumor of the stomach
LUQ mass	Tumor of the pancreas
Tender mass in the region of the sigmoid colon	Diverticulitis
Tender palpable sigmoid colon	Irritable-colon syndrome
Tender pulsatile mass	Aneurysm of the aorta
Epigastric tenderness	Peptic ulcer; also observed in nonulcer dyspepsia: pancreatitis, cholecystitis, gastric cancer, functional dyspepsia

Jaundice; palpable gallbladder; hepatomegaly	Liver, bile ducts, or pancreas disorder
Fever	Regional enteritis; chronic ulcerative colitis; diverticulitis; lymphoma; connective-tissue disease; tuberculosis
Fever; jaundice; RUQ tenderness	Biliary tract disease; chronic cholecystitis
Hepatomegaly; ascites; spider angiomas	Liver cirrhosis
Rectal and pelvic examination	May reveal: rectal mass; metastatic tumor; pelvic inflammatory disease; abnormalities of the uterus or adnexae; prostatic abnormalities

LABORATORY TESTS PERTAINING TO THE COMPLAINT

Procedure	*Finding*	*Diagnostic possibilities*
Blood Bilirubin	Elevated	Obstruction
Alkaline phosphatase	Elevated	of the biliary tract
Amylase	Elevated	Pancreatitis
Sickle cell preparation	Positive	Sickle cell crises
Urine Bilirubin	Positive	Biliary tract disease
Porphobilinogen	Positive	Porphyria
Stool Occult blood	Positive	GI mucosal lesion
Fat, muscle fibers	Present	Pancreatic disorders; malabsorption syndrome

Procedure	*To detect*
Plain abdominal film	Renal, pancreatic, cholecystic calculi; displaced gastric or colonic gas patterns by a mass
Upper GI barium series	Hiatus hernia; duodenal and gastric ulcers; gastric neoplasms; hypertrophic gastritis; displacement of the duodenum by abnormal pancreas; regional enteritis; partial obstruction
Cholecystogram	Cholelithiasis; nonfilling of the gallbladder
Barium enema Proctosigmoidoscopy	Tumor; diverticulitis; ulcerative colitis
Esophagoscopy* Gastroscopy*	Reflux esophagitis; gastric or duodenal ulcers; atrophic gastritis; bile reflux gastritis; duodenitis
Psychologic evaluation*	Depression reactions; anxiety; hysteria

* If appropriate.

USEFUL REMINDERS AND DIAGNOSTIC CLUES

Misleading Factors

From 5 to 10 percent of the patients with peptic ulcers present with colonic symptoms, and diverticulitis sometimes mimics cholangitis: the location of the symptom is not an infallible guide to the location of the involved organ.

Diagnostic Considerations

Esophagus

There seems to be little reason to attribute dyspepsia or abdominal pain to hiatal hernia.

Heartburn does not indicate esophagitis, for it occurs in the absence of inflammation and is caused by acid-induced esophageal motor abnormalities.

Stomach

Pain before breakfast is so infrequent with a peptic ulcer that this complaint suggests that the patient's dyspepsia is not caused by a peptic ulcer.

A good appetite is commoner in duodenal ulcer than in gastric ulcer, and is uncommon in gastric carcinoma.

A bedtime snack, by stimulating hydrochloric acid secretion, increases the likelihood of night pain in patients with peptic ulcer.

The presence of gastritis does not correlate with dyspeptic symptoms.

Gallbladder

Persistent dyspepsia in a patient who has had cholecystectomy for chronic cholecystitis is usually caused by one of the following conditions: an unrecognized peptic or functional gastrointestinal disease, stones remaining in the common duct or cystic duct, a partial obstruction of the common duct, associated pancreatitis.

Pancreas

The presence of mental symptoms of depression associated with abdominal complaints should prompt concern regarding a carcinoma of the pancreas.

Colon

Irritable colon can never be accepted as the cause for blood in the stool, anemia, or weight loss.

Irritable colon is the most common cause of chronic or recurrent abdominal pain.

SELECTED BIBLIOGRAPHY

Coghill NF: Dyspepsia. Br Med J 4:97–99, 1967

Isselbacher KJ: Indigestion, in Thorn GW et al (eds), *Harrison's Principles of Internal Medicine,* 8th ed, pp 205–207, New York: McGraw-Hill, 1977

Lasser RB, Bond JH, Levitt MD: The role of intestinal gas in functional abdominal pain. N Engl J Med 293:567–569, 1975

15
Dysphagia

DEFINITION AND PATHOPHYSIOLOGY

Dysphagia difficulty in swallowing experienced only during attempts at swallowing and during or within seconds after the act of swallowing.

The esophagus is separated from the pharynx by the upper esophageal sphincter (UES), which prevents air from filling the esophagus during inspiration, and from the stomach by the lower esophageal sphincter (LES), which prevents the reflux of gastric juice into the esophagus. The body of the esophagus, extending between these two sphincters, contains predominantly striated muscle in the upper half and smooth muscle in the lower half.

When a subject swallows and moves a bolus of food into the hypopharynx with the tongue, the nasopharynx is closed by the soft palate to prevent the movement of food into the nose; the larynx is elevated against the epiglottis, thereby preventing the aspiration of food into the respiratory passages; the UES relaxes, thus permitting the bolus to enter the esophagus from the hypopharynx; a peristaltic wave initiated in the upper esophagus is propagated to the lower esophagus, propelling food along the body of the esophagus; the LES relaxes and permits the esophageal contents to enter the stomach. The movement of the bolus from the mouth to the pharynx is voluntary; subsequent events are involuntary.

In some patients, dysphagia is related to difficulty in initiating the voluntary act of swallowing or to defects in the reflex coordination of oropharyngeal movements. Neuromuscular diseases that affect striated muscle may cause dysphagia referable to the upper half of the esophagus and the UES, where striated muscle is located. Diseases involving smooth muscle (scleroderma) produce impaired peristalsis in the lower half of the esophagus and decreased pressure and incompetence of the LES. Achalasia is characterized by absence of peristaltic activity and increased LES pressure with incomplete relaxation after deglutition. Dysphagia may also result from the narrowing of the lumen by a tumor or an inflammatory stricture.

ETIOLOGY

Oropharyngeal disorders

Neuromuscular disorders: cerebral vascular accidents with pseudo-bulbar palsy or bulbar palsy; poliomyelitis; motor system disease; diphtheritic polyneuritis; myasthenia gravis; myotonic dystrophies and restricted muscular dystrophies (oculopharyngeal and laryngoesophageal); dermatomyositis

Ulcerative lesions: pharyngitis; Vincent's angina; *Monilia* stomatitis; viral infections with herpetic lesions; retropharyngeal abscess

Sideropenic dysphagia: Plummer-Vinson syndrome

Mechanical obstruction: tumor; enlarged thyroid; hypopharyngeal pulsion (Zenker's) diverticulum

Esophageal dysphagia

Intrinsic narrowing: carcinoma; benign tumor; inflammatory strictures resulting from reflux esophagitis, ingestion of corrosive substances, instrumentation, foreign bodies; lower esophageal (Schatzki) ring

Extrinsic pressure: aortic aneurysm; vascular anomalies; mediastinal tumor; paraesophageal hiatal hernia; pericardial effusion; left auricular enlargement

Motility disturbances: diffuse esophageal spasm; achalasia; esophageal reflux; scleroderma

Causes of Chronic Esophageal Dysphagia According to Decreasing Frequency

Before age 50	*Age 50 and over*
Reflux esophagitis	Carcinoma
Achalasia	Reflux esophagitis
Benign tumors	Lower esophageal ring
Extrinsic pressure	Achalasia
Scleroderma	Diffuse spasm

Iatrogenic Causes of Dysphagia

Antibiotics can cause dysphagia due to esophageal candidiasis, especially in patients weakened by prolonged illness and receiving corticosteroids.

QUESTIONNAIRE

Possible *meaning of response*

1   Character of complaint
1.1   Do you feel a lump in the throat, in the absence of food or fluid ingestion?

Globus hystericus, with actually no dysphagia

1.1*a*   Can you swallow foods and liquids without difficulty?

1.2   Do you have difficulty swallowing

• *at the beginning of a swallow?*

Oropharyngeal dysphagia

• *after a swallow has begun?*

Esophageal dysphagia

1.3   Do you chiefly have difficulty swallowing

• *liquids?*

Oropharyngeal dysphagia

• *solid foods?*

Esophageal dysphagia

• solid and liquid foods?

Dysphagia due to motor dysfunction; achalasia; late stage of esophageal dysphagia

1.4   Do you have difficulty

• in initiating swallowing?

• when you try to swallow saliva?

Oropharyngeal dysphagia

2   Location of complaint

2.1   At what level do you feel the sticking sensation?

Fairly good correlation with level of responsible lesion

• at the level of the lower part of the sternum?

The most frequent site of esophageal disease

• higher in the chest?

Responsible lesion is situated higher in the esophagus

2.2 How long after swallowing do you feel the sticking sensation?
- 2 to 5 s after swallowing?

Lesion in thoracic esophagus: carcinoma; cicatricial stenosis; midesophageal diverticulum

- 5 to 15 s after swallowing?

Lesion in lower thoracic or abdominal esophagus: <u>carcinoma</u>; <u>reflux esophagitis</u>; hiatal hernia; esophageal ulcer

3 *Mode of onset and chronology*

3.1 How long have you had difficulty swallowing?

3.2 Was the onset of dysphagia
- sudden?

Foreign body; ingestion of corrosive agent

- gradual?

Carcinoma

3.3 Is the dysphagia
- intermittent?

Schatzki ring; intermittent motor dysfunction; esophageal spasm; hypertonic sphincter; achalasia, early stages; globus hystericus

- persistent, after having been at first intermittent?

Reflux esophagitis; esophageal ulcer; esophageal carcinoma (in some patients); achalasia

- constant and progressively worse?
  - over a period of months?

Less than 2 years: esophageal carcinoma

  - over a period of years?

Achalasia

4 *Relieving factors*

4.1 Does tilting the head and neck a certain way facilitate deglutition?

Oropharyngeal dysphagia

4.2 Do you

- limit your diet to semiliquid or liquid foods?
- masticate your food longer than usual?
- drink liquids in order to be able to swallow solid foods?

May satisfactorily compensate esophageal dysphagia for a time

5 Accompanying symptoms

5.1 Do you have pain on swallowing?

Odynophagia: irritated lesion of the esophagus (foreign body, chicken bone); reflux esophagitis; diffuse esophageal spasm, idiopathic or secondary carcinoma of esophagus; any painful or ulcerative lesion of pharynx; Plummer-Vinson syndrome

5.1a *Is the pain relieved by regurgitation of (undigested) food?*

Esophageal dysphagia

5.2 *Does fluid run out of your nose when you swallow liquids?*

Oropharyngeal dysphagia

5.3 Do you experience

- *regurgitation of food, minutes or hours after a meal?*

Achalasia, early stages; esophageal malignancy; esophageal diverticulum

- *particularly when lying down?*

Regurgitation of retained material provoked by change in position: achalasia; also in pulsion diverticulum

5.3a Did you experience regurgitation

- before the appearance of dysphagia?

Regurgitation is often an early manifestation in pulsion diverticulum: stagnant food in the diverticular sac

• after the appearance of dysphagia?	Late manifestation of the other esophageal diseases
5.4 Do you sometimes choke, gag, cough, when trying to swallow?	In oropharyngeal dysphagia: aspiration into the trachea of material accumulating in the pharynx

5.4*a* Do you cough

• *with each swallow of food or drink?*	Fistulous communication between esophagus and trachea: neoplastic erosion of the trachea
• some time after swallowing?	Aspiration of regurgitated food: achalasia; Zenker's diverticulum
• at night?	Tracheal aspiration of esophageal contents: Zenker's diverticulum

5.5 Do you have

• a sore throat?	Can make swallowing difficult
• a painful tongue? a sore mouth?	Iron-deficiency anemia with Plummer-Vinson syndrome
• any difficulty walking?	Pseudobulbar palsy of diffuse cerebrovascular disease; spasticity of amyotrophic lateral sclerosis; paralysis of poliomyelitis; myasthenia gravis
• speech difficulty?	Motor system disorder
• heartburn?	Gastroesophageal reflux; <u>reflux esophagitis</u>; hiatus hernia
• hiccups?	Lesion at the terminal portion of the esophagus: carcinoma; achalasia; hiatus hernia
• a swelling in your neck?	Enlarged thyroid
• *pain in your fingers when immersed in cold water?*	Raynaud's phenomenon (scleroderma, connective-tissue disease with dysphagia)
• a loss of weight?	Common in most causes of dysphagia interfering with adequate food intake; esophageal carcinoma; achalasia

• no loss of weight?	Lower esophageal ring with intermittent dysphagia

6 *Personal antecedents pertaining to the dysphagia*

6.1 Have you ever had an x-ray examination of the esophagus? the stomach? an esophagoscopy? gastroscopy? chest x-ray? When? With what results?

6.2 Do you remember having swallowed

• a corrosive agent? • a foreign body?	Dysphagia due to a caustic stricture

6.3 Do you have any of the following conditions:

- a hiatus hernia?

• anemia?	Iron-deficiency anemia with Plummer-Vinson syndrome
• frequent bouts of broncho-pneumonia?	Aspiration of regurgitated material; commonly observed in patients with achalasia

PHYSICAL SIGNS PERTINENT TO THE COMPLAINT

Finding	**Possible** *significance*
Ulcerative lesions of mouth and/or pharynx	Vincent's angina; oral moniliasis; herpetic lesions
Pharyngeal swelling	Retropharyngeal abscess; peritonsillar abscess
Abnormal neurologic examination; abnormal gag reflex; nasal speech; dysarthria	Oropharyngeal dysphagia due to neuromuscular disorder
Constricted skin around the mouth; joint deformities	Scleroderma
Unilateral wheezing	Mediastinal mass involving the esophagus and a main or large bronchus

Enlarged thyroid	Mechanical obstruction of the esophagus
Pallor; glossitis; brittle nails; spoon nail changes (rare)	Iron-deficiency anemia with sideropenic dysphagia (Plummer-Vinson syndrome)
Foul breath (halitosis)	Retained esophageal material: achalasia, pharyngoesophageal diverticulum
Weight loss	Cancer of the esophagus; achalasia

LABORATORY TESTS PERTAINING TO THE COMPLAINT

Procedure	*To detect*
X-rays: barium swallow, esophageal cineradiography	Mechanical obstruction; motor abnormality
Esophagoscopy with biopsy and/or exfoliative cytology	Peptic esophagitis; esophageal varices; inflammatory or neoplastic lesions; stricture
Manometric studies	Pharyngoesophageal or lower esophageal sphincter abnormality; diffuse esophageal spasm; achalasia; infiltrative diseases altering esophageal mobility

USEFUL REMINDERS AND DIAGNOSTIC CLUES

General Considerations

Dysphagia is a most reliable symptom and indicates the presence of disease or motor dysfunction; it should never be dismissed as an emotional disturbance.

Swallowing is ordinarily not impaired in unilateral involvement of the vagus.

Diagnostic Considerations

In scleroderma, dysphagia does not become a prominent symptom until reflux esophagitis has led to an inflammatory stricture. Carcinoma of the lower two-thirds of the esophagus are five times as common in men as in women; carcinoma of the upper esophagus is more common in women.

In case of	*Suspect*
Dysphagia with hoarseness	
Preceding the dysphagia	Primary lesion in larynx
Following the dysphagia, after an interval of some duration	Carcinoma of esophagus with involvement of the recurrent laryngeal nerve

SELECTED BIBLIOGRAPHY

Hawkins CF: Dysphagia. Brit Med J 4:663–667, 1967
Levine SM, Rubin W: Benign disorders of the esophagus: Presentation, diagnosis, and treatment. Med Clin North Am 57:1107–1116, 1973

Hematemesis and/or Melena

DEFINITIONS AND GENERAL CONSIDERATIONS

Hematemesis   vomiting of blood, whether fresh and red or digested and black.

Melena   passage of black, tarry stools containing digested blood.

Hematemesis without melena is generally due to lesions proximal to the ligament of Treitz; melena without hematemesis is usually due to lesions distal to the pylorus. In general, the patient who presents with hematemesis is more likely to have bled greater amounts than the patient with melena.

At least 50 to 100 mL blood must rapidly enter the upper gastrointestinal tract to produce a single black, tarry stool. Blood that arises from the duodenum or jejunum must be retained in the intestinal tract for about 8 h to become black. Gaiac-positive stools indicate a blood loss of at least 10 mL/day.

ETIOLOGY

Lesions of the gastrointestinal tract
Ulcerative lesions
  Peptic ulcer disease
  Erosive gastritis
  Ulcerative colitis
  Fissures and fistulas
  Acute necrosis due to chemical agents
  Neoplasms:
    Benign: polyps, leiomyomas
    Carcinoma (esophagus to rectum)
    Neurofibromatosis
    Lymphoma

Hiatus hernia; esophageal ulcer
Intussusception
Marginal ulcer
Steroid ulcer
Stress ulcer
Ischemic colitis

Infection: dysentery (amebic, bacillary); intestinal parasites; tuberculosis; typhoid fever

Congenital anomalies: Meckel's diverticulum; other diverticula; pancreatic rests

Hereditary anomalies:

With cutaneous manifestations: Osler-Weber-Rendu (hereditary telangiectasia); Peutz-Jeghers syndrome; pseudoxanthoma elasticum; neurofibromatosis; Ehlers-Danlos syndrome; Gardner's syndrome

Without cutaneous manifestations: familial polyposis

Others: volvulus; embolism and thrombosis of mesenteric vessels; leakage of aneurysm

Associated with rupture of esophageal varices secondary to portal hypertension

Hepatic causes: cirrhosis; hemochromatosis; syphilis; sarcoidosis; schistosomiasis; hepatolenticular degeneration

Extrahepatic lesions: thrombosis of hepatic vein (Chiari's syndrome); thrombosis of portal vein (infection, compression, tumor invasion, blood dyscrasia); congenital anomalies

Bleeding disorders

Thrombocytopenia; hemophilia; anticoagulant therapy; von Willebrand's disease; disseminated intravascular coagulation

Systemic diseases

Leukemia and lymphoma; polycythemia; Henoch-Schönlein purpura; scleroderma; systemic lupus erythematosus; polyarteritis nodosa; amyloidosis; sarcoidosis; scurvy

Relative Incidence of Lesions

The three major causes of upper gastrointestinal bleeding are: peptic ulcer disease (duodenal ulcer being more frequent than gastric ulcer), erosive gastritis, and esophageal varices. These lesions encompass 90 to 95 percent of all cases of upper gastrointestinal hemorrhage in which a definite diagnosis can be made.

Iatrogenic Causes of Gastrointestinal Bleeding

Alkylating agents	Coumarin derivatives	Phenylbutazone
Aminosalicylic acid	Heparin	Potassium chloride
Antimetabolites	Hydralazine	Reserpine
Aspirin	Indomethacin	Xanthine derivatives
Corticosteroids		

QUESTIONNAIRE

Possible *meaning of responses*

1 Mode of onset

1.1 When did the bleeding occur?

1.1*a* Have you
- vomited blood?

Bleeding proximal to the ligament of Treitz

- passed black, tarry stools?

Lesion not lower than the ileocecal valve

- had both hematemesis and melena?

Melena may occur independently of, or be associated with, hematemesis; bleeding of sufficient volume to produce hematemesis usually results in melena

1.1*b* Have you had, prior to the hematemesis,
- bleeding from the nose?
- bloody expectorations?
- a dental extraction?

Blood from these conditions, swallowed and subsequently vomited, or resulting in melena

- *retching and severe non-bloody vomiting?*

Mallory-Weiss syndrome: vertical laceration of the gastroesophageal junction

2 Character of the bleeding

2.1 What is the color of the vomited blood?

Depends upon the duration of contact of the blood with gastric acid in the stomach

- red?

Vomiting occurring shortly after the onset of bleeding; bleeding site above the level of the pylorus

- dark red? black? "coffee-grounds"?

Delay in vomiting; blood converted to hematin in the stomach in the presence of hydrochloride acid

- bright red and frothy?

Blood coming from the lungs

2.2   What is the color of the
      stool?

• bright red?   Lesion in terminal ileum, colon,
                                  rectosigmoid; may result from
                                  massive and rapid bleeding from
                                  an upper or gastric lesion, or
                                  even from esophageal varices
                                  (see Chap. 19)

• black, tarry?   The altered color of the blood
                                  results from prolonged contact
                                  with gastric juice to produce
                                  hematin; a lesion in the jejunum,
                                  ileum, or cecum may produce a
                                  black, tarry stool provided that
                                  transit through the bowel is slow

3   Extent and rate of bleeding

3.1   Have you vomited blood

• only once?

• several times?

3.1*a*   Has the bleeding been   **Variceal bleeding, peptic ul-**
         abrupt? massive?   **cer;** the patient should be con-
                                  sidered to have lost one-third
                                  to one-half of his or her blood
                                  volume

3.2   In the case of melena:

• Have you had more than   Usually associated with a loss
  one black, tarry stool within   of more than 25 percent of the
  a 24-h period?   blood volume

• For how long have the tarry
  stools persisted?

  • for 1 to 3 days?   At least a single-liter episode of
                                  hemorrhage; stools may remain
                                  tarry for 48 to 72 h after bleeding
                                  has stopped

  • for more than 3 days?   Severe hemorrhage

4 *Accompanying symptoms*

4.1   Did you notice just before,
      during, or after, the hemor-
      rhage:
      • *lightheadedness? nausea?*   Clinical manifestations of hypo-
      thirst? sweating?   tension; rapid hemorrhage of
                                        more than 500 mL blood

      • faintness
        • *when lying down?*   **50 percent loss of
                                        blood volume** ⎫ should be
        • *when standing?*   20 to 30 percent loss ⎬ assumed
                                        of blood volume ⎭

        • *syncope?*   Signifies a **blood loss of at least
                                        1000 to 1500 mL blood**

4.2   Following the hemorrhage,   Common in gastrointestinal
      did you have diarrhea?   bleeding: blood within the GI
                                        tract is irritating

4.3   Have you noticed
      • heartburn?   Esophageal lesion: inflammatory,
                                        ulcerous, or malignant

      • pain in the stomach? ⎫
        • *relieved by eating?* ⎬   Peptic ulcer lesion
        • *relieved by antacids?* ⎭

      • a decrease of appetite? ⎫   Carcinoma in upper or lower
      • a weight loss? fatigue? ⎭   gastrointestinal tract

      • a change in the bowel ⎫   Colonic neoplasm; inflammatory
        habits?   ⎬   bowel disease; ulcerative colitis;
      • diarrhea? pain in the ab- ⎬   regional enteritis; amebic colitis;
        domen?   ⎭   diverticulosis

      • jaundice? a distended ab-   Cirrhosis with ascites
        domen?

4.4   Do you bruise easily?   Hemorrhagic diathesis

5 *Iatrogenic factors* see Etiology

6 *Personal antecedents pertaining to the GI bleeding*

6.1   Have there been similar episodes in the past? When? Diag-
      nosis?

6.1*a*   Were you hospitalized on this occasion? Did you receive a transfusion?

6.2   Have you ever had an x-ray of your stomach? of your intestine? a gastroscopy? When? With what results?

6.3   Have you had, prior to the bleeding, a heavy alcohol intake?

Erosive gastritis; acute peptic ulcer

6.4   Do you have any of the following conditions: peptic ulcer? liver disease? alcoholism? bleeding tendency? colitis?

6.5   What was your blood pressure prior to the bleeding?

Knowledge of the previous blood pressure allows more accurate evaluation of the significance of the blood pressure immediately after the hemorrhage

7   *Family medical history pertaining to the GI bleeding*

7.1   Are there any other members of your family who have

• an intestinal disease?

Familial colonic polyposis

• a bleeding tendency?

Congenital deficit of a coagulation factor; Osler-Weber-Rendu disease

PHYSICAL SIGNS PERTINENT TO THE COMPLAINT

Finding	**Possible** *significance*
Clinical shock: restlessness; acute hypotension; tachycardia; thready peripheral pulse; pallor; cold clammy skin	Acute blood loss of about 40 percent of the blood volume; blood loss in excess of 1500 mL usually leads to cardiovascular collapse
Systolic blood pressure below 100 mmHg	Blood volume probably less than 70 percent of normal
Pulse rate of 100 or more per minute	Blood volume probably less than 80 percent of normal

Postural signs: with patient placed in the upright position: • **pulse rate increase of 20/min** • **systolic pressure decrease of 20 mmHg**	Significant hypovolemia; acute blood loss of more than 1000 mL
Pallor of the palmar creases	Loss of more than 20 percent of the blood volume
Mild fever (100 to 102°F)	May be present with GI hemorrhage
Jaundice; spider angiomas; palmar erythema; hepatomegaly; ascites	Cirrhosis with portal hypertension and varices, gastritis, or gastric ulceration
Abdominal tenderness or masses	Malignancy
Left supraventricular (Virchow's) node	Metastatic intraabdominal malignancy
Epigastric tenderness	Peptic ulcer (not specific)
Arthritis	Possible salicylate and other drug ingestion causing gastritis; ulcerative colitis
Emphysema	Increased risk for development of peptic ulcer
Abdominal scars of previous surgery	Bleeding stomal ulcer; recurrent malignancy
Melanin pigmentation of the lips, buccal mucosae, distal extremities	Peutz-Jeghers syndrome: small intestinal polyps with recurrent melena
Telangiectases on upper trunk and oral pharynx	Hereditary hemorrhagic telangiectasia
Diffuse pigmentation; hepatomegaly	Hemochromatosis and liver impairment
Multiple sebaceous cysts; soft-tissue tumors	Colonic polyposis (Gardner's syndrome)

Café-au-lait spots; cutaneous neurofibromas	May be associated with neurofibromas of the intestinal tract
Ecchymoses; petechiae; bleeding gums	Bleeding tendency
Lymphadenopathy	Malignancy; leukemia with bleeding tendency
Rectal examination	Malignancy; polyposis

LABORATORY TESTS PERTAINING TO THE COMPLAINT

Procedure	Finding	Diagnostic possibilities
Blood		
Hemoglobin	<11 g/100 mL	Blood loss greater than 1000 mL (in an otherwise normal patient)
	<8 g/100 mL	Massive hemorrhage
RBC morphology	Hypochromic, microcytic anemia	Chronic blood loss
WBCs	Elevated	May be observed with acute hemorrhage
Platelets	Elevated	
	Low	Bleeding tendency
Prothrombin time (PTT)	Prolonged	Bleeding tendency
BUN (N: 10 to 20 mg/100 mL)	Elevated	Common following GI hemorrhage
	>40 mg/100 mL	Blood loss greater than 1000 mL (in an otherwise normal patient)
Creatinine	Normal	Not affected by blood in the GI tract
Liver function tests	Abnormal	Liver cirrhosis

Procedure	*To detect*
Nasogastric tube	Amount and character of blood present
Barium studies of GI tract and/or esophagogastro-duodenoscopy	Esophageal varices; peptic ulcer; superficial erosive gastritis; neoplastic ulcerative lesion; Mallory-Weiss tear
Fiberoptic colon-oscopy	Site and nature of bleeding lesions proximal to the rectosigmoid area
Selective visceral arteriography	Site of bleeding; bleeding lesion in the small intestine

USEFUL REMINDERS AND DIAGNOSTIC CLUES

Misleading Factors

Not all black stools are due to blood: patients receiving iron or bismuth therapy have blackish-green stools; charcoal and licorice impart a jet-black color to the feces.

Diagnostic Considerations

Peptic ulcer

About 20 to 30 percent of patients with peptic ulcer will have at least one episode of significant gastrointestinal bleeding.

Melena alone occurs more often than hematemesis in patients with bleeding ulcer.

Bleeding from duodenal or gastric ulcer occurs without prior symptoms in 20 percent of patients.

The pain of peptic ulcer may disappear at the onset of bleeding, because blood in the stomach and duodenum buffers the highly acid gastric juice.

Cirrhosis of the liver

Hematemesis may be the first manifestation of the disease in about 10 percent of cases of cirrhosis of the liver.

The cirrhotic patient may bleed from: acute gastric erosions, peptic ulcer, or esophageal varices.

Carcinoma

Severe hemorrhage is seen only in a small percentage of patients with carcinoma of the stomach; chronic blood loss is a more frequent complication of gastric carcinoma.

The finding of anemia and occult blood in stools in an elderly patient should arouse suspicion of a carcinoma of the cecum and ascending colon.

Miscellaneous

If intestinal bleeding occurs in a patient who is receiving anticoagulant therapy, an underlying gastrointestinal lesion (benign or malignant) should be considered.

SELECTED BIBLIOGRAPHY

Isselbacher KJ, Koff RS: Hematemesis and melena, in Thorn GW et al (eds), *Harrison's Principles of Internal Medicine*, 8th ed, pp. 214–218, New York: McGraw-Hill, 1977

Law DH, Gregory DH: Gastrointestinal bleeding, in Sleisenger MH, Fordtran JS (eds), *Gastrointestinal Disease: Pathophysiology, Diagnosis, Management*, pp 195–215, Philadelphia: Saunders, 1973

Moody FG: Rectal bleeding. N Engl J Med 290:839–841, 1974

17
Jaundice

DEFINITIONS AND PATHOPHYSIOLOGY

Jaundice　yellow pigmentation of the skin or sclerae by bilirubin.
Cholestasis　reduced bile flow with reduced excretion of bile constituents.

In the normal adult, 80 to 90 percent of serum bilirubin is derived from the breakdown of hemoglobin from aged or injured red blood cells, presumably in the reticuloendothelial system. About 10 to 20 percent of serum bilirubin is derived from destruction of immature erythroid cells in the bone marrow (ineffective erythropoiesis) and from the breakdown of nonerythroid components (myoglobin and cytochromes). Bilirubin is released from hemoglobin breakdown as a water-insoluble unconjugated compound (free bilirubin). It is transported in serum as a bilirubin-albumin complex which is not filtered by the renal glomeruli. At the hepatic cell membrane, bilirubin and albumin become dissociated, with selective uptake of the bilirubin. In the liver cell, bilirubin is conjugated to bilirubin diglucuronide. The conjugated bilirubin is then secreted into the bile canaliculi by an active process. In the intestine, bacterial enzymes convert conjugated bilirubin to colorless urobilinogen, which is excreted in the feces. Some urobilinogen is reabsorbed in the ileum and colon and is either reexcreted in bile or excreted by the kidneys.

Hyperbilirubinemia with jaundice may be due to one or several of the following mechanisms:

Excessive bilirubin production, as occurs in hemolysis; hemolysis in a patient with a normal liver does not elevate the serum bilirubin level above 4 mg/100 mL, because of the ability of the normal liver to handle six times the usual 250 mg/day of bilirubin presented to it.
Reduced hepatic uptake of bilirubin.
Decreased glucuronide conjugation of bilirubin.
Decreased excretion of conjugated bilirubin into bile resulting from hepatocellular injury or from biliary obstruction, either intrahepatic ("medical jaundice") or extrahepatic ("surgical jaundice").

The water-soluble conjugated bilirubin is dialyzable; if conjugated bilirubin is regurgitated into the serum, it can be filtered by the renal glomerulus: the presence of bilirubin in the urine is evidence of conjugated hyperbilirubinemia.

ETIOLOGY

Predominantly unconjugated hyperbilirubinemia
Overproduction of bilirubin
   Hemolytic disorders: intra- and extravascular
   Ineffective erythropoiesis: increased destruction of red cells or red cell precursors in the marrow
Defective hepatic uptake of bilirubin
   Familial: Gilbert's syndrome
   Drugs, flavaspidic acid; prolonged fasting
Impaired glucuronide conjugation: decreased activity of glucuronyl transferase
   Hereditary absence or deficiency of transferase
      Crigler-Najjar syndrome, type I and type II
   Immaturity of transferase: neonatal jaundice
   Acquired transferase deficiency
      Drug inhibition
      Hepatocellular disease: hepatitis; cirrhosis

Predominantly conjugated hyperbilirubinemia
Impaired hepatic excretion of bilirubin
   Hereditary: Dubin-Johnson syndrome; Rotor syndrome; recurrent (benign) intrahepatic cholestasis; cholestatic jaundice of pregnancy
   Acquired:
      Hepatitis: viral, A and B; infectious mononucleosis; bacterial: leptospirosis; toxin- and drug-induced; alcoholic hepatitis
      Cirrhosis: alcoholic, postnecrotic, biliary, cardiac, hemochromatosis, Wilson's disease
      Hepatoma; metastatic tumor; abscess
      Granuloma: sarcoidosis; tuberculosis
Extrahepatic cholestasis: gallstones; carcinoma of the bile ducts, pancreas, ampulla of Vater; bile duct stricture; biliary atresia; choledocal cyst; enlarged nodes in the porta hepatis

Iatrogenic Causes of Jaundice (partial list)

Hepatocellular disease
Alphamethyldopa; antidepressants; antimetabolites; diphenylhydantoin; halothane; isoniazid; oxyphenisatin; penthrane; phenylbutazone; rifampin; tetracycline

Cholestasis

Anabolic steroids; antibacterial agents (sulfadiazine, nitrofurantoin, PAS, erythromycin estolate); organic arsenicals; chlorpropamide; chlorpromazine and other phenothiazines; oral contraceptives; methimazole; methyltestosterone; phenindione; propylthiouracil; thiouracil; tolbutamide

Fatty liver and cirrhosis   Methotrexate

Hepatic adenoma   Oral contraceptives

Hepatocellular carcinoma   Anabolic steroids

QUESTIONNAIRE

Possible *meaning of response*

1   Mode of onset and duration

1.1 How long have you been jaundiced?	Days to weeks: <u>hepatitis</u>; <u>obstructive jaundice</u> Months: chronic liver disease, <u>cirrhosis</u>; chronic active hepatitis; primary biliary cirrhosis (in middle-aged women)
1.2 Did the jaundice develop • rapidly? (hours to days)	<u>Hepatitis</u>, viral, toxic; <u>choledocholithiasis</u>
• slowly?	Cirrhosis; carcinoma; cholestasis; chronic active hepatitis; subacute hepatic necrosis; primary biliary cirrhosis

1.3   Was the jaundice preceded by

- *loss of appetite?*
- *nausea? vomiting?*   Viral <u>hepatitis</u> A
- *aversion to smoking?*

2   *Character*

2.1   Is the jaundice

- mild?   <u>Cirrhosis</u>; hemolytic jaundice
- intense?   <u>Obstructive jaundice</u>, intra- or extrahepatic
- of varying intensity?   Incomplete extrahepatic obstruction: <u>gallstone disease</u>; hemolysis; cirrhosis

3   *Precipitating or aggravating factors*

3.1   *Have you had in the past*   Viral <u>hepatitis</u> B
6 months any injections?
(subcutaneous, intramuscular, intravenous) blood tests? vaccinations? intradermal tests? transfusions? dental treatment? tatooing?

3.1a   *Do you inject any narcotic*   Viral hepatitis B
drugs?

3.2   Did you recently consume   Viral hepatitis A
oysters? mussels? raw or steamed shellfish? unclean water?

4   *Accompanying symptoms*

4.1   *What is the color of your*
urine?

- as usual?   Unconjugated hyperbilirubinemia
- *like beer? Coca-Cola?*   Bilirubinuria: hepatocellular or obstructive jaundice
- bloody?   Leptospirosis; toxic agent with renal and hepatic involvement

4.2 *What is the color of your stools?*
- pale? *clay-colored?* — Obstructive jaundice (intra- or posthepatic)
- well colored? — Hemolytic jaundice
- black, tarry? — **Gastrointestinal hemorrhage**

4.3 Do you have
- fever? — Cholangitis with extrahepatic cholestasis
Low grade: hepatitis, cirrhosis (fever that persists after jaundice has appeared is rare in viral hepatitis and infrequent in drug-induced jaundice)
  - *with chills?* — Cholangitis (gallstone obstruction)

4.4 Do you have
- pain in your abdomen?
  - colicky? — Gallstone obstruction; frank pain is rare in viral hepatitis
  - RUQ discomfort? — <u>Hepatitis</u> (viral, toxic); cirrhosis; tumor
  - chronic dull, boring? — Carcinoma of pancreas
  - epigastric pain radiating to the back? — <u>Pancreas</u> disease
- loss of appetite? nausea? vomiting? — <u>Hepatitis</u> (anorexia at the onset of viral hepatitis improves with fully developed jaundice); <u>cirrhosis</u> (with splanchnic congestion and/or ascites)
- *pain in your joints?* — Hepatitis B; <u>drug-induced hepatitis</u>
- headaches? — Viral hepatitis; meningitis in leptospirosis
- *itching?* — Extrahepatic jaundice; cholestatic drug reaction; in the female patient: primary biliary cirrhosis

• easy bruising?	Impaired hepatic production of coagulation proteins
• diarrhea?	May occur in viral hepatitis: due to the cathartic action of nonabsorbed fatty acids; pancreatic disease
• abdominal swelling?	Ascites: cirrhosis
• weight loss?	Underlying carcinoma; primary liver disease, tumor

4.5 Do you feel

• ill?	Hepatocellular jaundice: hepatitis
• relatively well?	Cholestatic jaundice

5 Iatrogenic factors see Etiology

6 Environmental factors

6.1 *What is your alcohol intake?*   Cirrhosis; alcoholic hepatitis

6.2 Have you recently had any contact with

• a jaundiced person?	Viral hepatitis
• toxic products? (spot remover, cleaning agent)	Hepatocellular jaundice (carbon tetrachloride present in various solvents)
• rats?	Leptospirosis

6.3 Have you traveled to other countries in the past 6 months?   Areas where hepatitis may be endemic; exposure to contaminated water as a vector of hepatitis

6.4 What is your occupation? What sort of work have you done in the past?   Hepatitis B more common in: infant nurseries, laboratory technology, work in dialysis units; increased incidence of cirrhosis in bartenders, brewery workers

6.4a What are your hobbies?   May reveal evidence of toxic exposure

7 *Personal antecedents pertaining to the jaundice*

7.1 Have you ever had liver tests? a liver biopsy? an x-ray of your gallbladder? When? With what results?

7.2 Have you ever had jaundice?	Cirrhosis; extrahepatic jaundice (stones); drug-induced hepatitis

7.3 Do you have any of the following conditions: a liver disease (cirrhosis)? gallstones? GI bleeding? alcoholism?

8 *Family medical history pertaining to the jaundice*

8.1 Does someone in your family have

• jaundice?	Hemolytic jaundice; congenital hyperbilirubinemia (Gilbert, Dubin-Johnson, Rotor syndrome); exposure to a common toxic agent
• anemia?	Hemolytic jaundice; hereditary spherocytosis
• a neurologic disease?	Wilson's disease: hepatolenticular degeneration

PHYSICAL SIGNS PERTINENT TO THE COMPLAINT

Finding	**Possible** *significance*
Jaundice:	
Pale yellow	Hemolytic jaundice
Orange yellow	Hepatocellular jaundice
Yellow green	Prolonged obstructive jaundice
Pallor	Anemia: hemolysis, malignancy, cirrhosis
Normal liver size	Intrahepatic, not posthepatic, disorder; hemolytic jaundice
Hepatomegaly	Alcoholic cirrhosis, fibrosis with regeneration; fatty infiltration; cholestasis (intra- or extrahepatic); inflammation (hepatitis); venous congestion; malignancy

Stony-hard liver	Hepatoma; hepatic metastases
Palpable liver nodules	Neoplasm; cysts; regeneration nodules; abscesses
Small liver	Acute and subacute hepatic necrosis; postnecrotic cirrhosis
Liver tenderness on palpation	Hepatitis; congestive heart failure with acute enlargement
Friction rub over the liver	Neoplastic infiltration of the liver capsule and peritoneum
Vascular bruit over the liver	May be heard over large regenerating nodules in cirrhosis; vascular tumor
Abdominal distention; shifting dullness; fluid wave	Ascites; in cirrhosis, due to portal hypertension, hypoalbuminemia, increased plasma aldosterone
Ascites, dilated periumbilical veins	Cirrhosis with portal collateral circulation
With venous hum at the umbilicus	In cirrhosis: significant portal hypertension
Spider angiomas; palmar erythema	Acute or chronic liver disease (local arteriovenous shunts?)
Dupuytren's contracture; parotid gland enlargement; gynecomastia; diminished axillary or pubic hair; testicular atrophy	In an alcoholic patient: cirrhosis
Splenomegaly	Medical nature of hepatic disease: cirrhosis; hepatitis; infectious mononucleosis; portal hypertension; hemolytic jaundice
Scratch marks over the body	Pruritus: obstructive jaundice (intra- or extrahepatic cholestasis); ascribed to retained bile acids, not related to the intensity of jaundice

Clubbing; xanthoma	Chronic cholestasis; biliary cirrhosis
Ecchymoses	Impaired hepatic synthesis of coagulation proteins; vitamin K malabsorption in obstructive jaundice
Purpura	Thrombocytopenia of cirrhosis
Palpable enlarged gallbladder (Courvoisier's sign)	Extrahepatic biliary obstruction; pancreatic cancer
Tender gallbladder; positive Murphy's sign	Cholelithiasis; choledocho-lithiasis
Fever; chills	Suppurative cholangitis
Flapping tremor (asterixis) Fetor hepaticus	Portal-systemic encephalopathy; impending hepatic coma
Extrapyramidal signs; *Kayser-Fleischer corneal ring*	Wilson's disease

LABORATORY TESTS PERTAINING TO THE COMPLAINT

Procedure	*Finding*	*Diagnostic possibilities*
Blood		
Hematocrit	Decreased	Hemolysis
Reticulocyte count	Elevated	
Total bilirubin (TB) (N: $<$1 mg/100 mL)	Elevated	Parenchymal or obstructive jaundice; hemolysis
Direct-reacting bilirubin (N: 0.1 to 0.3 mg/100 mL)	Normal	Hemolysis; Gilbert's syndrome
	Elevated ($>$30 percent of TB)	Hepatocellular jaundice; intrahepatic cholestasis; extrahepatic biliary obstruction

Indirect-reacting bilirubin (N: 0.2 to 0.7 mg/100 mL)	Elevated (>85 percent of TB)	Hemolysis; Gilbert's syndrome
Alkaline phosphatase (N: 2 to 4.5 Bodansky U)	Slight to moderate increase (6 to 10 BU)	Hepatitis; cirrhosis
	Markedly increased	Extrahepatic biliary obstruction; intrahepatic cholestasis
SGOT, SGPT (N: <40 Karmen U/mL)	>300 U	Hepatic necrosis; viral hepatitis
	<300 U	Cirrhosis; tumor; intra- or extrahepatic cholestasis
Cholesterol (N: 130 to 230 mg/100 mL)	Normal	Viral hepatitis; Dubin-Johnson syndrome; Gilbert's syndrome; hemolytic anemia
	Elevated	Cholestasis
Serum albumin (N: 3.5 to 5.5 g/100 mL)	Decreased	Hepatic necrosis; chronic active hepatitis; cirrhosis
Serum globulin (N: 2 to 3.5 g/100 mL)	Elevated	Cirrhosis; chronic active hepatitis
Prothrombin time (N: 11 to 14 s)	Prolonged	Hepatitis; cirrhosis; chronic biliary obstruction
	Corrected with parenteral vitamin K	Extrahepatic obstruction
Hepatitis B surface antigen (HB$_s$Ag)	Positive	Hepatitis B
Antimitochondrial antibodies*	Positive	Primary biliary cirrhosis

* If appropriate.

Antinuclear anti-bodies*	Positive	Chronic active hepatitis
Alpha-fetoprotein*	Positive	Hepatoma
Urine		
Bilirubin	Negative	Hemolysis; Gilbert's syndrome
	Positive	Conjugated hyper-bilirubinemia: hepatocellular jaundice, intrahepatic cholestasis; extrahepatic biliary obstruction
Urobilinogen (N: 1 to 3.5 mg/24 h)	Elevated	Hemolysis; viral hepatitis
	Decreased	Cholestasis

* If appropriate.

Procedure	*To detect*
Barium study of GI tract	Esophageal varices: cirrhosis Displacement of stomach: enlargement of left lobe of liver Displacement of duodenum: tumor of head of pancreas
IV cholangiography	Localization of obstructing lesions of the major biliary ducts
Percutaneous trans-hepatic cholangiography* Endoscopic pancreatocholangiography*	Extrahepatic vs. intrahepatic cholestasis
Ultrasonography	Dilated bile ducts; tumors in liver, pancreas
Liver scan	Intrahepatic masses
Computerized tomography	Hepatic masses; pancreatic carcinoma
Peritoneoscopy and liver biopsy*	Cirrhosis; focal lesions (biopsy contraindicated in obstructive jaundice)

* If appropriate.

USEFUL REMINDERS AND DIAGNOSTIC CLUES

Misleading Factors

Carotenoid pigments in the bloodstream resulting from the ingestion
of large amounts of carotene-containing foods may produce a yellow discoloration of the skin, but not of the sclerae.

A yellow discoloration of the skin may result from excessive consumption of tomatoes or tomato juice (lycopenemia).

Atabrine treatment may produce a yellow color of the skin and urine.

General Considerations

Jaundice can be clinically recognized when the total serum bilirubin
exceeds 2 to 2.5 mg/100 mL.

In deep jaundice, the skin may take on a greenish hue because of
the conversion of bilirubin to biliverdin, an oxidation product of
bilirubin. Oxidation occurs more readily with conjugated bilirubin,
and hence a greenish hue is seen more frequently in conditions
with conjugated hyperbilirubinemia.

Conjugated bilirubin preferentially stains tissues with high elastin
content such as the sclerae or mucous membranes. Unconjugated
bilirubin accumulates predominantly in adipose tissue and is best
seen in the subcutaneous fat of the abdomen or extremities.

Jaundice is less apparent in edematous areas, because of the low
protein and bilirubin content of the edema. Scar tissue is rarely
bilirubin-stained.

Diagnostic Considerations

Intrahepatic obstructive jaundice in its pure form resembles posthepatic obstructive jaundice, except for the details of its onset in
which malaise and anorexia precede the onset of jaundice,
whereas posthepatic obstructive jaundice develops without anorexia and malaise.

Cholelithiasis frequently complicates the hereditary types of hemolytic anemias.

Over 90 percent of the cases of jaundice are found among viral hepatitis, drug hepatitis, cirrhosis, gallstones, and malignant obstruction of the common duct.

In case of
Acute hepatic and renal disease

Suspect
Occupational or domestic exposure to halogenated hydrocarbons, to rats or dogs (leptospirosis)

SELECTED BIBLIOGRAPHY

Isselbacher KJ: Jaundice and hepatomegaly, in Thorn GW et al (eds), *Harrison's Principles of Internal Medicine*, 8th ed, pp. 218–223, New York: McGraw-Hill, 1977

Jeffries GH: Mechanisms of hepatic disease, in Beeson PB and McDermott W, *Textbook of Medicine*, 14th ed, chap. 694, pp 1324–1332, Philadelphia: Saunders, 1975

Ostrow JD: Jaundice in older children and adults. JAMA 234:522–526, 1975

Sherlock S: *Diseases of the Liver and Biliary System*, 5th ed., pp 258–259, Philadelphia: Davis, 1975

Zimmerman HJ: Liver disease caused by medicinal agents. Med Clin North Am 59:897–907, 1975

18
Nausea and Vomiting

DEFINITIONS AND MECHANISMS

Nausea   the feeling of the imminent desire to vomit, usually referred to the throat or epigastrium.

Vomiting   forceful expulsion of the gastric contents through the mouth.

Retching   the labored spasmodic respiratory movements that frequently precede vomiting.

During nausea, gastric tone is reduced and peristalsis in the stomach is decreased or absent; duodenal tone is increased, with or without reflux of duodenal contents into the stomach. Nausea often precedes or accompanies vomiting.

During vomiting, the gastric fundus and corpus are flaccid, the gastroesophageal sphincter is relaxed, the antrum and the proximal duodenum are strongly contracted. The glottis is closed, preventing pulmonary aspiration, and the larynx and soft palate are elevated, preventing the entry of the gastric contents into the nasopharynx. Forceful contraction of the diaphragm and abdominal wall brings about a sharp increase in intraabdominal pressure; this results in the squeezing of the flaccid stomach and the ejection of its contents.

All the activity of vomiting is triggered by the vomiting center in the floor of the fourth ventricle on chemical, humoral, reflex neural, labyrinthine, or psychic stimulation. The efferent pathways in vomiting are the phrenic nerves (to the diaphragm), the spinal nerves (to the abdominal musculature), and visceral efferent nerves (to the stomach and esophagus).

ETIOLOGY

Acute abdominal emergencies: acute appendicitis; acute cholecystitis; acute pancreatitis; intestinal obstruction; acute peritonitis

Chronic indigestion; biliary disorders; peptic ulcer

Acute infectious diseases: acute systemic infection; viral, bacterial, and parasitic infections of the intestinal tract; viral hepatitis

Disorders of the nervous system: increased intracranial pressure (brain tumor); acute meningitis; acute labyrinthitis; Ménière's disease; migraine headache; tabetic crisis

Diseases of the heart: acute myocardial infarction; congestive heart failure; digitalis intoxication

Metabolic and endocrine disorders: at the onset of diabetic acidosis; adrenal insufficiency; hyperparathyroidism; early pregnancy; uremia

Drugs and chemicals; alcohol

Psychogenic vomiting: emotional upset; anorexia nervosa; motion sickness

Iatrogenic Causes of Nausea and/or Vomiting

Any medication, especially:

Antimetabolites	Salicylates
Digitalis	Tetracycline
Morphine	Xanthine derivatives
Potassium chloride	X-ray treatment

QUESTIONNAIRE

Possible *meaning of response*

1 Duration

1.1 How long have you had nausea with vomiting?

For years: psychogenic vomiting (especially in females)

2 Character of vomiting

2.1 Does the vomitus contain
- yellow material?

Bile: often present whenever vomiting is prolonged; open connection between the proximal duodenum and the stomach; eventual obstructive lesion below the ampulla of Vater

- mucus?

In the morning: pregnancy; rhinopharyngitis, with postnasal drip

• undigested food?

Achylia gastrica; vomitus from the esophagus (achalasia) or from an esophageal diverticulum

• *food eaten 12 h earlier?*

Pyloric obstruction

• blood?

<u>Peptic ulcer;</u> Mallory-Weiss syndrome; **acute abdominal emergency**

2.2   Does the substance that you vomit have

• a characteristic pungent odor?

Vomitus from stomach secreting hydrochloric acid

• *a fecal odor?*

Low-intestinal obstruction; gastrocolic fistula; **peritonitis with ileus;** ischemic injury to the intestine; long-standing gastric outlet obstruction with bacterial overgrowth caused by stasis

• no odor?

Regurgitation; vomitus from an achylic stomach

2.3   Can you estimate the quantity of vomit produced at any time?

Useful in judging replacement therapy; the volume lost may be very large when pyloric obstruction is present

2.4   Do you vomit

• every day?

<u>Peptic</u> ulcer with obstruction; pylorospasm with hypersecretion; <u>psychogenic</u> vomiting

• *in the early morning?*

<u>Uremia; pregnancy;</u> rhinopharyngitis with postnasal drip; <u>alcoholism</u>; after gastric surgery; brain tumor (often before breakfast)

• late in the day?

Pyloric obstruction

• during the night?

<u>Duodenal ulcer</u>

2.5   Is the vomiting

• *forceful?* ("projectile"), *not preceded by nausea?*

Increased intracranial pressure: brain tumor

2.6 Do you have nausea without vomiting?

Obstructive and hepatocellular jaundice; carcinoma of the stomach; early stages of cardiac failure; chronic renal failure; pregnancy

3 Precipitating or aggravating factors

3.1 Do you vomit after meals?
- during or soon after a meal?

Psychogenic vomiting; pylorospasm

- 1 to 4 h after eating?

Gastric or duodenal lesion

- 4 to 6 h or longer after eating?

Gastric retention: pyloric obstruction; motility disorder of the stomach: diabetic neuropathy, postvagectomy state

- only after fatty meals?

Chronic biliary tract disorders (see Chap. 14)

- only after alcohol?

Patient receiving disulfiram (Antabuse)

3.1*a* Is vomiting unrelated to meals?

Drug reaction; metabolic disorder; intracranial tumor

3.2 Do you vomit only
- in certain places? under certain well-defined circumstances: stress? fear? depression?

Psychogenic vomiting (rarely in a public place)

- as a passenger in a car? aircraft? ship?

Motion sickness

3.3 For the female patient: When did you last have your menstruation?

Possibility of early pregnancy if last menstruation more than 6 weeks ago

4 Accompanying symptoms

4.1 Do you have
- pain in the abdomen?

Peptic disease; biliary tract disease; gastroenteritis; **intestinal obstruction; acute appendicitis; acute peritonitis;** pancreatitis

• diarrhea?	Acute gastroenteritis
• constipation?	**Intestinal obstruction**
• a loss of appetite? of weight?	Organic cause of vomiting; carcinoma of the stomach
• light stools? dark urine? jaundice?	Hepatitis
• excessive thirst?	Onset of diabetic acidosis
• acute chest pain?	Myocardial infarction accompanied by vomiting
• fever?	Infectious process
• trouble with hearing? vertigo? an unsteady gait?	Disorders of the labyrinthine apparatus and its central connections; Ménière's disease
• headaches?	Migraine; brain tumor

5 *Iatrogenic factors*   see Etiology

6 *Personal antecedents pertaining to the complaint*

6.1 Have you ever had an x-ray of your stomach? gallbladder? When? With what results?

6.2 Do you have any of the following conditions: a peptic ulcer? a renal disease?

• diabetes?	Onset of diabetic acidosis
• a cardiac disease?	In congestive heart failure: congestion of liver with nausea and vomiting; digitalis intoxication

PHYSICAL SIGNS PERTINENT TO THE COMPLAINT

Finding	**Possible** *significance*
Hypotension; soft eyeballs; dry skin	Dehydration: acute prolonged vomiting
Fever	Acute gastroenteritis; viral hepatitis; systemic infection; meningitis
Abdominal mass	Intraabdominal neoplasm; intussusception; abscess with intestinal obstruction

Distended abdomen; abdominal tenderness; hyperactive high-pitched bowel sounds	Intestinal obstruction
Abdominal direct and rebound tenderness; guarding; absent bowel sounds	Peritonitis; adynamic ileus

Succussion splash
- with visible gastric peristalsis — Pyloric obstruction
- without visible peristalsis — Gastric atony

Fever; jaundice; liver tenderness ⎱ Hepatomegaly ⎰	Viral hepatitis; biliary tract disorder
Abdominal tenderness; hyperventilation; dehydration; acetone odor of the breath	Diabetic ketoacidosis
Stiff neck; fever	Meningitis
Neurologic abnormalities	Central nervous system disorder with increased intracranial pressure
Nystagmus; disturbance of gait	Labyrinthine disorder
Pigmentation of skin and mucosae; hypotension; orthostatic hypotension	Adrenal insufficiency
Funduscopic examination	To detect papilledema

LABORATORY TESTS PERTAINING TO THE COMPLAINT

Procedure	*Finding*	*Diagnostic possibilities*
Blood		
Electrolytes	Metabolic alkalosis ⎱ Hypokalemia ⎰	Substantial vomiting; loss of gastric secretions

Electrolytes Glucose (N: 60 to 100 mg/100 mL)	Metabolic acidosis ⎫ Elevated ⎬	Diabetic acidosis
BUN (N: 10 to 20 mg/100 mL)	Elevated	Dehydration; chronic renal failure
Vomitus Free hydrochloric acid	Present	Peptic ulcer
	Absent	Gastric malignancy

Procedure	*To detect*
Abdominal film	Intestinal Obstruction
Barium studies of GI tract	Peptic ulcer; gastric carcinoma
Biliary tract x-rays	Biliary system disorder; cholelithiasis
Pregnancy test	Pregnancy
EEG, brain scan	Intracranial mass lesions
ECG	Acute myocardial infarction
Labyrinthine examination	Disorder of the vestibular system; Ménière's disease; acute labyrinthitis

USEFUL REMINDERS AND DIAGNOSTIC CLUES

Misleading Factor

Vomiting should be distinguished from regurgitation, which refers to the expulsion of food in the absence of nausea and without the abdominal diaphragmatic muscular contraction which is part of vomiting.

Diagnostic Considerations

Patients with vomiting due to emotional disorders maintain a relatively normal state of nutrition, because a relatively small amount of the ingested food is vomited.

The nausea and vomiting associated with obstruction of the common bile duct are usually more intense than when the gallbladder alone is involved.

In case of	*Suspect*
Persistent vomiting without metabolic alkalosis	Achlorhydria (e.g., chronic renal failure)
Severe nausea without any relation to food in a cardiac patient	Digitalis intoxication

SELECTED BIBLIOGRAPHY

Fordtran JS: Vomiting, in Sleisenger MH, Fordtran JS (eds), *Gastrointestinal Disease: Pathophysiology, Diagnosis, Management,* chap 11, pp 127–143, Philadelphia: Saunders, 1973

McGuigan JE: Anorexia, nausea, and vomiting, in Mac Bryde CM, Blacklow RS (eds), *Signs and Symptoms,* 5th ed, chap 21, pp 369–380, Philadelphia: Lippincott, 1970

19
Rectal Hemorrhage

DEFINITION AND GENERAL CONSIDERATIONS

Rectal hemorrhage (hematochezia)   passage of red blood per rectum

Bright red blood, either by itself or coating the stools, may originate from any portion of the lower ileum as well as from the colon. Red blood may also appear per rectum from an upper intestinal or gastric lesion with massive bleeding and hypermotility. Thus, the appearance of blood in the stool depends largely on the site of the lesion and the rate of blood loss.

ETIOLOGY

Anal lesions
Hemorrhoidal veins; anal fissures; anal fistulas

Rectum and colonic diseases
Carcinoma of the rectum
Ulcerative proctitis
Radiation proctitis
Carcinoma of colon (left)
Polyps
Ulcerative colitis
Behcet's syndrome

Infection: amebiasis, shigellosis
Diverticulosis, diverticulitis
Ischemic colitis
Meckel's diverticulum
Ectopic gastric mucosa
Miscellaneous: uremia; arteri-
    tides; telangiectasis; rupture
    of aortic aneurysm

Causes of Colonic Bleeding According to Frequency

Common (10 percent or more of cases):
    Cancer of left colon; diverticulosis and diverticulitis; ulcerative colitis; hemorrhoids or fissures; benign polyps
Less common (less than 10 percent of cases):
    Cancer of right colon; Crohn's disease of colon
    Undetermined

Iatrogenic Causes of Rectal Bleeding

Clindamycin, lincomycin   Anticoagulants
Enteric-coated potassium chloride tablets

QUESTIONNAIRE

Possible *meaning of response*

1 Onset and duration

1.1 How long have you noticed red blood in your stools?

2 Character of rectal hemorrhage

2.1 Do you see streaks of bright red blood
- on the surface of the stools?
- on the toilet paper only?
- in toilet water?

Lesion in anal canal or rectum; commonly bleeding from hemorrhoidal veins, anal fissures, anal fistula (rare in rectal carcinoma)

2.2 Is the blood mixed with the stool?

Colonic bleeding lesion; also in rectal carcinoma

3 Accompanying symptoms

3.1 Have you vomited blood?

Bleeding site usually above the ligament of Treitz

3.2 Did you notice after your bloody stool weakness? syncope?

Massive rectal bleeding: losses of at least 1000 to 1500 mL of blood (greater than 20 percent of the blood volume)

3.3 Have you recently noticed
- *a change in your bowel habits?*
- *a change in the caliber of the stools?*

Carcinoma of the left colon

- a sensation that evacuation is incomplete?

Tenesmus; carcinoma of the left colon

• diarrhea?	Bloody diarrhea: acute inflammation of the colon; amebic colitis; ulcerative colitis; ischemic colitis; rectal and colonic carcinoma; shigellosis
• pain in your abdomen?	Carcinoma of the colon; ischemic colitis; ulcerative colitis; amebic colitis
• anal pain?	External <u>hemorrhoids</u>
• fever?	Amebic colitis; ulcerative colitis; shigellosis

3.4   *Is defecation painful?* — Anal ulcer; fissure; external <u>hemorrhoids</u>

3.5   Is the bleeding associated with straining? with passage of hard stools? — Internal or external hemorrhoids

3.6   Have you noticed bleeding from other sites? — Bleeding diathesis with gastrointestinal hemorrhage

4   *Iatrogenic causes*   see Etiology

5   *Environmental factors*

5.1   Have you ever lived in, or traveled to, foreign countries? — Amebiasis (Mexico, Western South America; South Asia; West and Southwestern Africa)

6   *Personal antecedents pertaining to the complaint*

6.1   Have you ever had an x-ray of your intestine? a rectosigmoidoscopy? When? With what results?

6.2   Do you have hemorrhoids? diverticulosis? bleeding tendencies?

PHYSICAL SIGNS PERTINENT TO THE COMPLAINT

Finding	*Possible significance*
Shock; acute hypotension; tachycardia; pallor; cold clammy skin; restlessness	Losses of about 40 percent of blood volume

Systolic blood pressure below 100 mmHg Pulse rate above 110 beats per min	At least 20 percent volume depletion
Abdominal mass	Malignancy
Hepatomegaly; jaundice	Cirrhosis
Epigastric tenderness	Peptic ulcer (not specific)
Fever; abdominal muscle spasm; guarding; rebound tenderness	Acute diverticulitis with peritoneal irritation
Arthritis	Ulcerative colitis; ingestion of salicylates and other drugs causing gastritis
Arthritis; purpura	Henoch-Schönlein purpura
Erythema nodosum; uveitis	Ulcerative colitis
In a patient over 50 years of age: evidence of atherosclerotic disease	Ischemic colitis
Rectal examination	May reveal: internal or external hemorrhoids; anal fissures, fistulas; rectal polyps; carcinoma (approximately 50 percent of all rectal carcinomas lie within the reach of the index finger)

LABORATORY TESTS PERTAINING TO THE COMPLAINT

Procedure	*To detect*
Anoscopy, procto-sigmoidoscopy, with biopsy	Anal diseases; proctitis; tumor (60 percent of all tumors of the large intestine lie within the terminal 25 cm of the colon and within the reach of the sigmoidoscope); ulcerative colitis
Barium enema	Lesions above the reach of the sigmoidoscope

Fiberoptic colonoscopy	Site and nature of bleeding lesions proximal to the rectosigmoid area: tumor; polyps; diverticulitis; ulcerative colitis
Stool	
Microscopic examination	Polymorphonuclear leukocytes: ulcerative colitis; amebic colitis; bacillary dysentery
Examination for ova, parasites; culture	Infectious origin of bleeding; amebic colitis

USEFUL REMINDERS AND DIAGNOSTIC CLUES

Misleading Factors

Beets may impart a red color to the stools.
Red stools are occasionally seen following intravenous administration of sulfobromophthalein.

Diagnostic Considerations

Carcinoma
Bleeding from carcinoma in any area of the colon may result in the appearance of gross blood, whether on the stool or mixed with the fecal contents.
Bleeding occurs in left-sided colonic carcinoma in about 70 percent of cases.
Malignant lesions arising in the rectal ampulla are notably painless.
An anal pathologic condition (hemorrhoids or anal fissures) does not preclude other causes and sources of bleeding, such as carcinoma.

Miscellaneous
Profuse or recurrent rectal hemorrhage in adolescents and young adults may be due to ectopic gastric mucosa in Meckel's diverticulum.
Significant large bowel bleeding should be attributed to diverticulitis by exclusion only.

In case of	*Suspect*
Rectal bleeding that is dark, associated with clots, well mixed with mucus, or adherent to the stool	Carcinoma of colon
Rectal bleeding with abdominal pain occurring over several days or weeks in an elderly patient and without recurrence	Ischemic colitis
Rectal hemorrhage in a patient with a bleeding tendency	An underlying local cause (tumor)

SELECTED BIBLIOGRAPHY

Moody FG: Rectal bleeding. N Engl J Med 290:839–841, 1974

Genitourinary System

20
Acute Oliguria and Anuria

DEFINITIONS AND PATHOPHYSIOLOGY

Oliguria passage of a volume of urine not adequate to maintain life (usually urine output of less than 400 mL/day). A sustained urinary output of less than 15 mL/h in a patient with previously normal renal function is evidence of significant oliguria.

Anuria complete failure of the kidneys to excrete water and normal urinary solutes.

Acute renal failure a clinical syndrome characterized by a sudden decrease in glomerular filtration rate, often to values of less than 1 to 2 mL/min, and usually accompanied by oliguria.

Oliguria may be associated with inadequate renal perfusion due to depletion of total body salt and water or to intravascular volume depletion (prerenal failure). Under these circumstances, oliguria results from a reduced glomerular filtration rate (GFR). The renal tubule responds to the deficit of effective extracellular fluid volume with enhanced salt and water reabsorption. Urine has a high specific gravity (over 1015 to 1020), a low sodium concentration (less than 10 meq/L), and an unremarkable sediment; the ratio of urine to plasma creatinine is above 14.

Various intrinsic renal diseases producing sufficient renal paren-chymal damage result in acute oliguria. In acute tubular necrosis, renal cortical ischemia (due to preglomerular afferent arteriolar vasoconstriction perhaps mediated by the renin-angiotensin system) results in a marked decrease in GFR. Tubular obstruction due to cellular debris and cylindruria or to interstitial edema, and passive back diffusion of filtrate across injured epithelium, are possible potentiating mechanisms. Oliguria associated with glomerulopathies is due predominantly to a drastic reduction in filtration rate. In the patient with chronic or end-stage renal insufficiency, oliguria results from the destruction of renal cell mass. The oliguria of renal parenchymal disease is generally accompanied by both diminished GFR and impaired tubular reabsorption of water and salt. Urinary sodium concentration is greater than 30 to 40 meq/L, specific gravity is fixed at 1010 to 1012, and the creatinine urine to plasma (U/P) ratio is less than 10.

Acute oliguria due to obstruction of the lower part of the urinary tract is common, especially in elder men with obstruction at the bladder outlet.

ETIOLOGY

Prerenal failure
Severe water and electrolyte loss: vomiting; diarrhea; gastrointestinal drainage; ileus; excessive diuretic medication; fever; diabetic ketosis
Blood or plasma loss
Congestive heart failure
Shock; acute hypotension
Postoperative antidiuresis

Intrinsic renal diseases
Acute tubular necrosis: shock, hypotension, extensive trauma, intravascular hemolysis, myoglobinuria, crushing injuries
Generalized sepsis
Nephrotoxic agents: metals (arsenic, bismuth, gold, thallium, mercury, lead), organic solvents, glycols, insecticides
Glomerulitis: acute, rapidly progressive; lupus nephritis; polyarteritis nodosa; hypersensitivity angiitis; Henoch-Schönlein purpura; Goodpasture's syndrome; malignant nephrosclerosis
End-stage chronic renal disease
Bilateral cortical necrosis

Papillary necrosis: diabetes mellitus, severe pyelonephritis, phenacetin abuse, sickle cell anemia

Renal vascular obstruction: arterial embolus, venous thrombosis, disseminated intravascular coagulation

Miscellaneous: hypercalcemia, multiple myeloma, Reye's syndrome, hepatorenal syndrome, transplant rejection

Postrenal obstruction

Bilateral ureteral obstruction: calculi, cancer, retroperitoneal fibrosis, anomalies of the ureteropelvic junction, surgical (inadvertent ligation of the ureters)

Obstruction of the bladder outlet: benign hypertrophy of prostate, carcinoma of prostate, bladder-neck obstruction

Iatrogenic Causes of Acute Renal Failure (partial list)

Amphotericin B	Neomycin	Salicylates
Bacitracin	Paraaminosalicylic	Streptomycin
Cephaloridine	acid	Sulfonamides
Colistin	Phenacetin	Tetracycline
Gentamycin,	Phenylbutazone	Vancomycin
kanamycin	Polymyxin B	Zoxazolamine
Methicillin		

Sulfonamides, uricosuric agents, alkylating agents may cause obstructive uropathy (sulfonamides or uric acid crystals) in dehydrated patients.

Ganglionic-blocking agents and/or antihistamines may precipitate acute urinary retention in patients with prostatic hypertrophy.

QUESTIONNAIRE

Possible *meaning of response*

1 Mode of onset and evolution

Obvious causes of prerenal failure such as dehydration, diarrhea, vomiting, shock, hemorrhage, surgery are not discussed.

1.1 How long have you been urinating

• less than usual?

The oliguric stage of acute tubular necrosis usually lasts for 8 to 16 days

• *not at all?*

Early total anuria: **obstructive uropathy;** complete anuria (for more than 48 h) also in: bilateral renal arterial emboli or thrombosis, cortical necrosis, acute glomerulonephritis

1.2 Presently, how many times a day do you urinate?

Normal frequency of micturitions: five to six times a day

1.3 Can you estimate the amount of urine passed
• at each voiding?
• per day?

The persistence of urine flow of less than 20 mL/h in the face of adequate hydration is strong presumptive evidence of acute renal failure

2 Character of the urine

2.1 What is the appearance of your urine, if you are passing any?

Oliguria: prerenal or renal causes

• smoky?

Acute glomerulonephritis

• cloudy?

Urinary infection; papillary necrosis

• dark, reddish, bloody?

Hematuria: renal stone; acute vasoocclusion of renal arteries or veins

3 Precipitating or aggravating factors

3.1 Have you recently had
• a sore throat?

Group A beta-hemolytic streptococcal infection preceding acute glomerulonephritis

• a urinary infection?

May precipitate acute retention in a patient with prostatism

• an x-ray of your gall-
bladder? kidneys? aorta?

Acute tubular necrosis may
follow oral administration of
bunamiodyl (Orabilex), IV
urography in patients with
multiple myeloma (induced
dehydration in preparing for
this procedure), abdominal
aortography

3.2   How much fluid do you
drink a day?

Oliguria may occur in individuals with normal renal function
as a result of water restriction

4   Accompanying symptoms

Severe systemic symptoms during the first days of oliguria usually
result from associated conditions, not from renal failure

4.1   Do you have
• a constant urge to urinate?

Acute retention: obstruction to
the urethra

• no desire to urinate?

Obstruction to the outflow of
urine from the kidneys; failure of
secretion by the kidneys

• pain in your abdomen?

Distended bladder, acute retention; Henoch-Schönlein purpura;
acute renal artery embolism

• pain in the lumbar regions?

May occur in acute glomerulonephritis; papillary necrosis

• acute flank pain?

Renal stone (anuria if contralateral kidney has previously been
destroyed by obstruction or infection)

• fever? chills?

Urinary infection: may precipitate acute retention in a patient
with prostatism; subacute bacterial endocarditis with glomerulonephritis

• headaches? nausea?
vomiting?

In untreated patients symptoms
of uremia generally develop during the second week of oliguria;
end-stage of chronic renal disease with oligoanuria

- puffiness of your eyelids? face?
- swollen legs?

Edema of acute glomerulone-phritis or chronic renal disease

5   *Iatrogenic factors*   see Etiology

5.1   Do you regularly take drugs for chronic headaches?

A common cause of chronic abuse of drugs: phenacetin nephropathy, retroperitoneal fibrosis related to the taking of methysergide

6   *Environmental factors*

6.1   What is your profession?

6.2   Do you have any hobbies?

Possible nephrotoxic <u>acute tubular necrosis</u>

6.3   Have you recently used a cleaning agent? a spot remover?

Inhalation of carbon tetrachloride present in various solvents

7   *Personal antecedents pertaining to the oliguria and anuria*

7.1   Do you have
- a kidney disease?
- recurrent urinary infections?

Oliguria of end-stage chronic renal disease

- renal stones?

Bilateral ureteral calculi

- a prostate disease?

Acute retention: obstruction of the bladder outlet

- arterial hypertension?

Oliguria in malignant hypertension

- diabetes?

Diabetic nephropathies: inter-capillary glomerulosclerosis (Kimmelstiel-Wilson lesion), sclerosis of the intrarenal arteries, urinary infections, papillary necrosis

- gout?

Gouty nephropathy, obstructive uropathy

8   Family medical history pertaining to the oliguria and anuria

8.1   Does someone in your family have a renal disease?

Polycystic disease; Alport's syndrome

PHYSICAL SIGNS PERTINENT TO THE COMPLAINT

Finding	**Possible** *significance*
Dry skin and mucosae; sunken eyeballs; flat neck veins; hypotension	Dehydration: severe fluid and electrolyte imbalance with diminished renal blood flow
Peripheral edema	Overhydration due to administration of excess fluid; acute glomerulonephritis
Pulmonary edema	Acute left ventricular failure (possibly due to overhydration)
Suprapubic cystic swelling	Distended bladder: urinary retention; obstruction of the lower part of the urinary tract; prostatic enlargement
Abnormal abdominal palpation	Renal mass; hydronephrosis in obstructive uropathy
Diastolic hypertension	Observed in about 25 percent of patients during the second week of oligoanuria; hypervolemia; malignant hypertension with oliguria
Cardiac arrhythmias	Potassium intoxication
Precordial friction rub	Pericarditis may appear in acute tubular necrosis
Abnormal rectal examination	May reveal enlargement of the prostate, a large pelvic mass compressing the ureters

LABORATORY TESTS PERTAINING TO THE COMPLAINT

Procedure	*Finding*	*Diagnostic possibilities*
Blood		
BUN: creatinine ratio	10 to 15:1	Renal parenchymal disorder
	>15 to 20:1	Prerenal disorder
Urine		
Sodium (meq/L)	<10	Prerenal oliguria; volume depletion
	>40	Acute tubular necrosis
	10 to 40	Combined hypoperfusion and acute tubular necrosis
Osmolality (mosmol/kg of water)	>500	Prerenal or postrenal disorder
	Isoosmotic to serum	Acute tubular necrosis
U/P creatinine ratio	<10	Acute tubular necrosis
	>14	Extracellular fluid volume depletion; acute glomerulitides

Procedure	*To detect*
Bladder catheterization	Residual bladder urine; obstructive uropathy
Plain abdominal film	Size of the kidneys; radiopaque stones
IV or retrograde pyelography	Obstructive uropathy
Renal arteriography*	Vascular occlusion
Renal biopsy*	Specific forms of parenchymal renal diseases

* If appropriate.

USEFUL REMINDERS AND DIAGNOSTIC CLUES
Misleading Factor

In some patients with tubular necrosis the period of diminished urine flow may be so short as to pass unrecognized.

Diagnostic Considerations

A transitory period of total anuria followed by 24 h or more of increased urine volume and a sudden return to anuria is characteristic of obstructive uropathy and is sometimes observed during the initial period of acute tubular necrosis.

Total anuria is rare in acute renal failure due to parenchymal damage or to prerenal causes. Obstruction should be suspected in all patients who exhibit complete anuria early in their illness.

A chronically distended bladder does not appreciably reduce the total urine output.

Obstruction of a single ureter in the presence of two previously normal kidneys usually does not result in anuria.

In chronic renal failure, acute obstruction due to uric acid crystals is unusual because of the patient's inability to produce a concentrated urine.

In case of	*Suspect*
Oliguria with pain in the back or abdomen	An obstructive uropathy
Total anuria with radiologic evidence of normal or enlarged kidneys	An obstructive uropathy
Immediate anuria following surgery in the lower part of the abdomen	Bilateral ureteral injury

SELECTED BIBLIOGRAPHY

Bricker NS: Acute renal failure, in Beeson PB and McDermott W, *Textbook of Medicine,* 14th ed, chap 604, pp 1107–1113, Philadelphia: Saunders, 1975

Epstein FH: Acute renal failure, in Thorn GW et al (eds), *Harrison's Principles of Internal Medicine,* 8th ed, pp 1424–1428, New York: McGraw-Hill, 1977

Harrington JT, Cohen JJ: Acute oliguria. N Engl J Med 292:89–91, 1975

Merrill JP: Acute renal failure, in Strauss MB, Welt LG (eds), *Diseases of the Kidney,* 2d ed, pp 637–666, Boston: Little, Brown, 1971

21
Hematuria

DEFINITIONS AND GENERAL CONSIDERATIONS

Hematuria   bleeding, whether microscopic or gross, from the urinary tract.

Microscopic hematuria   repeated presence of more than two erythrocytes per high-power field or more than 1 million/24 h.

Macroscopic or gross hematuria   can be detected by the human eye; occurs when more than 1 million red cells are excreted per minute.

Vigorous exercise and certain febrile diseases may increase the number of red cells in the urinary sediment of otherwise normal subjects without implying serious renal disease. Microscopic or macroscopic hematuria generally results from diseases of the renal parenchyma or of the genitourinary tract. The presence of red blood cell casts is pathologic and identifies the nephron as the source of bleeding.

Red urine is not necessarily indicative of hematuria (presence of red blood cells); it may also be produced by hemoglobinuria (intravascular hemolysis) and myoglobinuria (skeletal muscle damage). In the latter two conditions, occult blood tests in urine are positive. Nonheme pigments (liver diseases, rare diseases such as acute porphyria, ochronosis, malignant melanoma) may impart a red to brown to black color to the urine (occult blood tests negative).

The actual color of the urine that contains heme pigments depends on the concentration of the red blood cells or pigment, the pH of the urine, and the duration of contact between the pigment and the urine. In an acid urine, the color is dark or smoky, while in an alkaline urine, the color will be more nearly red.

ETIOLOGY

Renal disease   Glomerulonephritis; stone; tumor; polycystic disease; malignant hypertension; renal infarction; renal vein thrombosis; pyelonephritis; tuberculosis; pyonephrosis; infected hydronephrosis;

polyarteritis nodosa; systemic lupus erythematosus; nephrotoxic agents; trauma (including renal biopsy); arteriovenous malformations

Genitourinary tract   Ureteral stone; vesical stone; cystitis (acute or chronic); ureteritis; tumor; benign prostatic hypertrophy; carcinoma of the prostate; prostatitis; posterior urethritis; polyp of urethra; foreign body; trauma; vesical varicosities; postradiation changes of the bladder

Miscellaneous   Hemorrhagic diathesis; leukemia; sickle cell trait; allergy; pelvic and rectal malignancy; endometriosis

Iatrogenic Causes of Hematuria

Anticoagulant therapy; large doses of aspirin; birth control pills
Chronic abuse of phenacetine predisposes to necrotizing papillitis
Cyclophosphamide may induce hemorrhagic cystitis

Iatrogenic Causes of Intravascular Hemolysis (with Hemoglobinuria)

Acetophenetidin
Aminopyrine
Cephalosporins
Levodopa
Methyldopa
Nitrofurans

Phenylhydrazine
Primaquine
Quinidine; quinine
Sulfonamides
Sulfones

QUESTIONNAIRE

Possible *meaning of response*

1   Mode of onset and duration

1.1   How long have you had reddish, dark, urine?

1.2   Is this the first time that you have had red urine?

2   Character

2.1   What is the color of your urine?

- reddish-brown? smoky brown? like Coca-Cola?

Small amounts of blood, acid urine: diffuse renal parenchymal disease; <u>acute glomerulonephritis</u>

• bright red?	Alkaline urine; renal stone; tumor; <u>prostatic hypertrophy</u>
• grayish-green?	Hematuria less prominent: color due to the mixture of small amounts of pigments from red cell destruction with the normal urochrome pigmentation of concentrated urine

2.2 Is the red color present

• *at the beginning of the micturition?*	Initial hematuria: lesion in the urethra, distal to the bladder neck
• *at the end of the micturition?*	Terminal hematuria: lesion in the bladder, commonly trigonitis
• *throughout the urinary stream?*	Total hematuria: the bleeding originates from either the kidney or the ureter; may also occur in diffuse bladder inflammation: hemorrhagic cystitis
• independently of micturition?	Bleeding from the distal urethra

2.3 *Does the urine contain clots?*	Rapid major bleeding: casts of the ureter; renal tumor (excludes glomerular bleeding, i.e., glomerulonephritis)

3 Precipitating or aggravating factors

3.1 Does the dark urine appear

• only in the morning?	Paroxysmal nocturnal hemoglobinuria (in 25 percent of cases)
• following	
• prolonged walking or running?	March hemoglobinuria
• exposure to cold?	Paroxysmal cold hemoglobinuria (urine dark brownish)

3.1a *Does the urine, of normal coloration when freshly passed, darken on standing?*	Hepatic porphyria

3.2   Have you recently had
  • a trauma to the lower part of the back? the abdomen?

Hematuria due to trauma to the kidney (hematuria often painless); contusion of the bladder with hematuria

  • a renal biopsy?

Traumatic hematuria

  • a urologic manipulation?

Traumatic; <u>urinary tract infection</u>

3.3   *Did you have, 2 to 3 weeks prior to the onset of red urine, a sore throat?*

<u>Acute glomerulonephritis</u> with preceding infection of group A beta-hemolytic streptococcus

3.4   In case of recurrent hematuria for months or years, does the rematuria occur
  • immediately (within a few hours) after a respiratory infection? a febrile illness?
  • following exercise?

Focal glomerulonephritis with recurrent hematuria (Berger's disease, essential or benign hematuria): affects males much more frequently than females

3.5   For the female patient: Do your episodes of hematuria occur simultaneously with your menstruations?

Endometriosis of the urinary tract; bleeding perhaps vaginal in origin, not from the urinary tract

4   Accompanying symptoms

4.1   Do you have
  • *back pain? flank pain? abdominal colicky pain?*

<u>Nephrolithiasis</u>; embolic phenomena (may be painless in subacute bacterial endocarditis); <u>urinary tract infection</u>

  • a dull loin pain?

<u>Acute glomerulonephritis</u>

  • difficulty, burning on urination?

Probable source of bleeding: lower urinary tract infection, passage of <u>stone</u> in urethra

  • frequent urination?
  • a constant urge to urinate

Bleeding due to <u>urinary tract infection</u>; acute hemorrhagic cystitis

  • no pain?

Painless total hematuria in: diffuse kidney disease; polycystic disease; tumor; infection, tuberculosis; <u>bladder tumor</u>

4.2   Do you have
- fever? and/or chills?   Urinary tract infection; renal tumor; papillary necrosis; acute glomerulonephritis; bacterial endocarditis with focal glomerulonephritis

- a decreased volume of urine?   Papillary necrosis; acute glomerulonephritis; obstructive lesion; chronic renal insufficiency, late stage

- a loss of weight?   Renal tumor; chronic renal insufficiency

- swelling of your eyelids? face? feet?   Edema in acute glomerulonephritis

- a loss of appetite? nausea? vomiting?   Uremia: acute or chronic glomerulonephritis

- deafness?   Alport's syndrome

- bloody expectorations?   Goodpasture's syndrome; Wegener's granulomatosis

- chronic sinusitis?   Wegener's granulomatosis

- pain in your joints?   Systemic lupus erythematosus; polyarteritis nodosa

- easy bruising?   Bleeding tendency; thrombocytopenia with hematuria

- pale stool?   Liver disease with bilirubinuria

5   Iatrogenic factors   see Etiology

6   Environmental factors

6.1   Have you ever lived in, or traveled to, a tropical area?   Schistosomiasis haematobia: Africa (Nile Valley), Middle East
Malaria: in areas of South and Central America; Africa; Asia

7   Personal antecedents pertaining to the hematuria

7.1   Have you ever had an examination of your urine? blood? an x-ray of your kidneys? any operation for a stone? When? With what results?

7.2   Have you ever had any of the following conditions: a kidney disease? a stone passed in your urine? a prostate disease? a urinary infection?

7.3   Do you have

• a cardiac condition?	Atrial fibrillation, mitral stenosis: hematuria due to embolic phenomenon
• gout?	Urolithiasis
• a blood disease?	Sickle cell anemia (or trait): papillary infarct; aplastic anemia, leukemia, with thrombocytopenia
• a bleeding tendency?	

8   *Family medical history pertaining to the hematuria*

8.1   Does someone else in your family have

• hematuria?	Polycystic disease; Alport's syndrome (with deafness)
• a blood disease?	Hemoglobinopathies (sickle cell anemia); Osler-Weber-Rendu disease

PHYSICAL SIGNS PERTINENT TO THE COMPLAINT

Finding	**Possible** *significance*
Abdominal mass	Renal tumor, cyst
Bilaterally enlarged kidneys	Polycystic disease
Costovertebral angle tenderness	Nephrolithiasis; renal inflammation
Fever	Urinary tract infection; connective-tissue disease
Hypertension; edema	Acute glomerulonephritis
Arthritis	Systemic lupus erythematosus; Henoch-Schönlein purpura
Atrial fibrillation } Mitral stenosis }	Renal embolism and infarction

Ecchymoses; petechiae	Bleeding tendency
Lymphadenopathy; spleno-megaly	Lymphoma, leukemia, with bleeding tendency
Jaundice	Hemolytic disease; sickle cell trait; bilirubinuria rather than hematuria
Abnormal rectal examination	Prostatic hypertrophy or carcinoma; prostatitis

LABORATORY TESTS PERTAINING TO THE COMPLAINT

Procedure	*Finding*	*Diagnostic possibilities*
Urine Sediment	RBCs, WBCs	Stone; tumor; interstitial cystitis
	RBCs, WBCs, bacteria	Urinary tract infection; hemorrhagic cystitis
	RBC casts	Glomerular bleeding
Blood RBCs	Anemia	Chronic renal failure; systemic illness
	Polycythemia	Hypernephroma; polycystic disease; renal cysts
Platelet count	Thrombocytopenia	Bleeding tendency
Prothrombin time	Prolonged	Bleeding tendency
Hemoglobin electrophoresis*	Abnormal	Sickle cell disease

Procedure	*To detect*
Plain abdominal film	Radiopaque stones
IV pyelogram ⎫ Nephrotomography ⎭	Stones; tumor; obstruction; polycystic disease; etc.

* If appropriate.

Cystoscopy	Site of bleeding; urethral or bladder lesions; cystitis; bladder tumor; vesical calculi; prostatic bladder disease; diverticula
Ultrasonography	Renal tumor vs. cyst
Arteriography	Tumors; cysts; renal infarction; arterio-venous malformations
Renal biopsy*	Specific forms of parenchymal disease

* If appropriate.

USEFUL REMINDERS AND DIAGNOSTIC CLUES

Misleading Factors

Female patients sometimes have difficulty in determining whether bleeding is from the urinary tract, vagina, or rectum.

Phenolphthalein contained in some laxatives may impart a red translucent appearance to the urine.

Patients treated with phenazopyridine hydrochloride have an orange-red urine.

Injection of phenolsulfonphthalein as a test of kidney function produces a red-violet urine.

Occasionally a patient with a harmless and rare congenital metabolic error will have a red-brown urine after beet ingestion.

Rifampin and its metabolites may color urine a bright red-orange.

Diagnostic Considerations

Gross hematuria with no or mild proteinuria and without casts indicates a localized disease of the collecting system, a bleeding disturbance, or an abnormal hemoglobin; hematuria with significant proteinuria usually indicates a diffuse renal lesion.

About 20 percent of the patients who come to the physician with hematuria have it as the only symptom of their urinary tract disease.

Tumors, urinary tract obstructions, calculi, and infections account for the bleeding in about 75 percent of patients with hematuria, tumors alone accounting for some 20 percent of all cases.

Hematuria without other symptoms must be regarded as a symptom of tumor of the bladder or kidney until proved otherwise. Less

common causes of silent hematuria are a staghorn calculus, polycystic disease, a solitary renal cyst, sickle cell disease, hydronephrosis, acute glomerulonephritis.

Hematuria with ureteral colic and no calcified density on an x-ray
film suggests radiolucent stones (uric acid, xanthine), necrotic
papillitis, blood clots, or fragments of tumor.

Only 55 percent of renal tumors give symptoms: hematuria occurs
in 60 percent of the symptomatic patients, a palpable mass in 70
percent, pain in the kidney region in 90 percent.

Hematuria is the presenting symptom in 30 percent of patients with
renal tuberculosis.

If microscopic hematuria is present during an acute streptococcal
infection, acute glomerulonephritis is more likely to develop than
if hematuria is absent.

Prostatic hemorrhage is more often due to a benign lesion than to
a malignant one.

Patients on anticoagulants who develop hematuria often have an
underlying lesion of the urinary tract.

In case of	*Suspect*
A red supernatant of centrifugated urine associated with	
Red plasma	Intravascular hemolysis with hemoglobinuria
Clear plasma	Skeletal muscle damage with myoglobinuria (the small myoglobin molecule is rapidly excreted into the urine, leaving the plasma uncolored)
A clear yellow supernatant of centrifugated urine with a red button of sediment	Hematuria

SELECTED BIBLIOGRAPHY

Berman LB: When the urine is red. JAMA 237:2753–2754, 1977

Levinsky NG: *The Interpretation of Proteinuria and the Urinary Sediment,*
Disease-a-Month, Chicago: Year Book, March 1967

22
High BUN and/or Proteinuria

DEFINITIONS AND PATHOPHYSIOLOGY

Uremia   term applied to the symptoms and signs which occur when the kidneys are unable to maintain a normal internal environment.

Proteinuria   presence of protein in the urine.

Many chronic renal diseases are inherently progressive and eventuate in uremia, a symptomatic state with disorders of various systems. According to the "intact nephron" hypothesis, there are two populations of nephrons in the diseased kidneys of chronic renal failure: nephrons that are nonfunctioning, because of significant destruction of any portion of the nephron, and intact, normally functioning nephrons which maintain excretory function. In these remaining nephrons the concentration of urea in the glomerular filtrate and the resulting increase in solute load provoke a solute diuresis. This causes a loss of concentrating ability of intact nephrons, with resulting polyuria and nocturia. The osmotic diuresis also limits the ability to reabsorb sodium from the tubular lumen adequately, with a resulting loss of sodium in the urine. Metabolic acidosis is due to a decreased ability to excrete ammonium and to renal bicarbonate leak. Hypocalcemia due to hyperphosphatemia, impaired intestinal absorption of calcium, and vitamin D resistance, is generally present in chronic renal failure. Resistance to vitamin D can give rise to osteomalacia, whereas hypocalcemia stimulates the parathyroid glands, resulting in secondary hyperparathyroidism. Some gastrointestinal, cardiovascular, neuromuscular manifestations of uremia are attributed to retention of toxic products of protein metabolism (? middle molecules of molecular weight 300 to 1800), or to adaptive overproduction of polypeptide hormones. The mechanisms of anemia in chronic renal failure are discussed in Chap. 43.

Some protein is filtered by normal glomeruli (40 to 100 mg/day). Abnormal proteinuria is present when the protein in the urine is greater than 150 mg/day or 60 mg/m² of body surface per 24 h. Orthostatic proteinuria (protein present in the urine produced when the patient is in the upright position and absent when the patient is recumbent) occurs in about 3 percent of adolescents and is usually benign; it is associated with a lordotic erect position which produces venous congestion and renal vasoconstriction. Persistent proteinuria is always pathologic. Heavy proteinuria, in excess of 4 g daily (nephrotic syndrome), results from a gross increase in glomerular permeability; diseases of the glomeruli produce a proteinuria in which albumin predominates. In tubular proteinuria (pyelonephritis) reabsorption of proteins from the tubular lumen is incomplete because of tubular damage; low molecular weight nonalbumin proteins are prominent in tubular proteinuria. Proteinuria is generally absent or scant in renal insufficiency due to dehydration.

ETIOLOGY

Chronic renal failure (proteinuria rarely exceeding 1 to 2 g/24 h)
Glomerulonephritis: proliferative; membranous
Chronic pyelonephritis; tuberculous pyelonephritis
Polycystic disease; medullary cystic disease
Congenital nephritis; renal hypoplasia
Renal calculi
Upper urinary tract obstruction: hydronephrosis, neoplasm, retroperitoneal fibrosis
Lower urinary tract obstruction: prostatic adenoma, neoplasm; urethral stricture; urethral valve; bladder-neck obstruction; neurogenic bladder
Renal tubular acidosis
Connective-tissue diseases: systemic lupus erythematosus; polyarteritis nodosa; Henoch-Schönlein purpura; Wegener's granulomatosis
Other systemic diseases: diabetes; gout; malignant hypertension; subacute bacterial endocarditis; amyloidosis; hypercalcemia; potassium deficiency; cystinosis; oxalosis; hemolytic-uremic syndrome; thrombotic thrombocytopenic purpura; Goodpasture's syndrome
Intoxications: lead; cadmium; analgesic abuse

Heavy proteinuria: nephrotic syndrome
Primary glomerular disease: minimal change disease; focal glomerulonephritis; proliferative glomerulonephritis; membranous glomerulonephritis; homograft rejection
Systemic disease: diabetic glomerulosclerosis; connective-tissue

diseases: systemic lupus erythematosus, polyarteritis nodosa; amyloidosis; multiple myeloma
Infectious diseases: secondary syphilis; malaria
Mechanical causes with increased renal venous pressure: renal vein thrombosis; obstruction of inferior vena cava; constrictive pericarditis; sickle cell anemia
Nephrotoxins and allergens: insect stings; poison ivy; snake bites; mercury, gold, bismuth; drugs

Iatrogenic Causes of High BUN and/or Proteinuria

Chronic analgesic abuse: phenacetin, salicylates(?): chronic interstitial nephritis, papillary necrosis
Amphotericin B, outdated tetracycline: renal tubular acidosis
Methicillin, other penicillin-related antibiotics, sulfonamides: acute tubulointerstitial nephritis
Tridione, paramethadione, probenecid, penicillamine, gold salts: nephrotic syndrome
Streptomycin, gentamycin, kanamycin, vancomycin, neomycin: proximal tubular necrosis
Diuretics and antihypertensive drugs may induce sodium depletion and produce an elevation of BUN.

QUESTIONNAIRE

Possible *meaning of response*

1   Mode of onset and duration

1.1   How long have you known that you have uremia (and/or proteinuria)?

1.1*a*   How was it detected?
- during a check-up examination?   Renal functional impairment may be asymptomatic
- because you were sick?

1.2   Since when have you felt sick?   The onset of chronic renal failure is insidious

2   Character of the urine

2.1   What is the appearance of your urine?
- clear?   Chronic glomerulonephritis

• cloudy?	Presence of phosphates, urates, pus, blood
• reddish? bloody?	Acute glomerulonephritis, nephrolithiasis, tumor may cause hematuria

3   Precipitating or aggravating factors

3.1   Have you recently had

• an infection? a urinary infection?	Infection, especially streptococcal, may seriously impair residual renal function
• an episode of vomiting? diarrhea?	May cause severe saline depletion, hypovolemia, and diminished renal perfusion
• black, tarry stools?	Bleeding into the intestine increases production rate of urea

3.2 What is your daily intake of fluid? salt? meat, fish?	In patients with chronic renal failure, administration of excessive amounts of water and sodium may contribute to hypertension, produce overhydration and "uremic lung"; excessive intake of protein may increase production rate of urea

4   Accompanying symptoms

4.1 Do you feel weak? unwell? easily tired?	Almost universal in symptomatic uremia; anemia (becomes a major cause of symptoms when hemoglobin falls below about 7 g/100 mL)

4.2   Do you have

• a loss of appetite?	Anorexia in uremia is one of the first symptoms of a low serum sodium concentration
• *nausea? especially upon arising in the morning?* vomiting?	Common in early stage of chronic renal failure

• diarrhea?	Last stages of chronic renal failure
• hiccups?	Common in advanced chronic renal failure
• headaches?	<u>Arterial hypertension</u>
• a dimmed, blurred vision?	Hypertension with lesions in the optic fundi
• a swelling of your eyelids? • a swelling of your face?	Nephrotic syndrome with hypo-proteinemia Parotitis: advanced uremia
• swollen legs?	Edema: <u>hypertensive heart fail-ure</u>, one of the most common complications of uremia; hypo-proteinemia: nephrotic syn-drome; oliguric phase of terminal renal insufficiency with excessive intake of fluid
• trouble breathing?	Metabolic acidosis with Küss-maul respiration in chronic renal insufficiency; congestive heart failure; "uremic lung"; anemia
• fever?	Systemic lupus erythematosus; polyarteritis nodosa
• chest pain?	Pericarditis (usually painless; BUN above 80 mg/100 mL)
• abdominal pain?	Pancreatitis, pericarditis may oc-cur in uremia
• nocturnal muscle cramps in the calves? thighs?	Common in early renal failure: a sign of dehydration or sodium depletion; peripheral neuritis
• numbness, tingling, burning of the toes? feet?	Peripheral demyelinating neu-ropathy; hypocalcemia
• twitchings of your muscles?	Late renal failure
• easy bruising?	Platelet defect of uremia: dis-turbed ADP-mediated platelet aggregation; thrombocytopenia
• itching?	Ascribed to calcium phosphate deposition in the skin; often as-sociated with secondary hyper-parathyroidism

• pain in your joints?	Lupus nephritis; gouty nephropathy; Henoch-Schönlein purpura
• bloody expectorations?	Goodpasture's syndrome; Wegener's granulomatosis

4.3 During the day, do you urinate

• as much as usual?	Normal frequency of micturitions: five to six times a day
• less frequently than usual?	Oliguria: acute glomerulonephritis; end stage of chronic glomerulonephritis; obstructive uropathy
• more frequently than usual?	
• without discomfort, and passing large amounts of urine?	Polyuria commonly accompanies isosthenuria; an early sign of chronic renal failure; hypercalcemia; hypokalemia; diuretic medication

4.3a Do you have to get up at night to urinate? how many times?	Nocturia: chronic renal insufficiency with a constant osmotic diuresis per nephron and reversal of diurnal rhythm
4.4 Are you more thirsty than usual?	Polydipsia balancing the polyuria of chronic renal failure

5 *Iatrogenic factors* see Etiology

5.1 Have you regularly taken any drugs for headaches?	Phenacetin nephropathy; methysergide-induced retroperitoneal fibrosis
5.2 Are you taking any drugs for an elevated blood pressure?	Drug-induced hypotension and/or salt depletion tend to reduce renal function and may worsen renal insufficiency
5.3 Have you taken any drugs for recurrent urinary infections?	Nitrofurantoin may cause neuropathy in the uremic patient

6   *Personal antecedents pertaining to the complaint*

6.1   Have you ever had blood, urine examinations? x-rays of the kidneys? When? With what results?

6.2   Have you ever had any of the following conditions: a kidney disease? acute glomerulonephritis? stones? recurrent renal infections? elevated blood pressure?

•gout?	Gouty nephropathy: uric acid stones and interstitial deposits of urate crystals in the kidney
• diabetes?	Intercapillary glomerulosclerosis, uncontrolled hypertension, urinary tract infections, pyelonephritis, papillary necrosis, renal artery arteriosclerosis may cause a rapid deterioration of renal function in the diabetic patient

7   *Family medical history pertaining to the complaint*

7.1   Does someone in your family have

• a renal disease?	Polycystic disease
• deafness?	Alport's syndrome

PHYSICAL SIGNS PERTINENT TO THE COMPLAINT

Finding	**Possible** *significance*
Skin pigmentation	Common in slowly progressive renal failure: due to melanin and urochromes
Scratch marks	Pruritus, particularly associated with secondary hyperparathyroidism
Hypertension	Present at some stage in more than 80 percent of patients with chronic renal failure; associated with sodium and water retention

Pulmonary edema; peripheral edema	Hypertensive heart failure (heart failure is one of the most common complications of uremia); impaired sodium and water excretion; nephrotic syndrome; acute glomerulonephritis; oliguric phase of terminal renal insufficiency with excessive fluid intake
Precordial friction rub	Pericarditis (calls for urgent treatment)
Hypotension; distended jugular veins; paradoxical pulse	Pericardial effusion with cardiac tamponade
Diminished to absent deep tendon reflexes; muscle weakness	Peripheral demyelinating neuropathy may occur in patients with chronic renal failure; diabetes
Asterixis; muscle twitching	Late renal failure (metabolic origin?)
Pallor	Anemia: low plasma erythropoietin; bone marrow depression; hemolysis (absence of anemia suggests acute renal failure)
Ecchymoses; epistaxis	A bleeding tendency is common in late renal failure; disturbed ADP-mediated platelet aggregation and platelet adhesiveness
Large kidneys	Obstructive uropathy; polycystic disease
Palpable liver or spleen	Amyloidosis with nephrotic syndrome
Arthritis; skin rash	Connective-tissue disease
Metastatic calcification in the cornea	Band keratopathy: disturbed calcium metabolism

Funduscopic examination	May reveal: hypertensive retinopathy; diabetic retinopathy (patients with diabetic glomerulopathy almost invariably have retinal complications)

LABORATORY TESTS PERTAINING TO THE COMPLAINT

Procedure	Finding	Diagnostic possibilities
Blood		
BUN: creatinine ratio (N: 10 to 15:1)	10 to 15:1	Renal parenchymal disease
	>10 to 15:1	Extrarenal disorder: dehydration, hypotension, hypovolemia, GI hemorrhage
Uric acid	Disproportionate elevation	Gouty nephropathy
Hematocrit	Decreased	Normocytic normochromic anemia in chronic renal failure
Electrolytes	Metabolic acidosis	GFR below 20 mL/min
	Hyperkalemia	Terminal renal failure
Calcium	Decreased	Low serum albumin level; hyperphosphatemia; impaired GI absorption of calcium; formation of complexes with phosphate

Fasting glucose	Elevated	Diabetic nephropathy
Cholesterol, triglycerides	Elevated	Nephrotic syndrome
Serum electrophoresis	Hyperproteinemia ⎱ Monoclonal peak ⎰	Multiple myeloma
	Hypoalbuminemia	Nephrotic syndrome
Antinuclear antibodies	Positive	Systemic lupus erythematosus (SLE)
Serum complement	Decreased	Acute streptococcal nephritis; lupus nephritis; membranoproliferative glomerulonephritis

Urine

Protein	>4 g/24 h	Nephrotic syndrome
	<2 g/24 h	Glomerulitides; tubular proteinuria; congestive heart failure; orthostatic proteinuria
Sediment	RBC casts	Active glomerulonephritis; SLE; arteritis; malignant hypertension
	WBCs, bacteria	Urinary tract infection
Culture	Positive	Urinary tract infection
Electrophoresis	Low molecular weight protein, absence of albumin ⎱	Tubular proteinuria
	Light chains	Bence Jones proteinuria: multiple myeloma

Procedure	To detect
IV pyelogram (size of normal kidneys: three and one-half vertebral bodies)	Large kidneys: obstruction; polycystic disease; amyloidosis
	Small kidneys: chronic renal disease; pyelonephritis
	Irregular renal outlines: chronic pyelonephritis
	Normal renal size: acute renal failure
Renal venography*	Renal vein thrombosis
Renal biopsy*	Specific forms of parenchymal disease; causes of nephrotic syndrome; amyloidosis; polyarteritis nodosa; etc.

* If appropriate.

USEFUL REMINDERS AND DIAGNOSTIC CLUES

Misleading Factors

A doubling of the plasma creatinine at any absolute level of plasma creatinine represents approximately a 50 percent fall in the creatinine clearance; a similar change in blood urea concentration may reflect only a doubling of urea production caused by increased protein consumption or some other cause of accelerated nitrogen turnover.

Plasma concentration of urea and creatinine show little absolute change until, functionally, the patient has lost one kidney.

Bence Jones proteins do not cause positive Albustix test.

Diagnostic Considerations

Exacerbations of chronic nephritis caused by streptococcal infection have a short latent period (a few days), whereas attacks of acute nephritis following the onset of infections occur 2 to 3 weeks later

In case of	Suspect
Uremia with Hypertension and hypertensive retinopathy, without anemia	A primary vascular disease

Hypertension and normal optic fundi	Pyelonephritis or glomerulonephritis
A virtually normal sediment	Obstruction; hypercalcemia
A normal hemoglobin	Acute renal failure; early stage of: urinary obstruction, renal artery stenosis, polycystic disease
Uremia without proteinuria	Polycystic disease, hypercalcemic or hypokalemic nephropathy, obstruction, stone, pyelonephritis, disease of the large or small blood vessels, congenital malformation, tumor
"Unexplained uremia"	Obstructive uropathy

SELECTED BIBLIOGRAPHY

Bricker NS: On the pathogenesis of the uremic state: An exposition of the "trade-off hypothesis." N Engl J Med 286:1093–1099, 1972

Epstein FH, Merrill JP: Chronic renal failure, in Thorn GW et al (eds), *Harrison's Principles of Internal Medicine,* 8th ed, pp 1428–1438, New York: McGraw-Hill, 1977

Kerr DNS: Chronic renal failure, in Beeson PB, McDermott W (eds), *Textbook of Medicine,* 14th ed, chap 603, pp 1093–1107, Philadelphia: Saunders, 1975

Merrill, JP: Glomerulonephritis. N Engl J Med 290:257–266, 313–319, 374–381, 1974

———, Hampers CL: Uremia. N Engl J Med 282:953–961, 1014–1021, 1970

Rennie ID: Proteinuria. Med Clin North Am 55:213–230, 1971

Schrier RW, Guggenheim S: Nephrotic syndrome, in Thorn GW et al, op cit, pp 1450–1457

23
Pain in the Flank

DEFINITIONS AND GENERAL CONSIDERATIONS

Local pain   pain felt in or near the involved organ.
Referred pain   originates in a diseased organ but is felt at some distance from the organ.

Pain in the flank commonly originates in urinary organs. A diseased kidney gives rise to local pain (T10 to T12, L1) in the costovertebral angle and in the flank, in the region of and below the twelfth rib. The pain is associated with renal diseases which cause sudden distention of the renal capsule (acute pyelonephritis, acute ureteral obstruction). Renal diseases with a slow progression are not associated with sudden capsular distention and are painless (cancer, chronic pyelonephritis, tuberculosis, staghorn calculus, mild ureteral obstruction with hydronephrosis).

Ureteral pain is due to acute obstruction (stone, blood clot). This produces capsular distention with back pain, and renal pelvic and ureteral muscle spasm and hyperperistalsis with severe colicky pain that radiates along the course of the ureter.

Renal or ureteral diseases are often associated with nausea, vomiting, and abdominal distention. These gastrointestinal symptoms may result from renointestinal reflexes (common autonomic and sensory innervation of the two systems), organ relationships, or peritoneal irritation.

ETIOLOGY

Flank pain of urologic origin

Nephrolithiasis:
   Hypercalciuria: hyperparathyroidism, hypervitaminosis D, milk-alkali syndrome, sarcoidosis, malignancy, bone disease, renal tubular acidosis, hyperthyroidism, idiopathic hypercalciuria
   Uric acid lithiasis: gout, lymphoproliferative and myeloproliferative disorders, chronic diarrheal states, ileostomy

Hyperoxaluria: primary; acquired (small-bowel disease)
Xanthinuria; cystinuria
Recurrent renal infections (with urea-splitting microorganisms)
Upper urinary infection; papillary necrosis; renal abscess
Renal arterial embolism or thrombosis; renal vein thrombosis
Bleeding into: renal tumor, polycystic disease, renal tuberculosis
Retroperitoneal fibrosis

Flank pain in nonurologic disease
Cardiovascular: abdominal aortic aneurysm; bacterial endocarditis
   with splenic embolism
Irritation of diaphragm: pleural effusion; pneumonia; pulmonary embolism; perinephric and subphrenic abscess
Gastrointestinal: colonic obstruction; irritable colon syndrome; hepatic and splenic flexure syndrome; acute gallbladder disease;
   acute appendicitis
Neurologic: herpes zoster; cord tumor; radiculitis syndrome (spondylosis; compression fracture, vertebral body)
Retroperitoneal: lymphoma; metastatic carcinoma; pancreatitic carcinoma; pancreatitis; psoas abscess; lumbar abscess; torsion,
   undescended testis
Trauma: fracture of transverse process, lumbar spine
Psychogenic: depression; anxiety reaction; malingering

Iatrogenic Causes of Renal Stones

Absorbable alkalis, magnesium trisilicates
Allopurinol: may cause hyperxanthinuria
Chronic use of acetazolamide
Vitamin D intoxication

Iatrogenic Causes of Hyperuricemia

Thiazides, chlorthalidone; furosemide; ethacrynic acid
Antineoplastic drugs
Aspirin (small doses)

QUESTIONNAIRE

Possible *meaning of response*

1 Location and radiation of the pain

1.1   Where did the pain begin?
- in the side? flank?
- in the back? (costovertebral angle? lumbar region?)

Renal pain: <u>stone</u>; <u>acute pyelonephritis</u>; renal tumor, pelvis or calyx (blood clot causing obstruction); papillary necrosis

- in the right hypochondrium?

<u>Gallbladder disease</u>; acute pancreatitis; penetrating duodenal ulcer; hepatic flexure syndrome

- in the right flank?

Right colon; acute appendicitis; renal pain

- in the left hypochondrium?

Splenic infarction; penetrating gastric ulcer; acute pancreatitis; splenic flexure syndrome

- in the left flank?

Diverticulitis; renal pain

1.2   Does the pain radiate from the costovertebral angle
- along the subcostal area toward the umbilicus?

Sudden distention of the renal capsule; acute ureteral obstruction with sudden renal back pressure; acute pyelonephritis with sudden edema

- *down toward the lower anterior abdominal quadrant?*

Ureteral pain

  - *into the testicle?*

Ureteropelvic stone; stone lodged in the upper ureter (the nerve supply to the testis and to the kidney and upper ureter is the same: T11 and T12)

- with maximum pain in the lower abdominal quadrant?

Stone in midportion of ureter (T12–L1)

- into scrotum? (vulva?)

Low ureteral stone: common innervation of the lower ureter and bladder, scrotum, or vulva

1.3 *Does the pain radiate from the right hypochondrium to the back? right shoulder?*

Gallbladder colic

1.4 Does the pain radiate from the left hypochondrium to the precordium?

Splenic flexure syndrome

2 *Mode of onset and evolution*

2.1 How long have you had pain in the flank?

2.2 Has the pain appeared

• suddenly?

Stone colic; vascular pain (dissecting aortic aneurysm); blood clot causing urinary tract obstruction

• gradually?

Inflammatory pain: acute pyelonephritis; renal abscess; lumbar abscess

2.2*a* Did the pain disappear abruptly?

Renal colic

2.3 How long did the pain last?

The duration of a renal colic is variable; it may subside within a few minutes or last for hours

2.4 Have you experienced in the past similar episodes?

Renal stones tend to recur; gallbladder stones

3 *Character and intensity of the pain*

3.1 Is the flank pain

• very severe? constant?

Obstruction and capsular tension: renal colic; acute pyelonephritis (renal colic is one of the most severe pains encountered in medical practice)

• with paroxysms of colicky, excruciating radiating pain? (like a sharp stabbing sensation?)

Renal colic: hyperperistalsis of the smooth muscles of the calyces, pelvis, and ureter; progression of calculus in the ureter

- a low-grade pain or a chronic persistent discomfort?

Chronic obstructive nephropathy (dull flank pain due to parenchymal and capsular distention): stone in the renal pelvis; stone impacted in the ureter; hydronephrosis; renal tumor; polycystic disease; nonurologic condition

4 Precipitating or aggravating factors

4.1 In case of chronic discomfort in the flank, is it increased by

- exertion?

In steady pain due to renal lithiasis or stone impacted in the ureter; polycystic disease

- movements of the spine? straining?

Radicular pain: compression vertebral fracture; cord tumor

5 Relieving factors

5.1 In case of acute flank pain, do you prefer, in order to relieve the pain, to

- *remain immobile or lie quietly in bed?*

Inflammatory type of pain; peritoneal irritation

- *pace the floor, move constantly, in an attempt to find a position that could give some relief?*

Characteristic of renal colic

5.2 In case of chronic discomfort, is it relieved by

- lying down?

Polycystic disease

- passage of gas?

Irritable colon; hepatic or splenic flexure syndrome; incomplete obstruction of the large bowel

6 Accompanying symptoms

6.1 During or after the attack, did you pass

• urine of normal color?	Probably nonrenal disorder
• dark urine?	Acute gallbladder disorder with bilirubinuria
• *bloody urine?*	Hematuria, almost always present in renal colic; <u>renal calculus</u>; renal tumor; massive infarction of the kidney
• cloudy urine?	<u>Acute pyelonephritis</u>; infection complicating a renal stone; papillary necrosis

6.2 During the attack, did you pass

• a decreased amount of urine?	Renal colic
• a normal amount of urine?	Probably nonrenal disorder

6.3 After the attack, did you

• urinate more than usual?	Polyuria frequently appears after a renal colic
• stop urinating?	**Anuria** associated with bilateral ureteral calculi; papillary necrosis

6.4 Do you have

• a frequent desire to urinate? • burning on urination?	Urgency, frequency: renal stone approaching the bladder: inflammation and edema of the ureteral orifice; urinary tract infection
• fever? chills?	Urinary tract infection; renal or perinephric abscess; infection in other system(s)
• nausea? vomiting?	Renal colic with renointestinal reflexes: both systems have common autonomic and sensory innervation; intestinal obstruction; hyperparathyroidism; chronic renal insufficiency
• abdominal distention?	Paralytic ileus may accompany renal colic

• pain in your joints? toes?	Gout with uric acid lithiasis
• pain in your bones?	Multiple myeloma, hyper-parathyroidism with hyper-calcemia and nephrolithiasis
• increased thirst? increased urinary output?	Hypercalcemia with polyuria and polydipsia: hyperparathyroidism; chronic renal insufficiency
• chronic diarrhea?	The incidence of hyperoxaluria with calcium oxalate kidney stone is significantly higher in patients with inflammatory bowel disease, malabsorption, ileal resection, jejunoileal anastomosis

7   *Iatrogenic factors*   see Etiology

8   *Environmental factors*

8.1   What is your

• daily intake of fluids?	The type of water may give relevant information as to calcium content; a low fluid intake may produce an increased urinary concentration of salts and organic compounds
• diet: milk? cheese?	The major calcium foods; hypercalciuria may be observed in some adults who drink a quart or more of milk per day

9   *Personal antecedents pertaining to the complaint*

9.1   Have you ever had an examination of your urine? blood? an x-ray of your kidneys? a chemical analysis of a stone? a treatment for renal stones? When? With what results?

9.2   Have you ever
   • had previous kidney stone? gravel?

- passed a stone ("gravel") in your urine?

  About 80 percent of stones which reach the ureter can pass spontaneously

- had recurrent urinary infections?

  Suggests infection as an etiologic or complicating factor of renal calculus

- had gout?
- had a long period of immobilization?

  May cause hypercalciuria

10   *Family medical history pertaining to the complaint*

10.1   Is there someone in your family who has (had) renal stones?

Idiopathic uric acid lithiasis; hereditary hyperoxaluria, cystinuria, xanthinuria

PHYSICAL SIGNS PERTINENT TO THE COMPLAINT

Finding	**Possible** *significance*
Restless patient changing position frequently	Renal colic
Tenderness in the costovertebral angle and flank	Ureteral stone; blood clot obstructing the ureter
Fever; costovertebral angle tenderness on deep pressure	Acute pyelonephritis; infection complicating urinary lithiasis; renal abscess
Palpable kidney	Acute hydronephrosis; renal tumor
Fever; tenderness of flank; palpable mass moving with respiration	Perinephric abscess
Left pleural effusion; splenic friction rub	Splenic abscess
Fever; tenderness along the costal margin; basilar rales	Subphrenic abscess; pleurisy with pain referred to the abdomen

Jaundice	Gallbladder disease; sickle cell disease with renal infarction
Abdominal distention; diminished peristalsis	Often present in acute renal colic
Atrial fibrillation; cardiac lesion	Renal or splenic embolic episode
Tophi; gouty arthritis	Uric acid nephrolithiasis
Calcification in the cornea	Band keratopathy; hyperparathyroidism

LABORATORY TESTS PERTAINING TO THE COMPLAINT

Procedure	*To detect*
Blood Calcium (N: 9 to 11 mg/100 mL)	Hypercalcemic states
Phosphorus (N: 3.0 to 4.5 mg/100 mL) Alkaline phosphatase (N: 2.0 to 4.5 Bodansky U)	High calcium, low phosphate in hyperparathyroidism (with high alkaline phosphatase when there is significant bone disease)
Electrolytes	Metabolic acidosis in renal tubular acidosis
Uric acid	Gouty nephropathy
Parathormone assay*	Hyperparathyroidism
Urine pH	High urine pH (7 or higher): infection; renal tubular disorder
Sediment	RBCs: renal calculus
Culture	Renal infection with urea-splitting bacteria: may promote the formation of magnesium ammonium phosphate stones

* If appropriate.

Calcium (N: <150 mg/24 h with a low Ca diet)	Hypercalciuria: in most patients with calcareous calculi: hyperparathyroidism, hypervitaminosis D, sarcoidosis, idiopathic hypercalciuria, etc.
Qualitative test for cystine	Cystinuria
Analysis of stone	Oxalosis, primary or secondary; uric acid stones; etc.
Plain abdominal film	Radiopaque stones
IV pyelography	Radiopaque or radiolucent stones; obstruction; nephrocalcinosis; anatomic abnormalities predisposing to calculus formation: obstruction, medullary sponge kidney, localized deformity
X-rays of hands, lateral heads of clavicles, skull, long bones, pelvis*	Subperiosteal bone resorption in hyperparathyroidism

* If appropriate.

USEFUL REMINDERS AND DIAGNOSTIC CLUES

Misleading Factor

The gastrointestinal symptoms commonly associated with stone in the ureter may be very severe and simulate an intraperitoneal lesion.

Diagnostic Considerations

Sudden onset of renal pain, fever, with leukocytosis and without pyuria, should suggest the diagnosis of renal abscess.

Ninety percent of all kidney stones contain calcium.

If a stone is not obstructive, it is not apt to cause injury or symptoms.

Sites of impaction of a ureteral stone: the ureteropelvic junction; where the ureter crosses over the iliac vessels; the ureterovesical zone.

The urinary inorganic salts are less soluble in an alkaline medium: calcium phosphate forms at a pH of 6.6 or higher; magnesium ammonium phosphate precipitates at pH of 7.2 or higher.

The urinary pH (mean value: 5.85) is increased by ingestion of alkaline medicaments (treatment of peptic ulcer), acetazolamide (treatment of glaucoma), urea-splitting bacteria (usually *Proteus mirabilis*) liberating ammonia.

The urinary organic substances (cystine, uric acid) are least soluble at a pH below 7.0 (maximum insolubility: pH 5.5).

The rate of renal calculi in patients with hyperparathyroidism varies between 50 and 80 percent, whereas 5 to 8 percent of patients with renal calculi have primary hyperparathyroidism.

The rate of uric acid stone disease is approximately 25 percent in patients with primary overproduction gout and about 40 percent in patients with hyperuricemia secondary to lymphoproliferative and myeloproliferative disorders.

Radiopacity and Frequency of Renal Stones

Degree of radiopacity	Stone	Frequency, %
Very opaque	Calcium phosphate ⎱	±66
Opaque	Calcium oxalate ⎰	
Moderately opaque	Magnesium ammonium phosphate	±15
Slightly opaque	Cystine ⎱	±10
Nonopaque	Uric acid ⎰	
	Xanthine	±9 (including stones made up of silicates, matrix, etc.)

SELECTED BIBLIOGRAPHY

Smith DR: *General Urology,* 8th ed, p 200, Los Altos, Lange, 1975
Williams HE: Nephrolithiasis. N Engl J Med 290:33–38, 1974

24
Polyuria

DEFINITION AND PATHOPHYSIOLOGY

Polyuria persistent increase in urine flow, greater than 2500 mL daily.

The normal daily urine output in adults varies between 700 and 2000 mL. When a normal subject ingests an appreciable volume of water, plasma solute concentration decreases. Hypothalamic osmoreceptors sense the fall in plasma osmolality and inhibit both thirst and release of vasopressin, the neurohypophyseal antidiuretic hormone (ADH). In the absence of ADH, the distal convoluted tubule and the collecting duct become impermeable to water and an increased volume of dilute urine is formed. With the loss of free water, osmolality of plasma increases, stimulating ADH secretion and thus preventing further water loss. The other major regulators of ADH secretion are intravascular volume (an increased plasma volume inhibits ADH release and produces a diuresis that corrects the hypervolemia, whereas hypovolemia stimulates the secretion of ADH), and stress, either physical or emotional, which stimulates ADH release. The failure of the kidney to concentrate urine in the presence of increased plasma solute concentration results in the syndrome of diabetes insipidus (DI) with polyuria.

Diabetes insipidus due to vasopressin deficiency may be caused by any type of lesion in the hypothalamus or pituitary region. Patients with central DI cannot concentrate their urine despite a rise in plasma osmolality after water deprivation, but they respond normally to exogenous vasopressin.

Nephrogenic DI is characterized by inability of the renal tubules to respond to endogenous or exogenous vasopressin. The high osmotic load per nephron which occurs in diabetes mellitus and chronic renal failure may also cause polyuria. In psychogenic DI, polyuria is secondary to compulsive water drinking (primary polydipsia). This condition, far more common than central DI, is seen in patients with psychologic disturbances.

ETIOLOGY

Reduced production of antidiuretic hormone (ADH)
Diseases involving the hypothalamic-neurohypophyseal system
　Diabetes insipidus
　　Idiopathic (spontaneous)
　　Intracranial lesions: pituitary tumor, primary brain tumor, metastatic tumor, head trauma
　　Systemic disorders: multifocal eosinophilic granuloma, sarcoidosis, infectious diseases
　　Iatrogenic: hypophysectomy, pituitary stalk section, cryohypophysectomy, implantation of radioactive materials into the sella turcica
　Reduced secretion of ADH secondary to increased thirst
　Psychogenic diabetes insipidus

Renal abnormalities
Impaired tubular responsiveness to ADH
　Congenital nephrogenic diabetes insipidus
　Multiple renal tubular functional abnormalities: Fanconi's syndrome
　Acquired tubular lesions: potassium deficiency (aldosteronism, primary or secondary; Cushing's syndrome; corticosteroid therapy; diuretics; renal tubular diseases); hypercalcemia (malignancy, with or without metastases; hyperparathyroidism; thiazides; multiple myeloma; sarcoidosis; vitamin D intoxication; milk-alkali syndrome); chronic renal diseases; sickle cell anemia; unilateral renal artery occlusion; multiple myeloma; amyloidosis; drugs: lithium carbonate, demeclocycline
Osmotic diuresis: diabetes mellitus; chronic renal insufficiency

Psychogenic diabetes insipidus　excessive water ingestion

Iatrogenic Causes of Polyuria

Excessive doses of corticosteroids
Diuretics: thiazides, ethacrynic acid, furosemide, carbonic anhydrase inhibitors
Vitamin D intoxication with hypercalcemia
Demeclocycline
Lithium carbonate

QUESTIONNAIRE

Possible *meaning of response*

1 Mode of onset

1.1 How long have you been passing large quantities of urine?

Idiopathic diabetes insipidus (DI) may become manifest at any age; nephrogenic DI manifests itself early in life

1.2 Has the onset of polyuria been
- *abrupt?*
- *gradual?*

Psychogenic DI
Idiopathic DI

2 Character

2.1 What is the usual volume of urine passed per day?
- less than 5 L?

Chronic renal failure; potassium deficiency; diabetes mellitus; hypercalcemia

- *more than 5 L?*

DI: idiopathic, psychogenic, nephrogenic

2.2 How many times a day do you urinate?

Normally, a much larger volume is excreted in the waking period

2.3 Do you pass at each urination
- *a large quantity of urine?*
- *a small quantity of urine?* }
- with pain on urination?

Polyuria
Dysuria with frequency (not polyuria)

2.4 How many times do you have to get up at night to urinate?

Patients with psychogenic DI are usually not troubled at night

2.5 Do you urinate more during the night than during the day?

Nocturia: may be an early complaint in chronic renal failure when urine is excreted at a uniform rate with loss of normal diurnal rhythm

2.6   Does your large urine flow
  • *remain constant?*   Spontaneous DI
  • *vary from day to day?*   Psychogenic DI

3   Accompanying symptoms

3.1   Do you have
  • *an excessive, insatiable*   Polydipsia: secondary to the
    thirst?   polyuria in: idiopathic DI,
                                        nephrogenic DI, diabetes mel-
                                        litus, chronic renal failure;
                                        primary disorder in psychogenic
                                        DI

  • with a preference for
    • *water?*   Patients with spontaneous DI
    • other beverages?   characteristically prefer water
                                        rather than other beverages
                                        and desire ice water

    • no preference?   Psychogenic DI

3.1*a*   How much do you drink
       a day?

3.1*b*   Are there periods (from
       weeks to months) during
       which you do not have   Psychogenic DI
       excessive thirst?

3.1*c*   If you are deprived of
       water, do you urinate
  • *less than usual?*   Psychogenic DI
  • *as much as usual?*   Spontaneous DI

3.2   Do you have
  • headaches?   Increased intracranial pressure
                                        due to tumor
  • a loss of vision?   Compression of optic chiasma
                                        by an intracranial tumor:
                                        craniopharyngioma, pinealoma,
                                        glioma, metastases

• a skin rash? an ear inflammation? eyes becoming prominent?	Multifocal eosinophilic granuloma
• an increase of your appetite?	Polyphagia of <u>diabetes mellitus</u>
• a decrease of your appetite? nausea? vomiting?	<u>Chronic renal failure</u>; hypercalcemia; hypokalemia; intracranial tumor
• muscular weakness?	Potassium depletion; hypercalcemia
• pain in your back? bones?	Multiple myeloma, hyperparathyroidism with hypercalcemia

4   Iatrogenic factors: see Etiology

5   Personal antecedents pertaining to the polyuria

5.1   Have you ever had an examination of your urine? blood? an x-ray of your kidneys? your skull? When? With what results?

5.2   Do you have any of the following conditions: diabetes (mellitus)? a kidney disease? urinary tract infection? a prostate disease?

• an emotional problem? anxiety? depression?	A previous history of psychologic disturbances is nearly always present in patients with psychogenic DI
• a high blood pressure?	Chronic renal failure; aldosteronism (potassium depletion)

5.3   Have you ever had

• a severe head injury?	A fracture in or near the sella may tear the stalk of the pituitary gland
• intracranial surgery?	Hypophysectomy (e.g., for advanced breast carcinoma)

6 *Family medical history pertaining to the polyuria*

6.1 Is there someone in your
family
  • who also passes large   Nephrogenic DI
    amounts of urine?
  • who has diabetes (mel-
    litus)?

PHYSICAL SIGNS PERTINENT TO THE COMPLAINT

Finding	**Possible** *significance*
Abnormal neurologic examination	Intracranial space-occupying lesion
Exophthalmos; skin rash	Eosinophilic granuloma (Hand-Schüller-Christian syndrome: skull osteolytic lesions, exophthalmos, diabetes insipidus)
Calcification in the cornea Proximal muscular weakness ⎫	Hypercalcemic states; hyperparathyroidism
Visual field defects	Craniopharyngioma
Funduscopic examination: papilledema diabetic retinopathy	 Increased intracranial pressure Diabetes mellitus with polyuria

LABORATORY TESTS PERTAINING TO THE COMPLAINT

Procedure	*Finding*	*Diagnostic possibilities*
Blood		
BUN, creatinine	Elevated	Chronic renal failure
Fasting glucose	Elevated	Diabetes mellitus

| Electrolytes | Hypokalemia | Potassium depletion or hypercalcemia resulting in impaired ability to concentrate the urine maximally |
| Calcium | Elevated | |

Urine

Glucose	Positive	Diabetes mellitus
Protein	Positive	Chronic renal failure
Osmolality	Above serum osmolality	Solute diuresis; glycosuria
	Below serum osmolality	Diabetes insipidus (DI)
After fluid restriction	Urine becomes concentrated	Psychogenic DI
	Unchanged osmolality	Idiopathic or nephrogenic DI
After vasopressin test	Increase in urine osmolality	Idiopathic DI (of central origin)
	Unresponsive	Nephrogenic DI

Procedure	*To detect*	
Skull x-rays		
Visual field examination	Intracranial lesion	

USEFUL REMINDERS AND DIAGNOSTIC CLUES

Misleading Factor

Polyuria must be distinguished from frequency, a common complaint in patients with urinary tract infection or benign prostatic hypertrophy; these patients void frequent small quantities of urine.

Diagnostic Considerations

Diabetes insipidus is a rare disease (10 to 16 cases per 100,000 hospital admissions) but is becoming much more prevalent with the advent of hypophysectomy for the treatment of advanced breast carcinoma.

Intracranial tumors account for 40 percent of the variety of causes of diabetes insipidus; 33 percent are so-called idiopathic, and the remainder are due to a variety of disorders, including trauma.

Of the metastatic tumors, breast cancer seems to have a special predilection for the hypothalamic area.

A space-occupying lesion is suspect when insufficiency of both posterior and anterior pituitary occurs.

Idiopathic diabetes insipidus affects both sexes. Nephrogenic diabetes insipidus occurs more often in males than in females. Psychogenic diabetes insipidus occurs more often in females than in males.

Patients with psychogenic diabetes insipidus usually do not complain of thirst and polyuria.

SELECTED BIBLIOGRAPHY

De Wardener HE: *The Kidney: An Outline of Normal and Abnormal Structure and Function*, chap 24, Polyuria, pp 328–339, Edinburgh and London: Churchill Livingstone, 1973

Leaf A, Coggins CH: The neurohypophysis, in Williams RH (ed), *Textbook of Endocrinology*, 5th ed, pp 80–94, Philadelphia: Saunders, 1974

Streeten DHP, Moses AM, Miller M: Disorders of the neurohypophysis, in Thorn GW et al (eds), *Harrison's Principles of Internal Medicine*, 8th ed., pp 490–501, New York: McGraw-Hill, 1977

25
Urinary Dysfunction

DEFINITIONS AND GENERAL CONSIDERATIONS

Dysuria difficulty or pain associated with voiding.
Frequency an urge to void every few minutes.
Urgency frequent or continuous sensation of the necessity to void. Urgency may be so severe as to result in incontinence.
Incontinence inability to restrain the discharge of urine through the urethra.

Micturition is normally a voluntary, painless act. The commonest cause of dysuria and frequency is infection in the bladder, urethra, or prostate. In acute inflammatory lesions of the bladder, the loss of elasticity which results from edema and the pain induced by even mild stretching of the bladder decrease the capacity of the organ (normal capacity of the adult bladder: 400 to 500 mL). Under these circumstances, an urge to void will occur when only a small quantity of urine is present in the bladder. Chronic inflammatory diseases (tuberculosis) that cause permanently diminished bladder capacity from scarring produce frequency of urination. Extrinsic compression or distortion of the lower part of the urinary tract may also cause dysuria. Extreme variations of urine pH can irritate the bladder and cause frequency. Urgency occurs as a result of trigonal or posterior urethral irritation by inflammation, stones, or tumor. Urgency incontinence may occur with acute cystitis, particularly in women, or in tense anxious women even in the absence of infection. Paradoxical (overflow or false) incontinence is a loss of urine due to chronic urinary retention or secondary to a flaccid bladder. Small involuntary voidings occur as the intravesical pressure of accumulating urine overcomes the urethral resistance. Incontinence may also be related to a neurogenic bladder resulting from upper and lower motor neuron lesions; associated neurologic signs are then present in the lower extremities.

ETIOLOGY

Difficulty in voiding, without pain
Obstructive uropathy
   Benign prostatic hypertrophy; carcinoma of prostate; urethral stricture; bladder-neck contracture
   Expanding masses in the pelvis: pregnancy, large ovarian cyst, uterine fibroid
Neurogenic bladder
   Spastic (reflex or automatic): upper motor neuron lesion: trauma; tumor; multiple sclerosis
   Uninhibited (mild spastic): lesion of the inhibitory centers of the cortex or pyramidal tracts: cerebrovascular accident; arteriosclerotic degeneration in the spinal cord; multiple sclerosis
   Flaccid: lesion of the sacral portion of the cord or of the cauda equina: trauma; tabes dorsalis; tumor; congenital anomalies

Difficulty in voiding, with pain on urination
Acute urinary tract infection: acute urethritis, cystitis, or prostatitis; acute pyelonephritis with cystitis
Chronic infection: chronic prostatitis; chronic interstitial cystitis; chronic posterior urethrotrigonitis (in women)
Vesical calculi; urethral calculi
Urethral caruncle
The conditions under "Difficulty in voiding, without pain" when complicated by infection or vesical calculi

Frequency
With dysuria
   Bladder: infection; stone; neurogenic bladder dysfunction; chronic interstitial cystitis; irradiation injury
   Prostate: infection, bacterial, nonspecific; tumor; hyperplasia; cancer
   Urethra: infection, gonococcal, nonspecific; stricture; meatal stenosis; caruncle; diverticulum
Without dysuria
   Renal (polyuria): excessive water ingestion; diabetes insipidus; nephrogenic diabetes insipidus; osmotic diuresis (diabetes mellitus with glycosuria, mannitol); upper urinary tract obstruction with loss of concentrating ability; chronic renal insufficiency; hypercalcemia; hypokalemia; early congestive heart failure with nocturia; drugs

Incontinence
Overflow (paradoxical) incontinence
 Obstruction to the outflow of urine; flaccid neurogenic bladder
Congenital incontinence: malformations; urinary fistulas
Incompetence of the urinary sphincter
 Total:
  Female: parturition; following repair of procidentia, cystocele, vaginal hysterectomy
  Male: following prostatectomy
 Partial: stress incontinence, common in females
Neurogenic bladder
Following surgical or radiation injury, with fistulas
Psychogenic incontinence

Iatrogenic Causes of Urinary Dysfunction

Anticholinergics: acute urinary retention
Ganglionic-blocking agents: impairment of the voiding contractions of the bladder
Antihistaminics, hydralazine, monoamine oxidase inhibitors: difficulty in urination
Diuretics: frequency with polyuria

QUESTIONNAIRE

	Possible *meaning of response*
1 Mode of onset and duration	
1.1 How long have you had difficulty in urinating?	
1.2 How many times a day do you urinate?	Micturition every 4 to 6 h during the day and once at night is considered normal
1.3 When did you last void?	If no urination in the last 12 h: exclude **acute urinary retention**
2 Character of the complaint	
2.1 When urinating, do you have	

• *a burning sensation, as if passing hot water?*

Dysuria, urethral pain: <u>acute inflammatory process</u> of urethra; urethral calculus; bladder infection

• persisting a few seconds or minutes after urination?

Terminal tenesmus: <u>acute cystitis</u>

2.2 Do you urinate more frequently than usual?

Frequency: acute or chronic inflammation of the bladder with decreased capacity and acute pain on distention; polyuria

• only during the day?

Psychogenic frequency

• also at night?

Nocturia: frequency or polyuria

2.2*a* in case of frequent micturitions: Do you pass
• a small amount of urine?
   • *without pain on urination?*

Partial obstruction of the bladder: <u>benign prostatic hypertrophy</u>, neurogenic (uninhibited) bladder

   • *with pain on urination?*

Severe <u>infection</u> of lower urinary tract

• a large amount of urine?
• without pain on urination?

Polyuria: diabetes mellitus; chronic renal insufficiency

2.3 Do you have at times a sudden urge to urinate?

Urgency: irritation of the trigone and the posterior urethra: inflammation, stone, tumor

2.3*a* Are you at times unable to initiate urination in spite of an urgent desire to do so?

Episodes of urinary retention

2.3*b* Is the urge at times so severe that you void involuntarily?

Urgency incontinence: acute cystitis; in upper motor neuron lesion; in tense, anxious women

2.4 Do you lose urine
• intermittently?

Urinary incontinence, uncontrolled urination

- on straining? stooping? sneezing? laughing? bending over? lifting heavy objects?

Stress incontinence: partial incompetence of the urinary sphincter (common in women)

- constantly?
  - with dripping of urine? especially when standing or sitting?

Total incompetence of the urinary sphincter; true incontinence, neurogenic (no residual urine); paradoxical (overflow) incontinence: chronic urinary retention, secondary to a flaccid (neurogenic) bladder (residual urine); congenital incontinence

2.5   Is the stream of urine
- *small?* (decreased in caliber)
- *split?* slow? varying in intensity? sprayed?

Urethral obstruction, usually <u>prostatic hypertrophy</u>; neurogenic bladder

2.6   Do you have to wait more than a few seconds before your urine begins to flow?

Hesitancy in urination: <u>obstructive uropathy</u>; neurogenic bladder

2.7   Do you feel that
- your urinations last longer than usual?

Obstructive uropathy

- you still have urine in your bladder when you have finished urinating?

Prostatic obstruction

2.7a   Do you have
- *difficulty in maintaining the stream?*
- to strain to initiate urination?
- to strain at the end of urination?
- dribbling, spraying of the urine stream?

Increasing severity of obstructive uropathy

2.7*b*   After having apparently emptied your bladder, are you still able, a few minutes later, to pass several milliliters or ounces more?

Significant vesical residuum; bladder diverticulum

3   Accompanying symptoms

3.1   Is your urine
- clear?

May occur in chronic urinary tract infection

- cloudy?

Pyuria; phosphaturia (in alkaline urine)

- dark or bloody?

Hematuria, occasionally in cystitis

3.2   Does your urine have a foul, fishy odor?

Urinary tract infection

3.3   Do you have a urethral discharge?

Acute anterior urethritis: nonspecific, gonorrheal

- appearing in the morning?

"Morning drop"; chronic prostatitis

- with spraying of the urinary stream?

Chronic urethritis, with or without urethral stricture

- with burning on voiding?

Chronic prostatitis with posterior urethritis

3.4   Do you have
- a painful distention of your abdomen?

Acute urinary retention with distended bladder

- a dull suprapubic pain? (low in intensity)

Bladder pain: infection, obstruction (if not related to the micturition: usually not of urologic origin)

- with pain at the tip of the penis?

Vesical calculus (referred pain to the distal urethra)

- a fullness, a vague discomfort in the perineal and rectal areas?

Prostatic pain; prostatitis

- flank pain?

Nephrolithiasis with urinary tract infection

• fever? chills?	Acute infectious process: <u>pyelonephritis, cystitis</u>
• pain in your joints? eyes?	Reiter's syndrome
• a skin rash?	Stevens-Johnson syndrome
3.5 Have you ever noticed the passage of gas during micturition?	Pneumaturia: fistula between bowel and bladder (diverticulitis, regional enteritis, rectosigmoid cancer); gas-forming infection in bladder (diabetes mellitus)
3.6 Do you have a loss of power in your lower limb(s)?	Neurologic disorder with neurogenic bladder
3.6a Do you lose involuntarily frequent small amounts of urine?	Complete spastic neurogenic bladder
3.6b Do you have an urgent desire to void frequently, with involuntary loss of urine?	Uninhibited neurogenic bladder; <u>cystitis</u> (the neurogenic bladder is usually secondarily infected)
3.6c Do you lack any sensation of bladder fullness?	Complete spastic neurogenic bladder; overflow incontinence: flaccid neurogenic bladder
3.6d *Do you have to pinch your skin, tap your abdomen, in order to start micturition?*	Stimulation of the reflex arc of micturition, in complete spastic neurogenic bladder
3.6e *Do you have to strain or apply manual pressure on the bladder during all the micturition?*	Overflow incontinence: flaccid neurogenic bladder
3.7 For the female patient: Do you lose urine from the vagina?	
• with normal voiding?	Ureterovaginal fistula
• with no normal voiding?	Vesicovaginal fistula

4 *Iatrogenic factors* see Etiology

5 *Personal antecedents pertaining to the complaint*

5.1 Have you ever had an examination of your urine? blood? an x-ray of your kidneys? a cystoscopy? When? With what results?

5.2 Have you ever had
- a urologic operation?
- a trauma during parturition?

May cause partial or total incompetence of the urinary sphincter

5.3 Do you have

A history of recurrent urinary tract infection suggests underlying anatomic or physiologic abnormality of the urinary tract

- kidney stones?
- urinary tract infections?

- a venereal disease?

Syphilis: neurogenic bladder in tabes; gonorrhea

- a neurologic disorder?

Neurogenic bladder

- a prostate condition?

Obstructive uropathy

PHYSICAL SIGNS PERTINENT TO THE COMPLAINT

Finding	*Possible significance*
Fever; suprapubic tenderness	Cystitis
Fever; costovertebral angle tenderness	Acute pyelonephritis
Distended bladder	Obstruction of the lower part of the urinary tract; prostatic hypertrophy; paradoxical incontinence
Rectal examination	May reveal: benign prostatic hypertrophy; prostatic carcinoma; prostatitis
Pelvic examination	May reveal: cystocele with stress incontinence; uterine fibroids, pelvic masses reducing the bladder capacity by external compression

Neurologic abnormalities in the legs

- spastic paralysis; hyperactive deep reflexes; Babinski response; normal or increased anal sphincter tone; normal or hyperactive bulbocavernous reflex; no evidence of a distended bladder; stimulation of the skin of the abdomen or thigh may initiate voiding

- flaccid paralysis; decreased to absent reflexes; loss of anal sphincter tone; absent bulbocavernous reflex; overdistended bladder

Neurogenic bladder dysfunction with incontinence

Spastic neurogenic bladder (upper motor neuron lesion)

Flaccid neurogenic bladder (lower motor neuron lesion)

LABORATORY TESTS PERTAINING TO THE COMPLAINT

Procedure	*Finding*	*Diagnostic possibilities*
Urine		
Sediment	Pyuria	Urinary tract infection
	Leukocyte casts	Renal parenchymal infection
Culture	>100,000 colonies of bacteria per milliliter	Urinary tract infection

Procedure	*To detect*
Urethral discharge:	
Gram's stain, culture	Gonorrhea; nongonococcal urethritis

IV pyelogram
Retrograde pyelo-
gram
Cystoscopy

Anatomic or functional abnormalities of the
urinary tract

Voiding cysto-
urethrography

Ureteral reflux; posterior urethral valves;
urethral stricture

Cystometry

Types of nervous system lesions causing
neurogenic vesical dysfunction

USEFUL REMINDERS AND DIAGNOSTIC CLUES

Misleading Factor

The commonest cause of a turbid urine is not pus but phosphaturia.

Diagnostic Considerations

Voiding symptoms suggest lower urinary tract obstruction.
The patient with an acute urinary retention has severe pain in the
bladder area; the patient with a chronically overdistended bladder
may experience little or no pain.
Infection of the kidneys alone does not cause dysuria.
Hesitancy in the initiation of urination may be one of the earliest
signs of multiple sclerosis.
Frequency may be an early presenting symptom of primary malignant disease of the bladder.

In case of	*Suspect*
Sterile, abacterial pyuria Pyuria in an acid urine Unexplained symptoms in the urinary tract	Renal tuberculosis
Frequency without nocturia	Psychogenic frequency; polyp in posterior urethra (frequency relieved by recumbency)

SELECTED BIBLIOGRAPHY

Leadel AJ, Carlton, Jr CE: Urologic diagnosis and the urologic examination, in Campbell MF, Harrison JH (eds), *Urology,* 3d ed, pp 197–293, Philadelphia: Saunders, 1970

Lytton B, Epstein FH: Dysuria, incontinence, and enuresis, in Thorn GW et al (eds), *Harrison's Principles of Internal Medicine,* 8th ed, pp 233–236, New York: McGraw-Hill, 1977

Smith DR: *General Urology,* 8th ed, Los Altos: Lange, 1975

26
Abnormal Vaginal Bleeding

DEFINITIONS AND PATHOPHYSIOLOGY

Hypermenorrhea (*menorrhagia*)   increase in duration and/or quantity of menstrual flow that occurs at normal cycle intervals.

Metrorrhagia   irregular flow at times other than the menstrual period.

Polymenorrhea   menstrual flow close to normal in quantity and duration but which recurs more often than at intervals of 24 days.

Hypomenorrhea   lessening of the flow either in quantity or in duration.

The normal menstrual cycle is commonly stated to be 28 days, but intervals of 24 to 32 days are still considered normal unless grossly irregular. The average duration of menstrual bleeding is 3 to 7 days. For the first 10 to 14 days after the onset of menstrual bleeding, during the period of follicular maturation, a rising estrogen level results in proliferative changes of the endometrium (proliferative phase). During the latter part of the menstrual cycle (luteal phase), from ovulation to the onset of menstrual bleeding, the secretion of progesterone by the corpus luteum induces secretory activity of the glands of the endometrium. Menstruation appears to result from a critical drop in the blood estrogen and progesterone levels. About two-thirds of the endometrium is presumed to be lost with each ovulatory menstruation. The interval between ovulation and menstruation is normally 14 days. In contrast, the preovulatory period (the interval from the first day of menstruation to the day of ovulation) may be variable. The variations in cycle length are thus related to changes in the duration of the follicular phase preceding ovulation.

Hypermenorrhea may be due to local causes (e.g., myoma), blood dyscrasias, and psychic problems. Polymenorrhea may result from a shorter proliferative phase (less than 10 days) or secretory phase (less than 14 days), or from physical or emotional stress with premature interruption of the bleeding cycle. In anovulatory cycles the maturation and differentiation of the endometrium by progesterone do not take place and the sequence of events is therefore abbreviated; bleeding occurs from a nonsecretory endometrium. Anovulatory bleeding is a frequent cause of an irregular menstrual bleeding in adolescence and toward the end of the reproductive years. Metrorrhagia may be caused by hormonal imbalance (e.g., with hormonal contraceptive agents), intrauterine devices, or various pelvic abnormalities (disturbed pregnancy, submucous myoma, cancer of the cervix or endometrium). Dysfunctional uterine bleeding is an abnormal, painless bleeding unassociated with tumor, inflammation, or pregnancy, with complete irregularity of the menstrual interval; ovulation does not occur.

ETIOLOGY

Anatomic causes   carcinoma of the cervix, corpus uteri, fallopian tubes, ovaries; myoma of uterus; salpingitis; endometritis; endometriosis; chronic cervicitis; cervical and endometrial polyposis; cervical erosions or ectropion; endometrial hyperplasia; anovulatory bleeding
Foreign bodies; intrauterine devices
Tuberculosis of the genital tract
Uterine displacements

Abnormal uterine bleeding in the pregnant patient   threatened abortion; incomplete abortion; tubal pregnancy; hydatidiform mole; chorioepithelioma

Blood dyscrasias   thrombocytopenic purpura; aplastic anemia; von Willebrand's disease

Endocrinologic and metabolic causes   hypothyroidism; hyperthyroidism; adrenal dysfunction; diabetes mellitus

Dysfunctional uterine bleeding

Postmenopausal bleeding   estrogen therapy; malignant tumors: corpus, cervix, vagina, fallopian tubes, ovaries; atrophic vaginitis; infections: vaginitis, endometritis; dysfunctional uterine bleeding; foreign bodies, pessaries
Cervical or endometrial polyps; submucous myoma
Postradiation injury; diseases of the blood

Iatrogenic Causes of Abnormal Vaginal Bleeding

Estrogens; progestogens; androgens
Corticosteroids; anticoagulants

QUESTIONNAIRE

Possible *meaning of response*

1   Duration

1.1   How long have you had
trouble with your men-
struations?

1.1*a*   At what age did your menstruations begin?

Normal menarche (between 12
and 13 years) indicates a normal maturation of the hypothalamic-pituitary ovarian axis;
in a woman of childbearing age:
possible anatomic cause of
bleeding

1.2   When was the date of
• *the first day of your last menstrual period?*
• *the preceding menstrual
period?*

(Inaccurate in many cases);
every woman of childbearing age
should be regarded as being
pregnant until proved otherwise

2   Iatrogenic factors   see Etiology

2.1   Do you use birth control
pills? other contraceptive
methods?

A common cause of abnormal
vaginal bleeding

3   Character of bleeding

3.1   How many days apart do
your periods occur?
• from 24 to 32 days?
• less than 24 days?

Normal duration
Polymenorrhea

3.2   What is the duration of
your periods?

• from 3 to 7 days?	Normal, or hypermenorrhea if excessive in amount
• more than 7 days?	Hypermenorrhea
3.3 How many napkins do you use	A rough (and inaccurate) estimate of blood loss
• per day?	Normal: four per day
• per period?	Normally: up to 12 per period; normal average loss: 25 to 70 mL
• more than four per day? • more than 12 per period?	Hypermenorrhea: conditions affecting the uterus rather than the ovary
3.3a *Can you control bleeding with an intravaginal tampon?*	A proprietary intravaginal tampon is never enough to contain abnormally heavy bleeding
3.3b Are there any clots in the menstrual flow?	Hypermenorrhea
3.4 In case of periods occurring at too frequent intervals, is the bleeding	
• excessive?	Polymenorrhagia: disturbance in both the ovary and the uterus; widespread inflammation of all pelvic organs; anxiety states
• normal?	Polymenorrhea: disease or functional disturbance of the ovary or disturbed pituitary-ovarian interplay; uterus likely to be normal
3.5 *Are you still able to identify regular menstrual intervals?*	No interference with the ovarian ovulatory mechanism; anatomic origin of the bleeding
3.6 In case of hypermenorrhea and/or metrorrhagia in a previously regularly menstruating woman of childbearing age:	Accidents of early pregnancy; pelvic inflammatory disease; benign neoplasms; malignant tumors; dysfunctional uterine bleeding; irregular shedding; hormonal contraceptive agents

3.6a Has your expected last menstruation been delayed?

Possible pregnancy

3.6a(1) Is your bleeding
- profuse?
- spotty?

Threatened abortion
Ectopic pregnancy

3.6b Do you notice, between your menstruations,

- an occasional spot of blood?
- a blood-tinged discharge?

Carcinoma of cervix; endometrial carcinoma; cervical polyp; contraceptive pill; vaginitis

  - *after sexual intercourse?*
  - *after douching?*

Contact bleeding: <u>cervical carcinoma</u>; cervical polyp

3.6c *Do you have "a period every 2 weeks"?: the untimely bleeding occurring periodically during the midinterval?*

3.6c(1) *Is the bleeding associated with cramplike pain?* (of less than 24 h)

Cyclic intermenstrual (ovulatory) pain: "Mittelschmerz"

3.7 In case of menorrhagia and/or metrorrhagia in a premenopausal or menopausal woman (between 40 and 50 years old):

Perimenopausal and menopausal bleeding should be considered as caused by a malignancy until proved otherwise; dysfunctional uterine bleeding; uterine malignancy, with or without leiomyoma

3.7a Do you ever skip a period? several periods?

3.7a(1) Do you have
- *hot flushes?*
- cold sweats?

3.7a(2) Is your abnormal bleeding painless?

<u>Dysfunctional uterine bleeding</u>, the harbinger of the coming menopause

3.8   In case of bleeding in a postmenopausal woman (fifth and sixth decade):

Malignancy; estrogen therapy; vaginitis

3.8*a*   Is your bleeding
  • *slight?*

Genital <u>neoplasm</u>, benign or malignant; endometrial carcinoma; carcinoma of cervix

  • copious?

Not characteristic of neoplasm

4   *Accompanying symptoms*

4.1   Do you have
  • pain in the lower abdomen?

In women of childbearing age: <u>pelvic inflammatory disease</u>; <u>ectopic pregnancy; threatened abortion</u>; in menopausal women: uterine <u>malignancy</u>; large leiomyoma

  • of gradual onset?

Chronic salpingitis; large leiomyoma

4.1*a*   Do you have pain with, or just prior to, your menstruations?

<u>Dysmenorrhea</u>, more common in ovulatory cycles; endometriosis

4.2   Do you have
  • fever?

<u>Pelvic inflammatory disease</u> (in young women)

  • a vaginal discharge?

In women of childbearing age: acute salpingitis (gonorrheal); vaginitis (*Candida, Trichomonas*)

  • easy bruising?
  • a blood condition?

Thrombocytopenic purpura, von Willebrand's disease, leukemia, may cause uterine bleeding

  • depression? anxiety?

Abnormal uterine bleeding of psychic origin

5   *Personal antecedents pertaining to the bleeding*

5.1   Do you have children?

Implies a normal maturation of the hypothalamic-pituitary ovarian axis: possible anatomic cause of bleeding

5.2   Have you ever had a pap test? a pelvic examination? an x-ray of your uterus? When? With what results?

5.3   Do you have any of the following conditions:

• diabetes? a thyroid condition? (hypothyroidism)	May cause dysfunctional uterine bleeding
• a recent pregnancy? abortion?	Retention of gestation products
• a liver disease? • excessive alcohol intake? }	May result in the failure of estrogen to be conjugated in the liver, with resulting increase of free estrogens and abnormal uterine bleeding

PHYSICAL SIGNS PERTINENT TO THE COMPLAINT

Finding	**Possible** *significance*
Pelvic examination	May reveal: tumors of uterus, adnexae, vagina; polyps of cervix or uterus; pelvic infection; pregnancy; threatened or incomplete abortion; ectopic pregnancy; endometriosis; atrophic vaginitis; foreign body in vagina
Abnormal abdominal examination	Tumor; ascites; intraabdominal inflammatory process
Ascites, hydrothorax	Meigs' syndrome (with ovarian tumors)
Dry coarse skin; periorbital puffiness; prolonged tendon reflex relaxation time	Hypothyroidism
Hirsutism (with or without obesity)	Stein-Leventhal syndrome (with polycystic ovaries)
Fever	Pelvic inflammatory disease
Ecchymoses, petechiae	Bleeding tendency
Pallor	Hypochromic anemia resulting from excessive blood loss; underlying malignancy

LABORATORY TESTS PERTAINING TO THE COMPLAINT

Procedure	*To detect*
Blood	
RBCs	Anemia due to excessive blood loss
WBCs	Infection; leukemia
Hemostasis tests	Bleeding tendency
Thyroid function tests	Thyroid dysfunction
Urinary estrogens	Ovarian dysfunction
Progesterone	Ovulation
Vaginal smear	Ovarian dysfunction; tumor cells; trophoblastic squamae from a uterine abortion
Scraping, biopsy of cervix, vaginal canal	Tumor cells
Endometrial biopsy	Ovarian dysfunction; endometrial hyperplasia; endometrial neoplasm, polyps
Leukorrheal discharge: examination, culture	*Trichomonas, Candida* organisms; *Neisseria gonorrhoeae; Hemophilus vaginalis;* acute vaginitis
Pregnancy test	Threatened or incomplete abortion; ectopic pregnancy; tumors of the placenta
Flat abdominal film	Tumors; fluid levels; distortion
Ultrasonography	Uterine cavity content, volume; tumors; etc.
Hysterosalpingography	Submucosal myomas; polyps

USEFUL REMINDERS AND DIAGNOSTIC CLUES

Misleading Factor

Bleeding from urethra or rectum may be interpreted by the patient as vaginal bleeding.

General Considerations

Any postmenopausal bleeding or mere staining from the genital
tract after an interval of a year or more should be considered as
caused by a malignancy until proved otherwise.

The mere presence of a hematologic disorder is not proof that it is
the cause of any associated uterine hemorrhage.

Anticoagulants do not necessarily increase the menstrual flow.

Diagnostic Considerations

Every cervical lesion is malignant until proved otherwise, even when
present in a pregnant woman.

Cancer of the cervix or endometrium accounts for 35 to 50 percent
of cases of postmenopausal bleeding.

Cancer of the cervix occurs more frequently during the fifth and sixth
decades of life, in women who have born children; however, no
age is exempt from cancer of the cervix.

More than two-thirds of all cases of carcinoma of corpus uteri occur
in women beyond the menopause.

Anovulatory dysfunctional bleeding seems more common in short,
obese women.

In case of Vaginal bleeding	*Suspect*
• in an adolescent	Dysfunctional bleeding
• in a woman under 40 years of age	Accident of pregnancy; pelvic infection; contraceptive methods
• in a perimenopausal woman	Functional disorder; uterine myoma; carcinoma of the cervix
• after the menopause	Carcinoma of the endometrium; carcinoma of the cervix; exogenous estrogen administration

SELECTED BIBLIOGRAPHY

Charles D (ed): Menstrual disorders. Clin Obstet Gynecol 12:691–827, 1969
Israel SL: *Diagnosis and Treatment of Menstrual Disorders,* 5th ed, New
York: Hoeber-Harper, 1967

27
Amenorrhea

DEFINITIONS AND PATHOPHYSIOLOGY

Primary amenorrhea failure of the menarche to occur.

Secondary amenorrhea absence of menses for at least 3 months in a patient who previously has had normal menstrual function.

Physiologic amenorrhea absence of menses existing prior to puberty, during pregnancy and the puerperium, and after the menopause.

Oligomenorrhea a reduction in the frequency of menses; the interval is longer than 38 days, but less than 3 months.

Cryptomenorrhea hidden menstruation; menstruation actually occurs but makes no external appearance because of some uterine or vaginal obstruction.

Normal menstrual cycles are regulated by gonadotropin secretion. During the period preceding ovulation, levels of blood follicle-stimulating hormone (FSH) and luteinizing hormone (LH) rise slowly. The FSH rise stimulates follicle growth, and the thecal cells of the developing follicle secrete increasing amounts of estradiol. As estrogen rises to a peak, it triggers the release of LH by the pituitary, probably through the releasing hormone secreted by the hypothalamus. The LH surge results in ovulation, 18 to 36 h later, which in turn produces corpus luteum formation and function. During the period from ovulation to the onset of menstruation, a corpus luteum formed at the follicular site synthesizes and secretes estrogen and progesterone. The secretion of progesterone reaches a peak 5 to 8 days after the LH surge. As the estrogen and progesterone again decrease toward lower levels, the uterine endometrium sloughs and signals the onset of a new cycle.

Gonadotropin secretion begins to rise between the ages of 8 and 9 years. This is followed by increasing amounts of estrogen, which are responsible for breast and genital development. At about age 13, puberty is signaled by the onset of periodic uterine bleeding. A large proportion of women with primary amenorrhea have a 45 XO karyotype, resulting in the typical Turner's syndrome (gonadal differentiation does not occur in the absence of a second X or a Y chromosome). Secondary amenorrhea may result from a lesion of the uterus and vagina, from ovarian dysfunction (estrogen and progesterone production), and from a lesion of the central nervous system. Most women with secondary amenorrhea have "psychogenic" amenorrhea; it appears that emotional stress can suppress the hypothalamic center responsible for cyclic variations in gonadotropin secretion. Amenorrhea may be an early sign of pituitary disease (tumor). Excess androgen production will suppress gonadotropin secretion and thereby induce amenorrhea. Amenorrhea following conception (the most common cause of secondary amenorrhea) is due to the rising titer of chorionic gonadotropin. Increased blood prolactin is a common occurrence in amenorrhea with or without galactorrhea.

ETIOLOGY

Ovary dysfunction
Ovarian dysgenesis (Turner's syndrome)
Ovarian insufficiency after surgery, infection, irradiation
Polycystic ovary syndrome (Stein-Leventhal syndrome)
Granulosa-theca cell tumor; masculinizing tumor

Pituitary dysfunction
Chromophobe adenoma; eosinophilic adenoma; basophilic adenoma
Simmonds' disease; postpartum necrosis (Sheehan's syndrome)
Empty sella syndrome

Hypothalamic-pituitary functional disorder
Stress; malnutrition; depressive psychoses; anorexia nervosa; schizophrenia

Thryroid   myxedema; Graves' disease

Adrenal   Addison's disease; Cushing's syndrome

Systemic disease   hepatic disease; renal disease; diabetes mellitus; anemia

Uterine, cervical, vaginal   congenital absence; intrauterine adhesions (Asherman's syndrome); endometrial destruction (tuberculosis); imperforate hymen

Pregnancy   lactation

Menopause

Iatrogenic Causes of Secondary Amenorrhea

Androgens
Corticosteroids
Oral contraceptives
Cyclophosphamide

Drug addiction of
  various types
Ganglion-blocking
  agents
Phenothiazine de-
  rivatives

Reserpine
Spironolactone
Sulpiride
Tranquilizers

QUESTIONNAIRE

Note: the following questions pertain to secondary amenorrhea.

Possible *meaning of response*

1 Duration

1.1 When did you last have normal menstruation?

1.2 How many menstrual periods have been missed?

If four to six: investigation is warranted

1.3 At what age did your first menstruation appear?

The normal menarche occurs between 12 and 13 years

1.4 What were your previous menstrual habits?

Oligomenorrhea frequently precedes amenorrhea

2 Precipitating factors

2.1 Is there any possibility that you are pregnant?

Pregnancy is the commonest cause of secondary amenorrhea

2.2 Have you recently had any emotional stress?

Nervous tension may cause amenorrhea

2.3 Has the amenorrhea appeared following
  • a childbirth?

Possible ischemic necrosis of the anterior pituitary: Sheehan's syndrome

  • a D and C (curettage)?

Intrauterine synechiae or adhesions: Asherman's syndrome

3 Accompanying symptoms

3.1 Do you have

- depression? anxiety?

  Amenorrhea is common in depressive mental disorders

- a loss of vision?

  Pressure on the optic nerves due to a **pituitary tumor**

- headaches?

  Present in more than 75 percent of the patients with pituitary tumor: traction on the diaphragm sellae by the tumor

- nausea? vomiting?

  Increased intracranial pressure: pituitary tumor

- a heavy growth of hair on your face? arms? legs? back?
  - with atrophy of your breasts?

  Virilism: overproduction of androgens: masculinizing tumors of the ovary; tumor of the adrenal cortex

  - without atrophy of your breasts?

  Stein-Leventhal syndrome

- a loss of axillary and pubic hair?

  Adrenal cortical failure; Sheehan's syndrome

- *a decreased skin pigmentation?*

  Hypopituitarism

- *an increased skin pigmentation?*

  Primary adrenal cortical failure

- episodes of irregular or profuse vaginal bleeding?

  Menometrorrhagia: polycystic ovarian disease

- *milk secretion from your nipples?*

  Galactorrhea: usually increased prolactin secretion (in at least a third of pituitary tumors)

- intolerance to heat?
- excessive sweating?

  Hyperthyroidism

- intolerance to cold?

  Hypothyroidism, primary or secondary to anterior pituitary disease

- purple striations on your skin? ⎫
- easy bruising? ⎬ Cushing's syndrome
  ⎭
- weakness? easy fatigability?

Cushing's syndrome; Addison's disease; panhypopituitarism; malignancy; chronic systemic illness; depressive state

- fever? cough?

Pulmonary tuberculosis

- a loss of weight?

Addison's disease; hyperthyroidism; diabetes mellitus; chronic systemic illness; malignancy; anorexia nervosa

- a gain in weight?

Cushing's syndrome; myxedema; acromegaly; polycystic ovarian disease; amenorrhea is often associated with obesity

- hot flushes? ⎫
- profuse sweating? ⎬
- night sweats? ⎭

Menopause; <u>premenopausal amenorrhea</u>; these symptoms exclude hypothalamic, pituitary, uterine amenorrhea, and anorexia nervosa

4   *Iatrogenic factors*   see Etiology

5   *Environmental factors*

5.1   What is your usual diet?

May reveal nutritional deficiencies or food faddism; undernutrition is a frequent cause of amenorrhea in adolescents; patients with anorexia nervosa often say that they are eating well

6   *Personal antecedents pertaining to the amenorrhea*

6.1   Have you ever had
  - a meningitis? an encephalitis? ⎫
  - a fracture (of the base) of the skull? ⎬

Disease or injury in the region of the midbrain causing disturbances in hypothalamic function

- your ovaries removed?
- radiation to your ovaries? When? Why?
- your uterus removed? When? Why?

} Ovarian amenorrhea with underproduction of estrogen and progestogen

PHYSICAL SIGNS PERTINENT TO THE COMPLAINT

Finding
Pelvic examination

Possible *significance*
May reveal: mechanical obstruction; pregnancy; ovarian tumor; agenesis of uterus and vagina

Primary amenorrhea with:

- sexual infantilism, absent secondary sexual characteristics; sparse hair growth; short stature; webbing of the neck; short metacarpals; coarctation of the aorta; multiple skin nevi

Gonadal dysgenesis (Turner's syndrome)

- normal secondary sex characteristics

Extragonadal extrapituitary cause; agenesis of uterus and vagina; cryptomenorrhea

Secondary amenorrhea
Loss of axillary and pubic hair; bradycardia; hypotension; atrophy of breasts

Panhypopituitarism; postpartum pituitary necrosis (Sheehan's syndrome)

Nonpuerperal galactorrhea

Hypothalamo-pituitary dysfunction, usually with hyperprolactinemia: pituitary tumor, chromophobe adenoma, craniopharyngioma; sarcoidosis; eosinophilic granuloma; drugs (phenothiazines, alpha methyldopa, reserpine)

Hirsutism; virilism

Masculinizing tumor; Stein-Leventhal syndrome (with polycystic ovaries)

Neurologic and ophthalmic abnormalities	Pituitary tumor; aneurysm of the internal carotid; tumor of the third ventricle; glioma of the optic chiasma
Obesity	May be associated with secondary amenorrhea
Signs of chronic illness	Renal or hepatic disease; hyperthyroidism; Cushing's syndrome; anemia; diabetes mellitus

LABORATORY TESTS PERTAINING TO THE COMPLAINT

Procedure	To detect
Pregnancy test	Pregnancy; hydatidiform mole; chorioepithelioma
Vaginal smear	Degree of estrogen stimulation
Endometrial biopsy	Ovarian dysfunction; ovulation; endometrial responsiveness to hormonal stimulation
Serum gonadotropins	Hypothalamo-pituitary failure (low or absent gonadotropin) Ovarian failure (high gonadotropins)
Urinary estrogens	Ovarian secretion
Progesterone	Ovulation
Testosterone	Androgen-producing tumor
Urine: 17-hydroxy-corticosteroids, 17-ketosteroids	Adrenal and ovarian disorders
Prolactin assay	Pituitary adenoma
Thyroid function tests	Thyroid dysfunction
Chromosomal studies	Ovarian dysgenesis

Ultrasonography	Uterine cavity; ovarian tumor, cyst; etc.
Hysterosalpingography	Uterine abnormalities (contraindicated if pregnancy or infection is suspected)
Sella turcica x-ray ⎫ Visual fields ⎬	Pituitary tumor
Culdoscopy ⎫ Laparoscopy ⎬	Anatomic ovarian abnormalities
LHRH test, clomiphene test	Hypothalamo-pituitary dysfunction

Procedure	*Finding*	*Diagnostic possibilities*
Progesterone test	Positive: withdrawal bleeding	Adequate estrogen secretion and functional endometrium; anovulation
	Negative: no bleeding	Lack of estrogen production; endometrial failure
Estrogen-progesterone test	Bleeding	Functional endometrium; lack of estrogen production; ovarian or pituitary failure
	No bleeding	Target organ or outflow tract failure

USEFUL REMINDERS AND DIAGNOSTIC CLUES

Primary Amenorrhea

The etiologic basis for primary amenorrhea appears to be gonadal in about 50 percent of the cases.

Primary amenorrhea is usually due to delayed puberty.

Diabetes mellitus which appears in childhood and adolescence is associated with amenorrhea in 50 percent of cases.

Secondary Amenorrhea

In patients with secondary amenorrhea, the first diagnosis to be considered is pregnancy.

The first menstrual periods are nearly always anovulatory; several years often pass before ovulation occurs.

The most common causes of secondary amenorrhea in adolescents are psychogenic, neurogenic, and nutritional disturbances which primarily affect hypothalamic function.

The average age at menopause is 48 to 49; only 5 percent of women cease to menstruate normally before age 40.

Suppression of menstruation may be the only symptom of endocrine dysfunction in the case of a chromophobe adenoma.

Four percent of women who lose more than 800 mL of blood in the third or fourth stage of labor suffer some degree of damage to the anterior pituitary; the figures rise to 8 percent for moderate, and 50 percent for severe postpartum hemorrhage and shock.

Patients with anorexia nervosa develop amenorrhea before the onset of weight loss.

The majority of women who seek advice for facial hirsutism have no gross endocrine disturbances.

SELECTED BIBLIOGRAPHY

Smith RA: Investigation and classification of oligomenorrhea and amenorrhea. Med Clin North Am 56:931–936, 1972

Wentz AC: Oligomenorrhea and secondary amenorrhea in the adolescent. Med Clin North Am 59:1385–1394, 1975

Neuromuscular System

28
Coma

DEFINITIONS AND PATHOPHYSIOLOGY

Lethargy a stage at which the patient is drowsy and uninterested in his surroundings.

Obtundation a stage at which the patient is duller, more indifferent, just a little more than awake.

Stupor a stage at which the patient can be aroused only by vigorous, usually noxious stimulation.

Coma a stage at which the patient appears to be asleep and is at the same time incapable of sensing or responding adequately to either external stimuli or inner needs.

Consciousness, a state of awareness of the environment, is dependent on the functional integrity of the ascending reticular activating system, an arousal system in the upper pons, midbrain, and diencephalon (thalamus, hypothalamus) which must interact effectively with one or both cerebral hemispheres. Coma results from a disturbance in this system.

Coma may be produced by supratentorial mass lesions (subdural or intracerebral hemorrhage, brain abscess, tumor) which, by increasing size, distort and compress the brainstem reticular formation. Lesions of one cerebral hemisphere do not produce coma unless they secondarily affect the brainstem reticular formation.

Coma may result from infratentorial mass or destructive lesions, directly compressing or destroying the brainstem reticular formation structures (brainstem infarction, cerebellar hemorrhage). Toxic metabolic encephalopathy (anoxia, hypoglycemia, drug overdose) interfering with metabolism of both brainstem and cerebral cortical structures also produces coma. In psychogenic "coma" the patient is physiologically awake but appears comatose by not responding to his environment.

ETIOLOGY

Structural brain pathology
Supratentorial lesions: cerebral hemorrhage; cerebral infarction; brain tumor; subdural hematoma; epidural hematoma; brain abscess (rare)
Infratentorial lesions: pontine or cerebellar hemorrhage; brainstem infarction; tumor; cerebellar abscess

Metabolic and diffuse lesions
Intoxications: drug overdosage; alcohol
Respiratory insufficiency: hypoxia; hypercapnia
Hyperthermia; hypothermia
Metabolic disturbances: diabetic acidosis; lactic acidosis; hyperosmolar coma; hypoglycemia; uremia; Addisonian crises; hepatic coma; myxedema coma; thyrotoxic coma; hypercalcemia; hypocalcemia; hypernatremia; hyponatremia
Central nervous system infections: meningitis; encephalitis
Severe systemic infections: pneumonia; malaria; typhoid fever
Circulatory collapse; cardiac decompensation in the aged
Subarachnoid hemorrhage; ruptured aneurysm; trauma; concussion; seizures; postictal states

Iatrogenic Causes of Coma

Antidepressants, sedatives and tranquilizers; anticonvulsivants; amphetamines; atropine, scopolamine, and other antiparkinsonism medications; insulin; oral hypoglycemic agents; salicylates; vitamin D (hypercalcemia)
Stopping:
corticosteroids: Addisonian coma
insulin: diabetic acidosis

thyroid extracts: myxedema coma
alcohol ⎫
narcotics ⎬ withdrawal syndrome
barbiturates ⎭

QUESTIONNAIRE

Note: Since the patient is inaccessible to questioning, contact should be made at once with whoever (family, relatives, friends, attendants, acquaintances, police, ambulance personnel) came with the patient, or with relatives and friends at home or elsewhere. Past physicians, pharmacists, employers should be contacted for questioning. Past medical records should be obtained. Patient should be interrogated during lucid intervals, if any.

	Possible *meaning of response*
1 Mode of onset and duration	

1.1 When was the patient found unconscious?

1.2 Where was the patient found?

- in a bar? — Acute alcoholism
- in a locked room? — Exposure to <u>toxic</u> chemical agents: carbon monoxide
- in a locked garage? with automobile running? — Carbon monoxide poisoning
- at work? — Exposure to industrial toxic fumes

1.2a If the patient was found in a room, were other persons found unconscious? — Carbon monoxide poisoning; common exposure to a <u>toxic agent</u>; narcotic abuse

1.3 Was the onset of the coma

- *abrupt?* — <u>Cerebrovascular accident</u>; subarachnoid hemorrhage
- gradual? — Metabolic cause (e.g., renal insufficiency, ketoacidosis); subdural hemorrhage; drug intoxication; systemic infection

1.4 *Has the patient's unconsciousness fluctuated?* — Subdural hemorrhage

1.5 Has the patient had repeated episodes of unconsciousness?	Syncopal attacks; epilepsy; cerebrovascular accidents

2 *Precipitating or aggravating factors*

2.1 Is there any suggestion of • head <u>trauma</u>? exposure to violence? riot?	<u>Subdural or epidural hematoma</u>; depressed skull <u>fracture; concussion</u>; trauma may precipitate, or be secondary to, coma from other causes: Addisonian crisis, myxedema coma, stroke
2.2 Was the patient exposed to • abnormally low temperature?	Hypothermia; myxedema coma
• abnormally high temperature? (during a heat wave)	Heat stroke
2.3 Were any of the following items found in the vicinity of the patient: • medications?	Chronic or acute intoxication; suicide attempt
• syringes?	Narcotic abuse
• alcohol?	<u>Alcoholic</u> stupor
• household products?	Pesticide taken in error
• a letter?	Suicide attempt
2.4 Has an attempt to arouse the patient been made by attendants • by injections?	Frequent in narcotic abusers
• by pouring milk down the patient's throat?	May cause pulmonary edema or massive aspiration of gastric contents

3 *Accompanying symptoms*

3.1 Has the patient recently had	

- severe headache?
  - for days or weeks before the onset of coma?

    Increased intracranial pressure; meningitis; chronic subdural hematoma

  - *just before losing consciousness?*

    (Without cranial trauma): subarachnoid hemorrhage

- *recurrent vomiting?*

  Increased intracranial pressure

- muscle weakness? speech difficulties?

  Intracranial mass-expanding lesion

- fever?

  Acute systemic infection; pneumonia; intracranial infection, bacterial meningitis; brain lesion disturbing the temperature-regulating centers

- change in mental state? behavior?

  Evolving intracranial process; in the elderly, may be the presenting manifestation of gram-negative septicemia, pneumonia, other localized bacterial infections

  - just before losing consciousness?

    Hypoglycemia

3.2   Has the patient had a convulsion?

Epilepsy; hypoglycemia; Stokes-Adams syndrome; rare in cerebral infarction

3.3   Has any witness noticed
- loss of urine? feces?

  Convulsive seizure

- bloody froth around the mouth?

  (Blood may have been swept away): epilepsy; <u>trauma</u>

- bleeding from the ear or nose?

  (May be secondary to a fall caused by a stroke)

4   Iatrogenic factors   see Etiology

5   Environmental factors

5.1   What is the patient's occupation?

Professional exposure to toxic products

6 *Personal antecedents pertaining to the coma*

6.1 Does the patient have any chronic disease? diabetes? convulsive disorders? alcoholism? depression, emotional problems? narcotic abuse? past attempted suicide? past psychiatric hospitalization?

A renal disease? a hepatic condition? arterial hypertension? a chronic pulmonary disease? a neurologic disease? a bleeding tendency?

PHYSICAL SIGNS PERTINENT TO THE COMPLAINT

Finding	**Possible** *significance*
Fever	Severe systemic infection; pneumonia, bacterial meningitis; brain lesion disturbing the temperature-regulating centers; lymphomatous neoplasm; heat stroke (41 to 44°C)
Hypothermia	Exposure to cold; drug poisoning (alcohol, barbiturates); peripheral circulatory failure; extracellular fluid deficit; myxedema; hypoglycemia; severe lower brainstem injury
Hypotension	Low peripheral resistance: depressant drug poisoning; internal hemorrhage; low cardiac output: myocardial infarction; gram-negative bacillary septicemia; Addison's disease
Hypertension	Cerebral hemorrhage; hypertensive encephalopathy; in a previously normotensive patient: may be a sign of subarachnoid hemorrhage
Bradycardia	Heart block and Stokes-Adams syndrome; myocardial infarction

Tachycardia (>160 beats per minute)	Ectopic arrhythmia with lowered cardiac output and impaired cerebral circulation
Hyperventilation	Metabolic acidosis: diabetic coma, uremic encephalopathy; pneumonia; central neurogenic hyperventilation
Slow respiration (hypoventilation)	Intoxication: morphine, barbiturates; hypothyroidism; chronic pulmonary disease with carbon dioxide retention
Periodic (Cheyne-Stokes) respiration	Bilateral deep-seated cerebral lesion (hemispheres or diencephalon)
Hypertension, bradycardia, periodic breathing	Increased intracranial pressure

Skin:
- cyanosis of lips and nail beds — Inadequate oxygenation
- cherry-red coloration — Carbon monoxide poisoning
- petechiae — Thrombocytopenic purpura; meningococcemia; bacterial endocarditis
- jaundice — Hepatic coma

Clubbing	Bronchogenic carcinoma, lung abscess, congenital heart disease, with brain embolism or abscess
Cardiac murmur	Bacterial endocarditis with focal embolic encephalitis
Wheezes, diminished breath sounds	Chronic pulmonary disease with CO_2 retention

Abdominal examination:
- enlarged kidneys — Polycystic kidneys: in 20 percent of cases, associated with intracranial aneurysm (possible subarachnoid hemorrhage)

• hepatomegaly	Hepatoma with hepatic coma
Meticulous examination of the head	May reveal: depressed skull fracture, concussion
• bruise or boggy area in the scalp	Cranial fracture
Stiff neck	Meningeal irritation: bacterial meningitis, subarachnoid hemorrhage; cerebellar tonsillar herniation
Asterixis, tremor, multifocal myoclonus	Metabolic brain disease (structural brain disease unlikely)
Generalized convulsions	Hypoxia; hypoglycemia; sedative drug withdrawal; uremia; hyponatremia; hypocalcemia
Focal neurologic abnormalities	Supratentorial lesion causing upper brainstem dysfunction; subtentorial lesion destroying or compressing the reticular formation
Pupillary light reactions	
• *retained*	Metabolic coma; drug intoxication (exception: glutethimide and atropine intoxication; severe anoxia or asphyxia)
• absent	Structural brain lesion
Eyes turned away from the paralysis	Large cerebral lesion (eyes looking at the lesion)
Eyes turned toward the paralysis	Unilateral pontine lesion (eyes looking away from the lesion)
Funduscopic examination	May reveal: diabetic retinopathy; tuberculosis; bacterial endocarditis
Papilledema	Increased intracranial pressure: brain tumor or abscess, brain hemorrhage; brain trauma; hypertensive encephalopathy
Subhyaloid hemorrhages	Subarachnoid hemorrhage

LABORATORY TESTS PERTAINING TO THE COMPLAINT

Procedure	Finding	Diagnostic possibilities
Blood		
RBCs	Anemia	Acute blood loss
WBCs	Leukocytosis	Bacterial infection; cerebral hemorrhage; brain softening
Glucose	Low	Hypoglycemia
	Elevated	Diabetic acidosis; diabetic hyperosmolar coma; massive cerebral lesion
BUN, creatinine	Elevated	Uremic coma
Electrolytes	Metabolic acidosis, anion gap	Diabetic ketoacidosis; uremic acidosis; intoxication (salicylate, methanol, ethylene glycol); lactic acidosis
Calcium	Abnormal	Hypercalcemic coma; hypocalcemia
Serum ammonia	Increased	Hepatic encephalopathy
P_{O_2}, P_{CO_2}, pH	Abnormal	Hypoxia; hypercapnia
Thyroid function tests	Abnormal	Myxedema coma; thyroid storm
Blood smear	Plasmodia	Malaria
Cultures	Positive	Septicemia
Urine		
Urinalysis	Proteinuria	Uremia; subarachnoid hemorrhage

	Glycosuria	Diabetic coma; massive cerebral lesion
Tests for toxic agents	Positive	Acute intoxication
Lumbar puncture (N: 0 to 5 mono-nuclear WBCs)	Bloody	Subarachnoid hemorrhage; brain hemorrhage; cerebral contusion
Protein: (N: 15 to 45 mg/100 mL) Glucose: (N: 40 to 80 mg/100 mL)	Pleiocytosis, elevated protein, low glucose }	Bacterial meningitis (tuberculous meningitis: lymphocytosis in CSF)
Procedure Chemical analysis of gastric contents	*To detect* Intoxication	
Skull x-rays	Fracture lines; densities; pineal shift	
EEG	Symmetric slowing: diffuse metabolic brain lesion Focal or unilateral slow activity: structural brain disorder	
Brain scan	Tumor; subdural or intracerebral hemorrhage	
Computerized tomography	Tumor; ventricular size and position; fluid collections; atrophy of cerebral cortex; abnormal masses; etc.	
Arteriography	Tumor; subdural hematoma; arteriovenous malformation; etc.	

USEFUL REMINDERS AND DIAGNOSTIC CLUES

Misleading Factors

An alcoholic odor of the breath in an unconscious patient does not always reflect alcoholic intoxication.

Vodka is odorless.

Unconsciousness in elderly patients should not be too hastily ascribed to a stroke.

A history of head trauma is frequently absent in subacute or chronic
subdural hematoma.

Even when the coma is the result of some other primary cause, the
loss of consciousness may lead to a fall, resulting in head injury
and subdural or epidural hematoma, depressed skull fracture, or
concussion.

Diagnostic Considerations

Unconsciousness appearing immediately after a head trauma may
be followed by recovery itself succeeded by progressive stupor
and coma. A short lucid interval (minutes to hours) suggests an
epidural hematoma, while a longer interval (days to months) of
consciousness suggests a subdural hematoma (subacute or
chronic).

In case of	*Exclude*
Coma in an alcoholic patient	Subdural hematoma; hypogly-cemia; delirium tremens; Wernicke's encephalopathy; ingestion of toxic alcohol sub-stitutes; drug intoxication; over-whelming infection
Coma in an epileptic patient	Postictal state; serious head injury with subdural or epidural hematoma; overdose of seda-tives
Hepatic coma	Subdural hematoma; septice-mia; intoxication with alcohol or alcohol substitutes
Coma in a uremic patient	Subdural hematoma; seizures; Wernicke's encephalopathy; dis-equilibrium syndrome (after rapid dialysis)

SELECTED BIBLIOGRAPHY

Adams RD, Victor M: Coma and related disorders of consciousness, in *Principles of Neurology,* pp 194–210, New York: McGraw-Hill, 1977

Plum F, Posner JB: *The Diagnosis of Stupor and Coma,* 2d ed, Philadelphia: Davis, 1972

Sabin TD: The differential diagnosis of coma. N Engl J Med 290:1062–1064 1974

29
Confusional State

DEFINITIONS AND GENERAL CONSIDERATIONS

Confusion incapacity of the patient to think with customary speed and clarity.

Delirium acute and transient type of confusional state characterized by gross disorientation, in the presence of alertness and vigilance, disorders of perceptions, and hyperactivity of psychomotor and autonomic nervous system functions.

Dementia deterioration of all intellectual or cognitive functions without clouding or disturbances of perception.

The most common cause of delirium is the withdrawal of alcohol, barbiturates, or other sedative drugs following a period of chronic intoxication. These drugs have a depressant effect on the high brainstem reticular activating system. Withdrawal of these drugs is followed by the release and overactivity of this area, which are the basis of delirium. The delirious state observed in bacterial infections and drug intoxication probably results from the direct action of the toxin or chemical agent on the same areas of the brain. The function of these neuronal formations may be disturbed by destructive neurologic diseases, with resulting delirium.

In acute confusional states associated with metabolic and nutritional disorders, direct interference with the metabolic activities of the nerve cells in the cerebral cortex and central thalamic nuclei of the brain appears responsible. Sedatives (barbiturates, phenothiazines) impair consciousness by their direct suppressive effect on the neurons of the cerebrum and diencephalon.

Dementia is usually associated with structural diseases of the cerebrum and the diencephalon.

ETIOLOGY

Acute confusional state associated with delirium
Neurologic diseases: vascular or neoplastic; cerebral contusion; bacterial meningitis; tuberculous meningitis; encephalitis; subarachnoid hemorrhage; postconvulsive delirium

Infections: septicemia; pneumonia; rheumatic fever
Endocrine condition: thyrotoxicosis
Postoperative and posttraumatic states
Abstinence states: withdrawal of alcohol, sedatives following chronic intoxication
Drug-induced state

Acute confusional state associated with reduced mental alertness and responsiveness
Neurologic disease: cerebral vascular disease; tumor; abscess; subdural hematoma; meningitis; encephalitis
Metabolic disturbances: hepatic stupor; uremia; hypoglycemia; hypoxia; hypercapnia; porphyria
Infections: typhoid fever
Congestive heart failure
Postoperative, posttraumatic, and puerperal psychoses
Drug-induced state

Dementia
Presenile, senile dementia (Alzheimer's disease); Pick's disease
Slow virus diseases: Creutzfeldt-Jakob disease; subacute sclerosing panencephalitis
Huntington's chorea; Hallervorden-Spatz disease
Cerebral arteriosclerosis
Brain tumor; brain trauma; chronic subdural hematoma; normal pressure hydrocephalus
Neurosyphilis
Metabolic and endocrine disorders: hypothyroidism; hypoglycemia; uremia; hepatic disease; Cushing's disease; hepatolenticular degeneration; cerebral hypoxia; hypercalcemia; adrenal insufficiency
Nutritional deficiency: Wernicke-Korsakoff syndrome; pellagra; vitamin B_{12} deficiency
Connective-tissue diseases
Heavy-metal intoxication (lead, mercury, manganese); drug intoxications

Iatrogenic Causes of Alterations in Consciousness

Psychotropic drugs (amphetamines, phenothiazines, lithium, LSD, monoamine oxidase inhibitors, tricyclic antidepressants)

Anticholinergics, atropine
Anticonvulsivants
Barbiturates, bromides

Cortisone, ACTH
Digitalis
Salicylates

QUESTIONNAIRE

Note: The history should always be supplemented by information obtained from a person other than the patient.

Possible *meaning of response*

1 Mode of onset and evolution

1.1 How long has the patient been confused?

If state of consciousness has recently become disordered: metabolic encephalopathy (interference with brain metabolism by extracerebral disease) Presenile dementia appears before age 65; Huntington's chorea between 35 and 50 years

1.2 Have similar episodes previously occurred?

Hypoglycemia; porphyria

1.3 Has the onset of confusion been

• acute? (hours to days)
• subacute? (weeks)

Extracerebral disease with exogenous metabolic encephalopathy; confusional psychosis or delirium

• gradual? insidious? (months to years)

Dementia, degenerative or symptomatic; chronic use of barbiturates

1.3*a* In case of gradual onset, has the mental impairment
• *fluctuated?*

Metabolic encephalopathy; chronic subdural hematoma; chronic barbiturate intoxication

• progressively worsened?

Senile dementia

1.4 *In the elderly patient: Has the mental deterioration been "stepwise"?*

Episodes of strokelike events suggest arteriosclerosis

1.5 Where has the patient been
found? From where has he
been brought?
- his home? the street?
- a locked room?

Exposure to toxic chemical
agents; carbon monoxide
poisoning

- a bar?

Acute alcoholism

1.6 Were any of the following
items found in the vicinity
of the patient:
- medications?

Chronic or acute <u>intoxication</u>

- prescriptions? syringes?

Suggest use of medications

1.7 What is his present mental
status?

See Chap. 32

2 *Precipitating or aggravating factors*

2.1 Has the patient recently
had
- a trauma, an operation?

Postoperative or posttraumatic
confusional state; an operation
or any hospitalization may induce a withdrawal syndrome in
a chronic abuser of alcohol or
barbiturates

- a head trauma?

Subdural hematoma (a negative
history does not exclude the
diagnosis); posttraumatic confusional state

- (female): a pregnancy?

Puerperal psychosis

- a heavy intake of
  - alcohol?

<u>Acute alcoholism</u>, particularly
in the elderly; chronic alcoholism: Wernicke-Korsakoff syndrome

  - drugs?

Chronic drug intoxication; delirium due to psychogenic drugs
(LSD, mescaline)

2.2   *Has the patient recently stopped a chronic alcohol or barbiturate habit?*

Withdrawal syndrome; alcoholic hallucinosis appears within 24 to 36 h, delirium tremens within 72 h of withdrawal; barbiturates: between second and fourth days of abstinence

2.3   Has the patient recently had an emotional, personal problem? a change of environment?

In the elderly patient: may be causal factors of altered mental status

3   Accompanying symptoms

3.1   What were the first signs of the patient's abnormal mental status?
- irritability? excessive activity?
- restlessness? insomnia?
- hallucinations?

Approaching attack of delirium

- reduced responsiveness? slow reactions? difficulty in sustaining a conversation?

Acute confusional state with psychomotor underactivity

3.2   Prior to the onset of confusion, did the patient have
- fever? chills?

Acute infectious disease (intra- or extracranial)

- headache?

Intracranial evolving process

- abdominal pain?

Porphyria

- a convulsion?

Postconvulsive delirium; hypoglycemia; Stokes-Adams episode with cerebral hypoxia

3.3   In an elderly patient, does the patient have
- loss of memory for recent events? depression? anxiety? an inappropriate behavior? urine, fecal incontinence?

Senile dementia; Alzheimer's disease

3.4 In a young or middle-aged adult, is the mental impairment associated with
- abnormal movements?
- odd postures?

} Huntington's chorea

4 *Iatrogenic factors* see Etiology

5 *Environmental factors*

5.1 What is the patient's occupation?

Professional exposure to toxic products; heavy metal intoxication (rare): manganese, mercury poisoning

6 *Personal antecedents pertaining to the confusional state*

6.1 Has the patient ever had an x-ray of the skull? an EEG? a brain scan? a lumbar puncture? When? With what results?

6.2 Did the patient have an abnormal mental status prior to the present episode?

Preexisting dementing brain disease, possibly complicated by a medical disease

6.3 Does the patient have
- alcoholism? drug abuse?
- depression?

The distinction between depression and dementia with mental deterioration may be difficult

- a previous psychiatric hospitalization? previous suicide attempts?

Preexisting dementia; depression

- a cardiac disease?
- chronic bronchitis? emphysema?

} Cerebral hypoxia

- a liver disease?

Hepatic encephalopathy

- a renal disease?

Confusional state of uremia

- a thyroid, an adrenal condition?

Medication may have become irregular or abandoned

- hypertension?

In the elderly patient: antihypertensive drugs may cause mental

	impairment by reducing the blood pressure below an optimal level
• Parkinson's disease?	Anticholinergic drugs may cause confusional states
• a past operation on the thyroid?	Resulting in myxedema

7   *Family medical history pertaining to the confusional state*

| 7.1   Are there similar cases in the patient's family? | Huntington's chorea; lipidoses of the nervous system; Pick's disease |

PHYSICAL SIGNS PERTINENT TO THE COMPLAINT

Finding	**Possible** *significance*
Fever	Acute infectious disease; gram-negative sepsis
Hyperthermia	
• with profuse perspiration	Most delirium states; delirium tremens; salicylate intoxication
• without perspiration	Anticholinergic drug ingestion; infection
Hypothermia	Myxedema; hypoglycemia; barbiturate intoxication
Hyperventilating delirious patient	Diabetic ketosis; uremia; lactic acidosis; methyl alcohol poisoning; pulmonary or cardiac disease; hepatic encephalopathy
Hypoventilating patient	Chronic pulmonary disease with CO_2 retention; depressant drug poisoning
Hypoventilation; obesity	Pickwickian syndrome
Fluctuations of mental status	Metabolic encephalopathy (also in chronic subdural hematoma)

Flapping tremor (asterixis)	Hepatic encephalopathy; uremia; ventilatory failure
Tremor, asterixis, multifocal myoclonus	Metabolic brain disease (rare in dementia); structural brain disease unlikely
Increased psychomotor activity	Delirium tremens; drug withdrawal states
Focal neurologic abnormalities	Structural brain disease
Rhonchi, wheezes; cyanosis; mental dullness; drowsiness	Hypercapnia (and hypoxia) in pulmonary disease
Jaundice; asterixis; fetor hepaticus	Hepatic encephalopathy
Sixth nerve palsy; nystagmus (horizontal and vertical); paralysis of conjugate gaze; ataxia of stance and gait; polyneuropathy; retrograde amnesia; confabulation	Wernicke-Korsakoff syndrome
Funduscopic examination: • papilledema	Increased intracranial pressure: brain tumor, chronic subdural hematoma; hypercarbic encephalopathy

LABORATORY TESTS PERTAINING TO THE COMPLAINT

Procedure	*To detect*
Blood RBCs	Pernicious anemia
WBCs	Infection
P_{O_2}, P_{CO_2}, pH	Hypoxia; hypercapnia

Glucose	Hypoglycemia; diabetic acidosis
BUN, creatinine, electrolytes	Uremia; electrolytes disorders with confusion
Liver function tests Serum ammonia	Hepatic encephalopathy
Thyroid function tests	Thyrotoxicosis; myxedema
Antinuclear antibodies	Systemic lupus erythematosus
Culture	Septicemia
Urine Urinalysis	Chronic renal failure; diabetic acidosis
Porphobilinogen	Porphyria
Tests for toxic agents	Intoxication
Lumbar puncture	Subarachnoid hemorrhage; cerebral contusion; bacterial meningitis; encephalitis
Skull x-rays	Fracture line; abnormal calcifications; pineal shift
EEG	Symmetric slowing: diffuse metabolic brain disease Seizure activity; focal depression of activity: structural brain disorder
Brain scan	Tumor; subdural or intracerebral hemorrhage
Echoencephalography	Shift of ventricular position
Computerized tomography	Ventricular size and position; abnormal masses; fluid collections; atrophy of cerebral cortex

USEFUL REMINDERS AND DIAGNOSTIC CLUES

Psychoneuroses rarely begin in middle or late adult age; it is safe to assume that all mental illnesses beginning during this period are due either to structural disease of the brain or to depressive psychoses.

When the cause of delirium is unclear, the first conditions to consider are: hypoxia, hypoglycemia, and metabolic acidosis.

Vitamin B_{12} deficiency may advance to a frank psychosis in the absence of anemia.

Personality changes and depression may signal the evolution of neoplasms involving the frontal lobes, long before signs of increasing intracranial pressure or focal neurologic deficits develop.

Mild disorientation and intellectual dysfunction may develop in patients with carcinoma, even though there is no evidence of metastasis to the nervous system.

Confusion in the elderly patient is frequent with bacterial pneumonia, other localized bacterial infections, bacteremia, posttraumatic and postoperative states, congestive heart failure, chronic respiratory failure, severe anemia, removal of cataracts, subarachnoid hemorrhage, subdural hematoma.

Confusional psychosis and delirium are reversible, whereas dementia is more or less irreversible.

In case of	*Suspect*
An episode of mental impairment associated with	
• abdominal pain	Acute intermittent porphyria
• arthralgias	Systemic lupus erythematosus
• auditory hallucinations	Psychotic illness: schizophrenia
• visual hallucinations	Metabolic encephalopathy

SELECTED BIBLIOGRAPHY

Adams RD, Victor M: Delirium and other acute confusional states; Dementia and Korsakoff's Psychosis, in *Principles of Neurology,* pp 259–280, New York: McGraw-Hill, 1977

Adler G: Acute psychosis. N Engl J Med 291:81–83, 1974

Barrett RE: Dementia in adults. Med Clin North Am 56:1405–1418, 1972

Posner JB: Delirium and exogenous metabolic brain disease, in Beeson PB McDermott W, *Textbook of Medicine,* 14th ed, pp 544–552, Philadelphia: Saunders, 1975

30
Fatigue

DEFINITION AND GENERAL CONSIDERATIONS

Fatigue (*tiredness, lassitude*) loss of that sense of well-being typically found in persons who are healthy in body and mind; it is a subjective feeling of lack of energy, not necessarily associated with physical activity. Fatigue must be distinguished from weakness of neural or muscular origin.

Fatigue is a normal physiologic reaction when associated with or occurring after sustained muscular exertion. Under these circumstances a rest period rapidly restores the subject's feeling of well-being and capacity for work. In a normal subject continuous muscular work results in depletion of muscular glycogen and an accumulation of lactic acid and other metabolites which reduce the power of muscular contraction. Fatigue may result from overwork. It also occurs in various infectious, metabolic, endocrine, and nutritional diseases. Fatigue may be associated with true weakness in thyroid dysfunction, adrenal insufficiency, or neurologic disorders. Anxiety and depression account for 85 percent of cases in which fatigue is the major presenting problem.

ETIOLOGY

Predominating symptom of an organic disease

Acute infection: influenza; hepatitis
Chronic infections: tuberculosis; infectious mononucleosis; brucellosis; subacute infectious hepatitis; subacute bacterial endocarditis; asymptomatic urinary tract infection; hookworm, parasitic infection
Autoimmune conditions: systemic lupus erythematosus; rheumatoid arthritis
Neurologic disorders: Parkinson's disease; multiple sclerosis; posttraumatic syndrome
Primary muscle disorders: polymyositis; muscular dystrophy; myasthenia gravis

Endocrine and metabolic diseases: adrenal insufficiency; aldosterone deficiency; panhypopituitarism; Cushing's disease; hypothyroidism; hyperthyroidism; hypogonadism; hyperparathyroidism; hypercalcemic and hypocalcemic states; hyperaldosteronism; potassium depletion; uncontrolled diabetes mellitus; hypoglycemic states; renal insufficiency

Anemia from any cause; other blood dyscrasias

Nutritional deficiencies; Crohn's disease

Circulatory disorders: "silent" myocardial infarction; impending congestive heart failure; cardiomyopathy

Pulmonary insufficiency: emphysema; chronic bronchitis

Neoplastic disorders: lymphomas; carcinomas; occult tumors

Persistent chronic pain causing lack of sleep; metastatic disease of bone

Chronic drug intoxication; alcohol

Psychologic
Anxiety neurosis; tension states; depression

Iatrogenic Causes of Fatigue

Antihistamines

Prolonged ingestion of barbiturates

Bromides

Large doses of corticosteroids

Morphine addiction

Tranquilizers; sedatives

QUESTIONNAIRE

Possible *meaning of response*

1 Mode of onset and duration

1.1 How long have you been feeling tired?

If the patient has "always' felt tired: psychogenic fatigue

1.2 Has the onset of the fatigue been

• sudden? (days)

Acute infection; disturbance of fluid balance, extracellular deficit; rapidly developing circulatory failure (outspoken objective phenomena present)

• gradual? (weeks to months)	<u>Psychogenic fatigue</u> or fatigue due to an organic disease

2   *Character*

2.1   Is the fatigue

• constant?	Muscular weakness; fatigue due to an organic disease (also: depression)
• intermittent?	Psychogenic fatigue; weakness: in periodic paralysis

2.2   Do you feel tired
• all day?
• on awakening? *in the morning?*
• at the end of the day?

Psychogenic fatigue (frequently worse in the morning)

Organic cause of fatigue; psychogenic fatigue

2.2a   *Do you feel just as tired when you awaken as you do later on in the day?*

<u>Psychogenic fatigue</u>

2.3   When do you feel at your best?

• in the morning?	Fatigue due to an organic factor
• *in the evening?*	<u>Psychogenic fatigue</u>

3   *Precipitating or aggravating factors*

3.1   Does your fatigue appear

• during exertion?	Weakness
• only after a strenuous physical effort?	"Normal" fatigue
• without any relation to physical effort?	Psychogenic fatigue

3.1a   Do you feel tired

• before a physical effort?	Psychogenic fatigue
• after a physical effort?	Fatigue due to an organic disease; psychogenic fatigue

3.2   Is the fatigue related
   • more to some activities
     than to others?   } Psychogenic fatigue
   • to unpleasant emotional
     experiences?

3.3   Do you have any job prob-   Possible overwork with fatigue;
      lem?   eventual psychogenic cause of
                                  fatigue

3.3*a*   Do you take any vacation?   May reveal an overworked pa-
      • How many weeks a year?   tient with no time for diversion
                                  and sleep

3.4   Do you feel more tired at
      home than on your job?   }
                                  Familial psychogenic factor
3.4*a*   Do you have any family
      problem?

3.5   For the female patient who
      is a housewife: What is the
      size of your family? of
      your house?   }
                                  The "tired-housewife" syndrome
3.5*a*   How many children are
      living at home? any in-
      fants? other persons?

3.6   What is your daily diet?   A nutritional deficiency may
                                  cause fatigue

4   *Relieving factors*

4.1   Is the fatigue relieved by
                                  Fatigue due to an organic dis-
   • rest?   ease; weakness (if not relieved:
   • additional sleep?   psychogenic fatigue likely)

5   *Accompanying symptoms*

5.1   Do you feel anxious?   Associated symptoms in <u>anxiety</u>
      depressed? irritable?   <u>neurosis</u> or <u>tension states</u>: ex-
      unable to concentrate?   tension of psychogenic fatigue
                                  to mental activities

5.2   Do you have
- headaches?
- any sexual problems? a lack of interest in sex?
- poor sleep?

Frequently observed in depression with psychogenic fatigue

- a loss of weight?

Thyrotoxicosis; chronic infection; tuberculosis; diabetes mellitus; Addison's disease; may occur in depressive reaction

- a decreased appetite?

Chronic infection; uremia; Addison's disease; panhypopituitarism; depression

- fever?

Chronic infection; tuberculosis; lymphoma

- cough? night sweats?

Pulmonary tuberculosis

- palpitations?

Fever; thyrotoxicosis (arrhythmias); psychogenic fatigue

- pain in your chest? abdomen?

Carcinoma of the lung, pancreas, or colon; also: psychogenic fatigue

- changes in your bowel habits?

Carcinoma of colon or pancreas; depression

- *double vision?* (*diplopia*)
- *difficulty in speaking?* (dysarthria), in chewing?

Myasthenia gravis with involvement of cranial nerves (never present in psychogenic fatigue)

6   *Iatrogenic factors*   see Etiology

7   *Personal antecedents pertaining to the fatigue*

7.1   Do you have any of the following conditions: anemia? any chronic disease? alcoholism? a psychiatric condition?
- a cardiac condition?

Fatigue due to congestive heart failure: related to the reduction of cardiac output

7.1*a*   Have you recently had
- a prolonged illness? an operation? influenza? infectious hepatitis?

Convalescing, postinfectious, and postoperative states responsible for fatigue

PHYSICAL SIGNS PERTINENT TO THE COMPLAINT

Finding	**Possible** *significance*
Reduced muscular power; neurologic abnormalities; muscle wasting	Primary myopathic or neurologic disorder
Cranial muscle weakness; nasal voice	Myasthenia gravis (excludes emotional fatigue states)
Lack of facial expression; paucity of movements; inertia; slow speech; paucity of ideas	Depression
Weight loss	Nutritional deficiency; malignancy
Pallor; tachycardia	Moderate to severe anemia (hematocrit < 25 percent)
Fever	Occult or chronic infection: pulmonary or disseminated tuberculosis, viral infection; neoplastic disease
Fever; cardiac murmur	Subacute bacterial endocarditis
Dry skin; bradycardia; delayed relaxation phase of the tendon reflexes	Hypothyroidism
Thyroid enlargement; tremor; sweating palms	Thyrotoxicosis
Hyperpigmentation of skin and mucosae; hypotension; postural hypotension; muscular weakness	Adrenal insufficiency
Cardiomegaly; gallop rhythm; bilateral basal rales; pulsus alternans	Left ventricular failure; silent myocardial infarction: decrease in cardiac output and inadequate tissue perfusion and oxygenation
Distended jugular veins; cardiomegaly; hepatomegaly; edema	Fatigue is common in right (and/or left) ventricular failure

Prolonged expiration; rhonchi, wheezes; cyanosis

Chronic pulmonary disease with chronic dyspnea and fatigue

Hepatosplenomegaly; lymphadenopathy

Chronic active hepatitis; lymphoma; leukemia; chronic infection

LABORATORY TESTS PERTAINING TO THE COMPLAINT

Procedure	*To detect*
Blood	
Hematocrit	Anemia: a possible cause for fatigue if hematocrit less than 30 percent
WBCs	Leukemia; infection
Erythrocyte sedimentation rate	Infection; connective-tissue disorders; etc.
Liver function tests	Liver disease
BUN, creatinine	Chronic renal failure
Fasting glucose	Uncontrolled diabetes mellitus
Electrolytes	Endocrinopathies: Addison's disease, hyperaldosteronism; renal tubular acidosis; diuretic intake
Calcium	Hyperparathyroidism; other hypercalcemic states
Iron	Iron-deficiency anemia
Thyroid function tests	Thyrotoxicosis; myxedema
Cortisol*	Addison's disease
Stool	
Occult blood tests	Gastrointestinal tumor
Chest x-ray	Pulmonary tuberculosis; lung tumor; chronic pulmonary disease

* If appropriate.

ECG	Atherosclerotic heart disease with decreased cardiac output and resulting fatigue; silent myocardial infarction
Psychologic evaluation*	Depression or anxiety states

* If appropriate.

USEFUL REMINDERS AND DIAGNOSTIC CLUES

Misleading Factors

Fatigue is frequently ascribed to overwork when it actually reflects a psychoneurosis or depression.

Even when fatigue is associated with an organic lesion, it may not be attributable to it, but rather to independent or related psychogenic disturbances.

Diagnostic Considerations

Fatigue associated with weight gain suggests a depressive syndrome.

Neoplasms are seldom manifested primarily by fatigue; however, carcinoma of the lung, pancreas, or right colon in particular may be introduced by fatigue.

Mental symptoms of depression and anxiety occur in many patients with pancreatic carcinoma.

Fatigue may be produced by iron deficiency without any anemia at all.

Mild anemias are usually asymptomatic and any associated fatigue is probably attributable to some other condition.

More than 25 percent of the patients referred by physicians with the presumptive diagnosis of disease of the neuromuscular system have proved to have fatigue of emotional origin.

SELECTED BIBLIOGRAPHY

Adams RD: Lassitude and asthenia, in *Harrison's Principles of Medicine*, 8th ed, pp 72–75, New York: McGraw-Hill, 1977

Rhoads JM: Overwork. JAMA 237:2615–2618, 1977

31
Headache

DEFINITION AND GENERAL CONSIDERATIONS

Headache   painful or unpleasant sensations in the region of the cranial vault.

Structures sensitive to pain in the region of the head and face include all extracranial tissues, especially the arteries, the basal dura mater, the venous sinuses and their tributary veins, the arteries within the dura mater and piarachnoid, and nerves with sensory afferents (fifth, ninth, tenth cranial nerves, first three cervical nerves).

Headache may originate from extracranial or intracranial structures. Vascular headaches are principally due to painful dilatation and distention of extracranial branches of the external carotid artery. Most of the pain of migraine is attributed to dilatation of the temporal arteries, with stretching of surrounding sensitive structures. During the migraine attack plasma serotonin levels have been found to be low; serotonin constricts large vessels and dilates small ones, and it has been postulated that a fall in plasma serotonin level permits the dilatation of large vessels of the scalp and contraction of small arterioles during the headache phase of migraine. In cluster headache no decrease of plasma serotonin is observed, but plasma histamine levels have been found to be increased during the headache period; edema of the wall of the internal carotid may be responsible for the syndrome. The headache associated with febrile states or some cases of hypertension is probably due to dilatation and distention of intracranial arteries. Tension headache is ascribed to long-sustained contraction of skeletal muscle about the face, scalp, and neck; it usually coincides with anxiety and depression. Pain of infection or blockage of paranasal sinuses is due to changes in pressure and irritation of pain-sensitive sinus walls. Headache of ocular origin is believed to be caused by ocular muscle imbalance. Intracranial mass lesions may cause headache by deforming, displacing, or exerting traction on vessels and dural structures at the base of the brain. Headache of meningeal irritation is ascribed to increased intracranial pressure, and dilatation and congestion of inflamed meningeal vessels. The pain of trigeminal neuralgia (over the distribution of one or more branches of the fifth cranial nerve) can occur spontaneously or may be brought on by stimulating a trigger zone, which may exist in any part of the face.

ETIOLOGY

Extracranial headache
Vascular headaches of migraine type: classic migraine; common migraine; cluster headache; hemiplegic or ophthalmoplegic migraine
Muscle contraction headache (psychogenic)
Sinus headache
Nonmigrainous vascular headaches: systemic fever; carbon monoxide poisoning, lead, nitrates; acute pressor reaction; pheochromocytoma; arterial hypertension
Ocular headache: glaucoma; inflammation; excessive contraction of ocular muscles
Aural headache
Dental headache
Headache due to spread of pain from other structures of cranium and neck: periosteum, joints, ligaments, muscles, cervical nerve roots
Cranial neuritides
Extracranial arteritis; temporal arteritis (polymyalgia rheumatica)

Intracranial headache
Traction headache:
   Primary or metastatic tumors of meninges, vessels, or brain
   Hematomas, abscesses (epidural, subdural, or parenchymal)
   Headache following lumbar puncture
   Pseudotumor cerebri
Inflammation of cranial structures: meningitis, subarachnoid hemorrhage, arteritis, phlebitis

Cranial neuralgias
Trigeminal and glossopharyngeal

Headaches of a delusional or conversion reaction (rare)

Iatrogenic Causes of Headache

Nitrites, nitrates, nitroglycerin; caffeine withdrawal; reserpine

QUESTIONNAIRE

Possible *meaning of response*

1   *Location of headache*

1.1   Where do you have pain?

1.1*a*   Can you point to the painful area?

Local disorder: frontal sinus;
ear; temporal arteritis

1.2   Is the pain
  • *unilateral?*

<u>Migraine</u>; cluster headache
(male preponderance); one-
sided intracranial lesion; trigeminal neuralgia

  • *temporal?*

Temporal arteritis

  • *recurrent and always on the
    same side of the head?*

Intracranial vascular anomaly;
<u>migraine</u>; cluster headache

  • *orbital or supraorbital?*

Cluster headache; glaucoma

  • bilateral?
    • bitemporal? frontal?

<u>Tension headache</u>

  • occipitonucchal?

<u>Tension headache</u>; arterial hy-
pertension; cervical disease; if
in deeper structures: intracranial lesion in posterior fossa

  • moving from one side to
    the other?

May occur in migraine

1.3   Does the pain spread to
the
  • face?

Trigeminal neuralgia

  • face, neck, shoulder?

May occur in cluster headache
and in pain referred from lesions
of the upper cervical portion of
the spinal column; subarachnoid
hemorrhage

2   *Mode of onset and chronology*

2.1   How long have you had
headaches?

If many years: benign, tends to
eliminate intracranial or inflammatory lesion; probably <u>vascular</u>
or <u>muscle contraction</u> mechanism

2.2   Was the onset
- *sudden (over a period of minutes) and violent?*   Subarachnoid hemorrhage

- acute?   Meningitis; epidural hematoma; glaucoma; purulent sinusitis

2.3   Is your headache
- continuous?   <u>Tension headache</u>, functional problem

- recurrent?   Organic: <u>migraine</u>, cluster headache; trigeminal neuralgia

2.3*a*   In case of recurrent headache, what is the frequency of the episodes?
- a single attack every few weeks?   Migraine

- several attacks per week?   Usually combination of migraine and tension headaches

- once to several times daily, for several weeks?   Cluster headache

2.3*b*   Are the headaches becoming more frequent and severe over a period of months?   Expanding intracranial lesion; **brain tumor; subdural hematoma;** aneurysm

2.3*c*   What is the duration of your headaches?
- 1 to 2 s?   Uninterpretable; no serious underlying disease

- a few minutes to hours?   Intracranial tumor
- dissipates within an hour?   Cluster headache
- lasts for several hours up to 1 to 2 days?   <u>Migraine</u>
- may last for
  - days or weeks?   Temporal arteritis; sinusitis
  - weeks or months with fluctuations?   <u>Tension headache</u>

2.3*d*   At what time in the day does your headache appear?

• *upon awakening in the morning?*	Hypertensive headache (occipital)
• in the morning?	Migraine; brain tumor; frontal sinusitis
• in the early afternoon?	Maxillary sinusitis
• at night? *2 to 3 h after onset of sleep?*	Cluster headache
• at any time of day or night?	Intracranial tumor; the onset of tension headache is generally not related to time of day

2.3*e* How quickly does your headache reach a maximum?

• abruptly, rapidly peaking?	5 to 10 min: cluster headache
• gradually?	Over ½ to 1 h: migraine

3 *Character of the pain*

3.1 Is the pain

• sharp? stabbing?	Trigeminal neuralgia
• throbbing? *pulsatile?*	Vascular, migraine headaches
• persistent? (and intense?)	Subarachnoid hemorrhage; cluster headache
• tight? *bandlike? pressing? nonthrobbing?*	Tension headache (psychogenic)

3.2 Does your pain seem

• deep located?	Pain arising from structures deep to the skin: extracranial, subdermal, intracranial
• superficial?	Localized to the skin

4 *Precipitating or aggravating factors*

4.1 Is your headache caused or worsened by

• stooping? straining? coughing? sneezing? lifting? exertion?	**Intracranial mass lesion;** subarachnoid hemorrhage; infection of nasal sinuses
• sudden head movement?	Cervical disease; sinus headache

• alcohol?	Migraine; cluster headache; sinusitis
• prolonged reading? watching movies, TV?	Eyestrain headache
• anxiety? fatigue? emotional upset?	Psychogenic (tension) headache; vascular, migraine, hypertensive headache
• sudden temperature changes?	Sinusitis
• *touching a trigger point?*	Trigeminal neuralgia
• a period of inactivity?	Headaches of cervical arthritis
4.2 *Does your headache occur during weekends?*	Migraine may occur at the time of relaxation following a stressful situation

5 *Relieving factors*

5.1 Is your headache relieved by

• recumbency?	Brain tumor
• neck massage?	Cervical disease
• heat? aspirin?	Tension headache
• ergot preparations? sleep?	Migraine
• Tegretol?	Trigeminal neuralgia

6 *Accompanying symptoms*

6.1 Do you have

• fever?	**Meningitis; subarachnoid hemorrhage;** headache of febrile illness; temporal arteritis
• nausea? vomiting?	Migraine; brain tumor
• *nasal congestion? rhinorrhea? lacrimation? ipsilateral conjunctival injection?*	Cluster headache
• blurred or decreased vision?	**Malignant hypertension; temporal arteritis**
• muscle aches?	Temporal arteritis; febrile illness
• weakness in (a) limb(s)?	Organic intracranial involvement

6.2 *Are there any warnings minutes or hours before your headache? scintillating scotomas?* depression? fatigue? nausea? vomiting?

Migraine; vasodilating headaches

7 *Iatrogenic factors* see Etiology

8 *Environmental factors*

8.1 What is your profession?

Exposure to occupational toxins (nitrates, carbon monoxide); stress

9 *Personal antecedents pertaining to the headache*

9.1 Have there been similar episodes in the past? When? Diagnosis?

9.2 Have you ever had a skull x-ray? an EEG? a brain scan? When? With what results?

9.3 Have you had during the preceding weeks or months
  • a head injury?

Subdural hematoma

  • an infection?

Brain abscess

9.4 Do you have an ear infection? a sinus disease? glaucoma?
  • a personal, familial, professional problem?

Psychogenic headache

10 *Family medical history pertaining to the headache*

10.1 Are there other members of your family who have headaches?

A family history of migraine is present in about 65 percent of patients with migraine

PHYSICAL SIGNS PERTINENT TO THE COMPLAINT

Finding
Fever

Possible *significance*
Headache accompanying febrile illnesses; meningitis; temporal arteritis; subarachnoid hemorrhage

Stiffness of neck on bending forward	Meningeal irritation: infection, hemorrhage
Severe diastolic hypertension, (>120 mmHg)	Headache related to hypertension; intracerebral hemorrhage
Fever; pallor (anemia); *tender thickened temporal artery*	Temporal arteritis
Homolateral lacrimation, rhinorrhea, nasal congestion, conjunctival injection, flush and edema of the cheek, myosis, ptosis	Cluster headache
Neurologic abnormalities	Intracranial space-occupying lesion: brain tumor, chronic subdural hematoma
Painful active and passive movements of the cervical spine	Disease of ligaments, muscles, and apophyseal joints of the cervical spine
Tender contracted muscles of head, neck, upper part of back; localized tender areas or nodules	Muscle-contraction headache
Sinus tenderness	Infection or blockage of nasal and paranasal sinuses
Funduscopic examination: Papilledema	Intracranial lesion with increased intracranial pressure
Hypertensive retinopathy	Arterial hypertension
Subhyaloid hemorrhages	Ruptured saccular aneurysm

LABORATORY TESTS PERTAINING TO THE COMPLAINT

Procedure	Finding	Diagnostic possibilities
Blood ESR	Elevated	Temporal arteritis (in elderly patients)
Hemoglobin	Anemia	

Procedure	To detect
EEG*	
Skull x-rays*	
Brain scan*	Space-occupying lesion; primary or metastatic neoplasm; abscess; subdural hematoma
Computerized tomography*	
Echoencephalogram*	
Sinuses: x-rays, transillumination	Purulent sinusitis
Eyes:	
Intraocular pressure	Glaucoma
Refraction	Refraction errors
Visual fields	Intracranial mass lesion
Biopsy of temporal artery*	Temporal arteritis
Thermography*	Supraorbital spotted areas of dense coolness, ipsilateral to the patient's headache: cluster headache
Lumbar puncture*	Subarachnoid hemorrhage; meningitis; encephalitis
Psychologic evaluation*	Underlying anxiety or tension state

* If appropriate.

USEFUL REMINDERS AND DIAGNOSTIC CLUES

As a rule, the most intense cranial pains are those associated with subarachnoid hemorrhage, meningitis, migraine, and cluster headache.

Positive evidence of neurosis must be present before any headache is ascribed to functional causes; even positive evidence of neurosis does not rule out brain tumor or other organic disease.

More than 90 percent of all headaches seen in office practice are of the muscle-contraction or migraine type.

Characteristic	Organic headache	Psychogenic headache
Duration	Usually short (exception: temporal arteritis)	Chronic
Isolated events, with a definite beginning and an end	+	—
Periods with complete freedom from pain	+	Patient reluctant to admit
Usually described by the patient in fairly definite terms	+	—
Secondary symptoms (nausea, vomiting, etc.)	+	Not impressive
Pharmaceutical influence	+	Insignificant

In case of	Suspect
Headache in older persons associated with pain on mastication, impairment of vision, muscular aches, fever, weight loss	Temporal arteritis
Attacks of severe headache with palpitations, sweating, pallor	Pheochromocytoma
Episodic headache occurring for the first time after age 50, associated with neurologic disturbances	Basilar or carotid artery insufficiency
Headache with fluctuating level of consciousness over months, especially in alcoholics	Subdural hematoma

SELECTED BIBLIOGRAPHY

Adams RD, Victor M: Headache and other craniofacial pains, in *Principles of Neurology*, pp 95–111, New York: McGraw-Hill, 1977

Friedman AP (ed): Symposium on headache and related pain syndromes. Med Clin North Am, 62:427–623, 1978

Mayo Clinic and Mayo Foundation: Headache, in *Clinical Examinations in Neurology*, p. 11, Philadelphia: Saunders, 1971

Plum F: Headache, in Beeson PB, McDermott W, *Textbook of Medicine*, 14th ed, chap 350, pp 614–619, Philadelphia: Saunders, 1975

32
Mental Status Examination

QUESTIONNAIRE

1 Insight

1.1 What are your complaints?

1.2 When did your illness be-gin?

1.3 Do you recognize the need for treatment?

Possible *meaning of response*
The patient's understanding of the illness may guide the physi-cian's therapeutic planning

2 Orientation

2.1 What is your name?

2.2 What is your occupation?

2.3 Where do you live?

2.4 Are you married?

2.4*a* Do you have children?

2.5 How long have you been in your present home?

2.6 Orientation for place

2.6*a* What is the name of the place where you are now?

2.6*b* How did you get there?

2.6*c* What floor is it on?

2.7 Orientation in time

2.7*a* What is the date today? (year, month, day)

2.7*b* What time of day is it?

Test the patient's knowledge of personal identity and present situation

The passage of time is the most sensitive of all the components involved in orientation; disorien-tation in time usually appears first, followed in more severe

2.7*c*   When was the last holiday?

2.7*d*   If defects are suspected: Would you please estimate the duration of a minute?

disturbances by disorientation for place and persons in that order

A normal estimate is within plus or minus 10 s

3   *Memory*

3.1   Memory for remote past events

3.1*a*   Tell me your birth date

3.1*b*   When were you married?

3.1*c*   What was your mother's maiden name?

3.1*d*   When did you graduate from school?

3.1*e*   What jobs have you held?

Disorders of memory are indicative of cortical disturbance of a permanent nature (brain atrophy or other gross destructive lesion), or of a transient nature (delirium, marked disorders of thinking of the affective and schizophrenic type); memory defects appear early in organic diseases of the brain which cause dementia; memory for distant events may remain relatively unaffected until the dementia becomes gross

3.2   Memory for recent past experiences (in the past 24 h)

3.2*a*   What did you have for breakfast today?

3.2*b*   What were the headlines in the newspaper today?

3.2*c*   What is my name?

3.2*d*   When did you see me for the first time?

In dementia, recent memory is most affected, with faulty recall of day-to-day happenings

3.3   Short-term memory: recall of immediate impressions

3.3*a*   Please repeat these numbers after me:
   • series of 3, 4, 5, 6, 7, 8 digits

A normal person can repeat seven to eight digits without errors

3.3*b*   Please repeat backward the series of numbers I give you now

Normal limit: five to six digits

3.3*c*   Please listen to the three following (unrelated) words: X; Y; Z; I shall ask you after 3 min to repeat them

4   *General intellectual evaluation*

4.1   General information

The intellectual functions are invariably impaired when there is brain damage, whether focal or generalized, e.g., cerebrovascular disease, cerebral tumor, damage from head injury, generalized cortical atrophy; similar disturbances occur transiently in association with toxic or inflammatory disease of the brain

4.1*a*   What are the five largest cities in the United States?

4.1*b*   What are the five largest rivers in the United States?

4.1*c*   What is the name of the capital of: this state? the United States? England? France? Italy?

4.1*d*   What is the name of the last four presidents? their political parties?

4.2   Calculations

4.2*a*   Test ability to add, subtract, multiply, divide

Capacity for sustained mental activity

4.2*b*   Please subtract 7 from 100 and continue subtracting until you can no further

A good test of calculation as well as of concentration; average time: 40 to 50 s

4.2*c*   If 5 times x equals 20, how much is x?

4.3   Discrimination and judgment

4.3*a* Can you state the difference or similarity between:
  • a dwarf and a child?
  • a lie and a mistake?
  • a tree and a bush?

Abstract thinking: commonly disturbed in organic mental disease

4.3*b* Please explain the meaning of the following proverbs:
"A stitch in time saves nine."
"People who live in glass houses should not throw stones."

Patients with organic brain disease often treat such proverbs entirely literally and seem unaware of their underlying meaning

5 *Mood and feeling patterns*

5.1 Inadequacy

5.1*a* Do you get nervous when approached by a superior?

5.1*b* Is it always hard for you to make up your mind?

5.1*c* Do you wish you always had someone at your side to advise you?

5.2 Depression

5.2*a* Do you usually feel unhappy and depressed?

5.2*b* Do you often cry?

5.2*c* Does life look entirely hopeless?

5.2*d* Have you ever contemplated suicide?

Depressed patients do not resent this question and are often relieved to be able to admit their feelings

5.3 Anxiety

5.3*a*   Do you worry about minor matters?

5.3*b*   Does worrying continually get you down?

5.3*c*   Are you considered a nervous person?

5.4   Sensitivity

5.4*a*   Are you extremely shy or sensitive?

5.4*b*   Are your feelings easily hurt?

5.4*c*   Do people usually mis-understand you?

5.5   Anger

5.5*a*   Do you always do things on sudden impulse?

5.5*b*   Are you easily upset or ir-ritated?

5.5*c*   Do little annoyances make you angry?

5.6   Tension

5.6*a*   Do sudden noises make you jump?

5.6*b*   Do you become afraid with sudden movements or noises at night?

5.6*c*   Do you often become sud-denly afraid for no good reason?

6   *Special preoccupations and experiences*

6.1   Obsessions, compulsions, and phobias   Neurotic manifestations

6.1*a*   Are there any thoughts that come to your mind over and over again and which you feel are abnormal?

Obsessions: uncontrollable thoughts

6.1*b*   Do you need to wash your hands very frequently to be clean?

6.1*c*   Do you return time after time to assure yourself that the light has been turned off? the door has been locked?

Compulsions: uncontrollable acts: in obsessive-compulsive neurosis; minor variations of this neurosis are extremely common

6.1*d*   Do you have irrational fears of animals? darkness? elevators? closed places?

Phobias: in phobic neurosis (mild phobias are frequent); the irrational nature of the uncontrollable thoughts, acts, or phobias is recognized by the neurotic patient

6.2   Hallucinations and

Perceptions of visual, auditory, olfactory, or tactile sensations without apparent external stimulation

   illusions

Misinterpretations of sounds, sights, smells, and other stimuli

May arise in states of altered consciousness, in sleep (dreaming); delirium; diseases of the sensory pathways or of the CNS; in certain psychotic states; in some disorders of the temporal lobes of the brain

6.2*a*   Do you hear (imaginary) voices or noises?

Hallucinations in schizophrenia are typically auditory (rarely visual)

6.2*b*   Do you sometimes hear things when other people do not?

6.2c Do you see things which you know are not there?

6.2d Have you ever had any unusual visions?

In organic mental syndromes

6.2e Do you have any unusual skin sensations?

May be attributed by the patient to worms, ants, bugs, etc (illusions)

6.3 Delusions

False belief in which the patient persists in spite of demonstrations of its falseness

6.3a Do you believe that people are trying to harm you?

6.3b Are people laughing at you or talking about you?

Paranoid schizophrenia syndrome

6.3c Do you believe that you have a great mission in life?

SELECTED BIBLIOGRAPHY

Cornell Medical Index: Health Questionnaire (C.M.I.), 1960
Mackinnon RA, Michels R: *The Psychiatric Interview in Clinical Practice,* Philadelphia: Saunders, 1971

33
Seizures

DEFINITION AND GENERAL CONSIDERATIONS

Seizure any abnormal motor, sensory, or psychic phenomenon which is abrupt in onset, of short duration, and followed by a return to normal. The term *epilepsies* encompasses convulsive disorders with loss of consciousness as well as nonconvulsive seizures with only slight alterations in awareness.

A seizure results from a sudden, excessive, disorderly discharge of neurons in either a structurally normal or diseased cortex. This arises from an instability of the neuronal membrane caused by an excess of excitation or a deficiency of normal inhibitory mechanisms.

Epilepsy may be due to various cerebral and systemic diseases (secondary or acquired epilepsy), or it may occur without demonstrable cause (idiopathic epilepsy). Focal (partial) seizures occur when there exists involvement of a specific region of the brain; they are typical of acquired epilepsy. Lesions involving any of the motor regions of the brain produce focal motor seizures. Focal sensory seizures are due to a lesion involving the sensory cortex. Autonomic seizures are caused by focal lesions in the deep temporal, limbic, and diencephalic areas. Psychomotor (temporal lobe) seizures are produced by lesions in the temporal lobe, the amygdala and hippocampus, and their associated limbic system structures. A focal-onset seizure can occasionally spread extremely rapidly throughout the brain to become generalized.

In idiopathic epilepsy, seizures are generalized from the onset, seemingly without focal origin; they begin with a loss of consciousness, presumably because of involvement of subcortical centers. Grand mal, petit mal, myoclonic seizures, and akinetic seizures are forms of generalized seizures. Status epilepticus is the rapid repetitive recurrence of seizures without recovery of consciousness between attacks.

ETIOLOGY

Idiopathic epilepsy
Severe birth trauma

Metabolic disorders: hypoglycemia; uremia; hypocalcemia; hypo-
natremia; water intoxication; alkalosis; hypoxia; liver coma;
porphyria; thyrotoxic storm; pyridoxine deficiency; alcoholism;
phenylketonuria
Intracranial infections: bacterial meningitis; encephalitis; cerebral
abscess; parasitic brain diseases (hydatid cyst, cysticercosis)
Cerebral traumatism, concussion of the brain
Subdural hematoma
Hypertensive encephalopathy; eclampsia; systemic lupus erythema-
tosus; polyarteritis nodosa
Intracranial neoplastic diseases: primary and metastatic tumors
Intracranial hemorrhage
Cerebral degenerative and developmental diseases: Alzheimer's dis-
ease; tuberous sclerosis; Sturge-Weber disease; hydrocephalus
Toxic substances: drugs; drug withdrawal; carbon monoxide poison-
ing; acute lead encephalopathy; immunizations
Syncopal attacks: Stokes-Adams syndrome; carotid sinus syndrome

Iatrogenic Causes of Seizures

Amphetamines	Lidocaine
Atropine	Penicillin
Imipramine, amitriptyline	Phenothiazines
Insulin	Tolbutamide
Isoniazid	Xanthine derivatives

Withdrawal from: barbiturates, other sedatives and tranquilizers; alcohol

QUESTIONNAIRE

Note: If the patient has amnesia for portions of the attack and is unable to
report what has occurred, careful questioning of the family and/or witnesses
to the attack is mandatory.

Possible *meaning of response*

1 Duration of the seizures

1.1 When did your seizures
appear for the first time?

• in childhood?   Birth injury; trauma; infections

- in adolescence? (age 10 to 18)

Idiopathic epilepsy; trauma; congenital defects

- in early adulthood? (18 to 35)

Trauma; neoplasm; idiopathic epilepsy; alcoholism; drug addiction

- in middle age? (35 to 60)

Neoplasm; trauma; vascular diseases; alcoholism; drug addiction

- in late life? (over 60)

Vascular disease; degenerative lesions; tumor

1.1*a*   What is the frequency of the seizures?

Important for treatment program; grand mal seizures may occur once or twice yearly to many times daily; in women, the seizures may appear with or immediately before the menstrual periods

2   *Location, spread, and character of the seizures*

2.1   Does the seizure consist of
- sudden twitching in the fingers or toes? the arm, or the leg, the face, on one side?

Focal motor seizure: initial cortical discharge in motor Rolandic cortex, area 4 on the opposite side

2.1*a*   Do these movements spread to the muscles of the extremity, the face, on the same side of the body?

"March" of epileptic discharge into adjacent parts of the cortex; the focal seizure may remain limited to the extremity

2.1*b*   Does this spread terminate in a general convulsion with loss of consciousness?

The focal seizure may spread rapidly to become generalized

2.2   Does the seizure consist of
- forced turning of the head and eyes?

Focal motor seizure, "adversive seizures": origin in the contralateral eye-turning fields (area 8)

2.2*a*   Does it terminate in a
general convulsion with
loss of consciousness?

2.3   Does the seizure consist of
- chewing, smacking of the
lips, swallowing, profuse
salivation?

Focal motor seizure; origin in
lower part of the motor strip
subserving mastication and salivation

2.3*a*   Does it terminate in a
general convulsion with
loss of consciousness?

2.4   Does the seizure consist of
- a tingling numbness of the
fingers? lips? toes?
some other part of the
body?

Focal sensory seizure; attack
arises in the sensory region:
post-Rolandic convolution of the
parietal lobe

2.4*a*   Does this sensation
spread to adjacent
parts of the body?

2.4*b*   Does it terminate in a
general convulsion with
loss of consciousness?

Any partial or focal seizure may
occur without further symptoms
or progress to a generalized
convulsion

2.5   Does the seizure consist of
- paroxysmal nausea,
vomiting?
- abdominal discomfort?
- excessive salivation?
sweating? trouble
breathing? palpitation?

Visceral (autonomic) seizures;
foci in frontotemporal, midfron-
tal, parasagittal, or insular areas
(mesial temporal)

2.5*a*   Does it terminate in a
general convulsion with
loss of consciousness?

2.6   Does the seizure consist of

• forced, compelled thinking?	Psychic seizure; lesion in the frontal lobe
• olfactory hallucinations?	Lesion near the uncus of the hippocampal gyrus, uncinate fits
• visual ("déjà vu") hallucinations?	Lesion in the occipital area
• auditory, vertiginous hallucinations?	Superior temporal area
• peculiar sensations of taste?	Lesion in upper surface of the temporal lobe

2.6*a*   Does it terminate in a general convulsion with loss of consciousness?

2.7   Does the seizure consist of activities being carried out in a state of impaired consciousness? out of contact with other people?

Psychomotor seizure with automatic behavior: temporal lobe, limbic system

2.8   Does the seizure consist of

• brief "absences" (10 to 45 s)?

• chewing, blinking movements? (three per second)

• without warning, convulsions, or fall?

Petit mal (minor motor) seizure (childhood and adolescence); origin in mesodiencephalic regions

2.9   Do you at times suddenly lose consciousness and fall motionless to the ground? (without convulsions)

"Akinetic attacks," closely related to petit mal; pronounced loss of muscle tone

2.10   Do you have a sudden loss of consciousness and generalized convulsions (without any of the warnings in 2.1 to 2.7)?

Grand mal seizure; may occur alone or may be preceded by a focal convulsive attack ("aura"); idiopathic epilepsy

2.10*a*   Have you been told that the seizure begins with
- a forceful fall to the ground?
- a cry?

"Tonic stage": contraction of diaphragm and chest muscles with forced expiration of air from the lungs

- *biting of the tongue?* inside of the cheeks?

The tongue is frequently caught between the teeth during the tonic stage

- *loss of urine? feces?*

Bladder and bowel may be emptied during the tonic stage

2.10*b*   How long does your attack last?

Habitual duration of convulsions ("clonic stage") less than 5 min

2.10*c*   How long does your period of unconsciousness last?

The coma may last for many minutes to ½ h

3   Precipitating or aggravating factors

3.1   Are your seizures precipitated
- by adjusting the TV? driving through trees in the sunshine? flickering lights?
- by sounds? music?

"Reflex" epilepsy, sensory-induced

- emotional tension? alcoholic drinks? menstrual periods?

Seizures may be related to these factors

4   Relieving factors

4.1   Do you take any drug for your seizures?

4.1*a*   How does medication influence your seizures?

With adequate therapy, most patients with occasional generalized and psychomotor seizures achieve complete or nearly complete reduction of seizures

5 *Accompanying symptoms*

5.1 Do you have any warning, minutes to hours before a seizure?
- apathy? depression?
- irritability? headache?

A prodromal phase of altered emotional reactivity may precede generalized seizures

5.2 *Do you have any warning (see 2.1 to 2.7) immediately prior to the attack?*

"Aura": provides the most reliable clue to the location of the underlying disease

5.3 After the attack, do you have
- mental confusion? headache? muscular pain?

Postictal symptoms

- a transitory (minutes to hours) weakness of an extremity?

Todd's postictal paralysis: seizure arising in a motor strip; focal brain lesion

- a transitory disorder of speech?

Postictal aphasia: attack occurring in the dominant hemisphere

5.4 When you awaken, are you aware of
- the eventual aura?
- your attack?

Patient may remember prodromal phase or aura, but is usually not aware of his attack

5.4*a* Do you regain full consciousness
- *slowly?* (minutes to hours)
- *promptly?*

Usual duration in epilepsy
Syncope

5.5 Do you have
- headaches? vomiting?
- disorders of speech? gait?
- weakness of an extremity?

Increased intracranial pressure: expanding intracranial mass; meningitis

- fever?

Brain abscess; meningitis; encephalitis

- blurred vision?

Hypertensive encephalopathy with altered fundi

• cough? bloody expectorations?	Bronchogenic carcinoma with cerebral metastases

6 *Iatrogenic factors*   see Etiology

7 *Environmental factors*

7.1 What is your occupation?	Occupational exposure to toxic products; patient's disease may require job alteration
7.2 Do you have any problems due to your seizures with your family? at school? professionally?	Patients with convulsive seizures have often emotional problems, usually in response to environmental restrictions

8 *Personal antecedents pertaining to the seizures*

8.1   Have you ever had an x-ray of your skull? an EEG? a brain scan? a lumbar puncture? When? With what results?

8.2 Did you ever hurt yourself from the fall during a seizure?	Injury may be sustained during the fall or may result from violent muscular contraction (crushed vertebra)

8.3   Have you had any of the following conditions: a birth trauma? a head trauma? meningitis? encephalitis? a cerebral vascular accident? (stroke)

• febrile seizures during childhood?	30 percent of those children may develop epilepsy later, without fever

8.4   Do you have any of the following conditions: arterial hypertension? a renal disease? drug abuse?

• diabetes?	Hypoglycemia: overdose of insulin
• alcoholism?	Alcohol withdrawal seizures in addicted individuals occur within 36 to 48 h after alcohol is stopped

9 *Family medical history pertaining to the seizures*

9.1 Are there other members of your family who have	The relatives of patients with idiopathic epilepsy have a 3 to 5

epilepsy? other neurologic disorders?

percent incidence of epilepsy (incidence in the ordinary population: 0.5 to 1.0 percent)

PHYSICAL SIGNS PERTINENT TO THE COMPLAINT

Finding	**Possible** *significance*
Focal neurologic deficit(s)	Localizing value; intracranial mass lesion: tumor, abscess; cerebral vascular lesion
Sixth nerve paralysis	Often associated with increased intracranial pressure
Fever	Brain abscess; meningitis; encephalitis
Stiff neck; fever	Bacterial meningitis
Ear infection	Brain abscess
Congenital heart disease with a right-to-left shunt	Brain abscess
Heart murmur; fever	Subacute bacterial endocarditis with cerebral embolism
Clubbing; abnormal lung examination	Bronchogenic carcinoma or lung abscess with metastatic tumor or abscess
Café-au-lait spots; pedunculated tumors	Von Recklinghausen's disease with intracranial glioma or neurofibroma
Sebaceous adenomas of the face; white spots over the trunk and limbs	Tuberous sclerosis
Craniofacial nevus	Sturge-Weber syndrome (with venous hemangioma of the leptomeninges and cerebral calcifications)
Funduscopic examination: Papilledema	Increased intracranial pressure: tumor, abscess
Papilledema, hemorrhages	Hypertensive encephalopathy

LABORATORY TESTS PERTAINING TO THE COMPLAINT

Procedure	To detect
Blood	
Fasting glucose	Hypoglycemia
Calcium	Hypocalcemic states
BUN, creatinine	Kidney disease
Electrolytes	Metabolic disturbances; dilutional hyponatremia
EEG	Petit mal; focal or generalized abnormalities of cortical activity (EEG may be normal in epilepsy)
Skull x-rays	Erosion of the clinoid processes (increased intracranial pressure); hyperostoses; abnormal vascular markings; intracranial calcifications
Brain scan	Intracranial mass lesions
Computerized tomography	Hemispheric mass; ventricular size and position; cerebral atrophy
Chest x-ray	Primary carcinoma of lung, frequently associated with cerebral metastases
Cerebral arteriogram	Ventricular size and position; position of cerebral vessels; abnormal vessels; herniation
Lumbar puncture*	Elevated cell count: CNS infection Increased pressure and protein: tumor

* If appropriate.

USEFUL REMINDERS AND DIAGNOSTIC CLUES

Misleading Factors

Generalized seizures may be confused with hysteria.
Akinetic seizures may be confused with syncope.
Temporal lobe seizures may be difficult to separate from acute psychotic episodes.

Diagnostic Considerations

Epilepsy
The various motor, sensory, or psychic phenomena may be combined in many different sequences, indicating the spread of a seizure discharge from one cortical area to another.
Seizures are one of the few motor disturbances which occur in sleep.
The appearance of impaired mental function in an epileptic patient should suggest: recurrent subclinical seizures not controlled by medication, drug intoxication, postseizure psychosis, subdural hematoma, or brain disease causing both dementia and seizures.

Miscellaneous

Between 30 and 40 percent of all patients with cerebral tumors have seizures; the seizure is the first symptom in 15 to 20 percent of cases.
Cerebral trauma gives rise to seizures in about 20 to 40 percent of cases; the average interval between the head injury and the first seizure is about 9 months.
Brain abscesses are followed by seizures in nearly 40 percent of cases.
Thrombotic strokes are rarely followed by recurrent seizures, in contrast with embolic cortical infarcts, where they occur in more than 20 percent of patients.
Thrombotic occlusions of cerebral arteries are almost never convulsive in the evolving phases of the stroke.
Convulsions appearing initially in adult life are likely to be manifestations of an intracranial neoplasm.

SELECTED BIBLIOGRAPHY

Adams RD, Victor M: Epilepsy and the convulsive states, in *Principles of Neurology*, pp 211–230, New York: McGraw-Hill, 1977
Glaser GH: The epilepsies, in Beeson PB, McDermott W, *Textbook of Medicine*, 14th ed, pp 723–734, Philadelphia: Saunders, 1975
Schmidt PP, Wilder BJ: *Epilepsy*, Philadelphia: Davis, 1968
Singer HS, Freeman JM: Seizures in adolescents. Med Clin North Am 59: 1461–1472, 1975

34
Sleep Disorders

DEFINITIONS AND GENERAL CONSIDERATIONS

Sleep a state of physical and mental inactivity from which the patient may be aroused to normal consciousness.

Insomnia any impairment in the duration, depth, or restorative properties of sleep.

Hypersomnia excessive sleepiness.

There are two kinds of sleep: the REM sleep and the NREM (non-REM) sleep. The REM sleep is characterized by tumultuous brain activity, rapid eye movements (REM), and simultaneous muscular paralysis (paradoxical sleep). The NREM sleep lacks rapid eye movements; it is divided into four separate stages on the basis of the EEG record; during NREM sleep the brain is resting. In a normal individual NREM sleep always comes first. The first NREM period lasts for about 60 min and then is followed by about 10 min of REM sleep, making a "sleep cycle" of one NREM period and one REM period totaling about 70 min. The subsequent cycles are longer (90 to 120 min). Five sleep cycles represent an average night's sleep. About three-fourths of the night are spent in NREM sleep. Cerebral oxygen metabolism, which is always depressed with coma or anesthesia, remains equivalent to waking levels during natural sleep.

In idiopathic (primary) insomnia, there appears to be a primary disturbance of the normal sleep mechanism. Patients with this condition sleep for shorter periods than normal subjects, awaken more often, and spend less time in REM sleep and more in stage 2 NREM sleep than the good sleepers. The majority of cases of insomnia are secondary to psychologic disturbances or are associated with another disease, including any condition in which pain and physical discomfort are important symptoms.

Narcoleptic patients are subject to either complete or partial sleep attacks which begin with REM sleep rather than with the usual NREM sleep observed in normal subjects. In contrast to narcolepsy, the excessive sleep of hypersomnia is not irresistible but is usually much longer (hours to days). The sleep-stage pattern of hypersomniac patients resembles normal sleep except in terms of duration. Hypersomnia may be primary or, more often, secondary to organic neurologic or metabolic diseases.

ETIOLOGY

Insomnia
Primary (idiopathic)
Secondary to psychologic disorder: anxiety, fear, depression
Associated with medical disorders or physical discomfort: acute infection, coronary artery disease, duodenal ulcer, bronchial asthma, hyperthyroidism, pregnancy, cluster headache, acroparesthesias, restless-leg syndrome, nocturnal myoclonus
Sleep apnea
Drug dependency; drug withdrawal

Hypersomnia
Primary (idiopathic)
Periodic: narcolepsy; Kleine-Levin syndrome (in adolescent males); Pickwickian (obesity-hypoventilation) syndrome; sleep apnea
Chronic:
  Central nervous system lesion: head injury, brain tumor, encephalitis, cerebrovascular disorder
  Metabolic disorders: obesity, carbon dioxide retention, hepatic encephalopathy, hypothyroidism, uremia, pituitary insufficiency, drug dependency, surreptitious taking of drugs

Conditions causing sleep disorders
Night terror; nightmares; enuresis; nocturnal epilepsy; somnambulism

Iatrogenic Causes of:

Insomnia: caffeine; analeptics, amphetamine
Drug-dependent and drug-withdrawal insomnia: barbiturates; gluthetimide; methyprylon; ethchlorvynol
Hypersomnia; barbiturates; hypnotics; tranquilizers

QUESTIONNAIRE

Possible *meaning of response*

Insomnia

1   *Duration*

1.1   How long have you been unable to sleep at night?

Lifelong history: primary insomnia

2   *Character of insomnia*

2.1   How many hours do you sleep at night?

Insomniac's description of amount of sleep is a poor indication of the situation

2.2   Do you have difficulty in
• falling asleep? ⎫
• staying asleep? ⎬

Frequent in <u>anxiety</u> and fear states; also in debilitating or painful illness

2.3   *Do you fall asleep easily but wake up in the early morning?*

Has been said to be typical of <u>depression</u> (this rule is undependable); also in the elderly: frequently reflects a declining need for sleep

(Note: The patterns 2.2 and 2.3 may appear singly or in combination.)

3   *Precipitating or aggravating factors*

3.1   Do you engage in strenuous physical activity during the day?

Excessive fatigue may give rise to abnormal muscular sensations which delay the onset of sleep

3.2   Do you engage in vigorous mental activity late at night?

A cause of difficulty in falling asleep

3.3   Do you drink much coffee? tea? alcohol? in the afternoon? before retiring?

Stimulants producing insomnia

3.4   At night, do you have
• pain?

The pain may keep the patient awake

• in the spine?

Vertebral lesion

• in the abdomen?	Patients with duodenal ulcer secrete 3 to 20 times more gastric acid at night during REM sleep than normal subjects do
• in the chest?	Nocturnal angina pectoris (during REM sleep)
• shortness of breath?	Unrecognized orthopnea due to heart disease; asthmatic attack
• frequent disturbing dreams? • cough? pruritus? diarrhea? tinnitus? nocturia?	Any of these conditions may awaken the patient

3.5 *Are you awakened about 2 to 3 h after falling asleep by headaches?* (unilateral? orbital?)

Cluster headache

3.6 Do you take naps frequently during the day?

Frequent in senile and arteriosclerotic patients

3.7 Are you sometimes aroused by twitching in your legs?

Nocturnal myoclonus

3.8 At night, do you feel tired, aching legs?

3.8*a* Does this sensation disappear on moving about?

"Restless-legs syndrome": may delay the onset of sleep

4 Accompanying symptoms

4.1 Do you feel
  • anxious? depressed?
  • a loss of sex drive?

Insomnia secondary to psychologic disorder

4.2 Do you have
  • heat intolerance? palpitations? weight loss? excessive sweating?

Hyperthyroidism: may produce insomnia

5 Iatrogenic factors   see Etiology

6 *Personal antecedents pertaining to the insomnia*

6.1 Do you have
- personal, familial, professional problems?
- a psychiatric condition?

Psychoneuroses and psychoses commonly produce sleeplessness

Hypersomnia

1 *Duration and character*

1.1 How long have you felt sleepy all day?

Of recent onset: structural nervous system disease

1.2 *Do you have recurrent attacks of irresistible sleep?*
- at any time of the day?
- since adolescence?

1.2*a* Do you awaken refreshed after the attack of sleep?

Narcolepsy

2 *Accompanying symptoms*

2.1 Do you sometimes experience
- a sudden loss of muscle power provoked by strong emotions? anger? laughter?

Cataplexy: in about 70 percent of narcoleptic patients

- when falling asleep:
  - an inability to move or speak?
  - visual or auditory hallucinations?

Sleep paralysis in narcolepsy (25 to 30 percent)

Hypnagogic hallucinations in narcolepsy (25 to 30 percent)

2.2 Do you have
- attacks of excessive sleepiness

• with excessive eating?	Kleine-Levin syndrome (in adolescent males)
• with obesity?	Pickwickian (obesity-hypoventilation) syndrome
• headaches? vomiting? loss of muscular strength in a limb?	Brain tumor (a central nervous system lesion may produce chronic hypersomnia)
• intolerance to cold?	Hypothyroidism, if severe, may cause hypersomnia

3 Personal antecedents pertaining to the hypersomnia

3.1 Have you ever had a head injury? a brain inflammation? encephalitis?	CNS lesion producing hypersomnia

4 Family medical history pertaining to the hypersomnia

4.1 Are there similar cases in your family?	Narcolepsy has a genetic basis (single dominant)

PHYSICAL SIGNS PERTINENT TO THE COMPLAINT

Finding	**Possible** *significance*
Enlarged thyroid; warm, moist skin; tachycardia; proptosis	Hyperthyroidism with insomnia
Periorbital puffiness; cold coarse skin; delayed relaxation phase of the tendon reflexes	Hypothyroidism with sleepiness
Obesity; cyanosis; periodic respiration; drowsiness	Hypoventilation-obesity ("Pickwickian") syndrome with somnolence
Neurologic abnormalities	Structural brain lesion causing hypersomnia
Funduscopic examination: papilledema	Increased intracranial pressure: CNS lesion with hypersomnia

LABORATORY TESTS PERTAINING TO THE COMPLAINT

Procedure	*To detect*
Polygraphic sleep recording*	Sleep apnea; idiopathic insomnia; narcolepsy
EEG	Structural brain lesion producing hypersomnia
Psychologic evaluation*	Anxiety state; depression

* If appropriate.

USEFUL REMINDERS AND DIAGNOSTIC CLUES

In healthy adults sleep has a mean duration of about 8 h; women sleep more than men.

The pattern of insomnia helps relatively little in estimating its seriousness as a symptom.

Direct observation on patients suffering from insomnia almost always reveals that they are less wakeful than they think.

There is little evidence that chronic insomnia takes any physical toll.

SELECTED BIBLIOGRAPHY

Adams RD, Victor M: Sleep and its abnormalities, in *Principles of Neurology*, pp 241–255, New York: McGraw-Hill, 1977

Dement WC, Guilleminault C: Sleep disorders: The state of the art. Hosp Pract 8:57–71, 1973

Kales A, Kales JD: Sleep disorders. N Engl J Med 290:487–499, 1974

35
Syncope

DEFINITIONS AND PATHOPHYSIOLOGY

Syncope (faint)   generalized weakness of muscles with inability to stand upright and impairment of consciousness, of brief duration and with complete recovery within a few minutes.

Faintness (incomplete faint)   lack of strength with a sensation of impending faint.

Syncope results from a transient impairment in cerebral metabolism as a consequence of essential energy substrates (oxygen and glucose) deprivation. This deprivation may be due to a decrease in cerebral blood flow or to insufficient concentration of oxygen or glucose in the blood perfusing the brain. Decreased cerebral blood flow may be caused by arterial hypotension, diminished cardiac output, or obstruction to cerebral blood flow. A decrease in blood pressure may result from a decrease in peripheral resistance induced by decreased sympathetic stimulation (vasodepressor syncope, orthostatic hypotension) or by vasodilator drugs. In the ordinary vasodepressor syncope the loss of consciousness usually occurs when the systolic pressure falls to 70 mmHg or below. Cardiac output may be reduced as a consequence of decreased stroke volume (diminished cardiac contractility, decreased cardiac filling), arrhythmias, or anatomic obstructive lesions (aortic stenosis, pulmonary hypertension). Cerebral arterial obstruction generally due to arteriosclerosis is one of the less common causes of syncope. An inadequate oxygen or glucose concentration in the blood delivered to the brain may cause loss of consciousness which generally persists longer than in the other types of syncope. More than one mechanism may be involved in syncope. Hyperventilation with resulting hypocapnia simultaneously produces cerebral vasoconstriction and peripheral vasodilation. Carotid sinus hypersensitivity may occur in a cardioinhibitory (bradycardia) type, a vasodepressor (hypotension without bradycardia) type, and a possible rare central (without bradycardia) type.

Syncope is usually due to processes external to the central nervous system. Vasovagal (vasodepressor) syncopes, cardiac arrhythmias, and postural hypotension are the commonest causes.

ETIOLOGY

Circulatory
Reduced quantity of blood to the brain

Decreased total peripheral resistance (defective vasoconstrictor mechanisms)
  Vasovagal (vasodepressor) syncope
  Postural hypotension: idiopathic orthostatic hypotension; post-sympathectomy, drugs; prolonged standing; micturition syncope; disease of peripheral and central nervous system (diabetes, tabes dorsalis, syringomyelia); carotid sinus hypersensitivity
Hypovolemia: bleeding, external or internal; sodium loss
Arrhythmias
  Bradyarrhythmias: atrioventricular block (Stokes-Adams attacks); tachycardia-bradycardia syndrome; sinus bradycardia; carotid sinus hypersensitivity
  Tachyarrhythmias: supraventricular and ventricular tachycardias
Reduced cardiac output
  Obstructive lesions: aortic stenosis; idiopathic hypertrophic subaortic stenosis; atrial myxoma; pulmonary stenosis; pulmonary hypertension; pulmonary embolism
  Myocardial infarction
  Cardiac tamponade
Obstruction to cerebral blood flow
  Cerebrovascular accident (thrombosis, embolus); transient ischemic attacks
  Tussive (cough) syncope; hypertensive encephalopathy

Defective quality of blood to the brain
Hypoxia; anemia; hypoglycemia

Emotional disturbances
Hyperventilation, anxiety states; hysterical seizures

Iatrogenic Causes of Syncope

Anticoagulants: acute internal hemorrhage
Antihypertensive drugs: guanethidine, alpha methyldopa, reserpine, propranolol, diuretics (sodium loss and hypovolemia)
Digitalis: heart block, drug-induced tachyarrhythmia
Insulin, oral hypoglycemic agents; L-dopa
Nitrites, nitrates; tranquilizers: vasodilating
Quinidine: episodes of ventricular tachycardia or fibrillation

QUESTIONNAIRE

Note: The following questions apply to recurrent syncopes as well as to a single episode of unconsciousness.

	Possible *meaning of response*
1　Mode of onset and duration	
1.1　When did your syncope occur?	
1.1*a*　What precisely were you doing?	Most syncope occurs when the patient is in the upright position (exception: Stokes-Adams attacks)
1.2　Do you have recurrent episodes of syncope?	See p. 377.
1.2*a*　In case of recurrent episodes of unconsciousness: How long and how frequently have you had syncopes?	Several per day, per month: epilepsy, Stokes-Adams attacks
1.3　Is the onset of the syncope	
• abrupt? (a period of a few seconds)	**Stokes-Adams attacks;** carotid sinus syncope; chronic orthostatic hypotension; epilepsy; cerebrovascular disease
• gradual? (several minutes)	Vasodepressor syncope; hyperventilation; **hypoglycemia**
1.4　Do you lose consciousness?	True syncope

1.5 Do you feel faint, without loss of consciousness?	Faintness: <u>anxiety</u>; hyperventilation; hypoglycemia; cerebral ischemic attacks; hysteria
1.6 What is the duration of the unconsciousness?	
• a few seconds to a few minutes?	<u>Vasodepressor syncope</u>; carotid sinus syncope; <u>postural hypotension</u>
• more than a few minutes? (but less than 1 h)	Aortic stenosis; hysteria; hypoglycemia; hyperventilation

2 *Precipitating or aggravating factors*

2.1 Does the syncope occur	
• *in an upright position?*	<u>Postural syncope</u> and most others
• in a standing, sitting position?	Syncopal attacks characteristically occur in erect position; <u>vasodepressor syncope</u>; paroxysmal tachycardia; carotid sinus attack
• *upon suddenly arising from a recumbent to a standing position?* • *after prolonged standing?*	Postural hypotension; chronic orthostatic hypotension
• *in the recumbent position?* • independently of your position? • in any body position?	Most probably not vasodepressor syncope; cardiac origin of the syncope, Stokes-Adams attacks; hypoglycemia; hyperventilation; hypertensive encephalopathy; akinetic epileptic seizure
• *when leaning over?* (as to tie a shoe lace)	Left atrial myxoma; ball-valve thrombus
• *during or immediately after exertion?*	Aortic stenosis; idiopathic hypertrophic subaortic stenosis; primary pulmonary hypertension; tachycardia; in elderly subjects: postural hypotension
• in the fasting state?	Hypoglycemia

• 2 to 5 h after eating?	Reactive hypoglycemia (faintness)
• *following an emotional stress?* (fright, anxiety, pain)	Vasodepressor syncope; hyperventilation
• during micturition?	A form of postural syncope, usually seen in the elderly
• after a paroxysm of coughing?	In overweight men with chronic obstructive lung disease: "tussive syncope" (increased intrathoracic pressure interfering with the venous return to the heart)
• on sudden movements of the head? • when wearing a tight collar? shaving the neck?	Carotid sinus syncope

3   Relieving factors

3.1   Can you avert an impending faint by

• *promptly lying down?*	Vasodepressor syncope; postural syncope
• eating?	Hypoglycemia

4   Accompanying symptoms

4.1   Is the syncope preceded by

• *nausea? sweating?* yawning? giddiness? dim vision? ringing in the ears?	Autonomic hyperactivity preceding <u>vasodepressor syncope</u>
• palpitations?	Arrhythmia; hypoglycemia; hyperventilation
• chest pain?	Cardiac origin of syncope
• deep sighing? • numbness, tingling in the extremities?	Hyperventilation
• a sensation of hunger? weakness? mental confusion? sweating?	Hypoglycemia (faintness rather than true syncope)

• aphasia? unilateral weakness? confusion?	Cerebrovascular disease
4.1a *Do you have no warning of any sort before the fainting spell?*	Stokes-Adams syndrome; arrhythmia; aortic stenosis; idiopathic orthostatic hypotension; carotid sinus syncope; epileptic attack
4.2 After the beginning of the unconsciousness	
• do you lie motionless?	Usually in syncope
• do you have	
• convulsive movements?	Epilepsy; heart block; hypertensive encephalopathy
• loss of urine? feces? • biting of the tongue?	Frequent in epilepsy, rare in syncope
4.3 Do you regain full consciousness	
• *promptly?*	Syncope
• slowly?	Epilepsy
4.4 Following a syncopal attack, do you have	
• headache? drowsiness? mental confusion?	Common in epilepsy; may occur in the postsyncopal state; slight confusion in Stokes-Adams attacks
• a slurred speech? transitory paralysis?	Epilepsy; may occur in Stokes-Adams syndrome; cerebral arterial occlusive disease
4.5 Prior to, or after the faint, did you notice the passage of black, tarry stools?	**Acute gastrointestinal hemorrhage** with syncope

5 *Iatrogenic factors*   see Etiology

6 *Personal antecedents pertaining to the faint*

6.1 Did you ever sustain injury when falling to the ground during a fainting spell?	May occur in epilepsy; rare in syncope; absent in hysteria

6.2   Do you have any of the following conditions: epilepsy? any
      neurologic disease? hypertension? a cardiac disease?

• diabetes?	Iatrogenic hypoglycemia; diabetic neuropathy may cause postural hypotension
• Parkinson's disease?	Shy-Drager syndrome with chronic orthostatic hypotension

7   *Family medical history pertaining to the complaint*

7.1 Are there members of your family who have epilepsy?	The relatives of patients with idiopathic epilepsy have a 3 to 5 percent incidence of epilepsy (incidence in the ordinary population: 0.5 to 1.0 percent)

PHYSICAL SIGNS PERTINENT TO THE COMPLAINT

Finding	**Possible** *significance*
Pallor without cyanosis	An early finding in all types of syncope, except chronic orthostatic hypotension and hysteria; disorder of the peripheral circulation
Pallor, cyanosis, dyspnea, distended jugular veins	Disorder of cardiac function with reduced cerebral blood flow
Bradycardia	Complete atrioventricular (AV) block (heart rate <40 beats per minute) with Stokes-Adams attacks; sick-sinus syndrome; vasodepressor syncope
Bradycardia, variable intensity of first sound	Complete AV block
Tachycardia (>160 beats per minute)	Ectopic cardiac rhythm; paroxysmal tachycardia
Response of blood pressure and pulse rate to standing:	

Orthostatic hypotension
With unchanged pulse rate   Dysfunction of the autonomic nervous system; chronic orthostatic hypotension

With increased pulse rate   Hypovolemia: diuretics, salt and water deprivation, adrenal insufficiency

Heart murmurs   Aortic stenosis; idiopathic hypertrophic subaortic stenosis; tetralogy of Fallot; primary pulmonary hypertension; left atrial myxoma; ball-valve thrombus

Muscle weakness; depressed or absent deep-tendon reflexes   Neuropathy with chronic orthostatic hypotension

Focal neurologic deficits, dysarthria, carotid bruits   Cerebral arterial occlusive disease with ischemic attacks

Tremor, ataxia, rigidity, pupillary paralysis, anhydrosis   Shy-Drager syndrome with chronic orthostatic hypotension

Tachycardia, sweating, tremulousness   Hypoglycemia

Rectal examination   May reveal gastrointestinal hemorrhage

Voluntary hyperventilation   May reveal hyperventilation

Carotid sinus massage (with caution)   May reveal carotid sinus hypersensitivity

LABORATORY TESTS PERTAINING TO THE COMPLAINT

Procedure	Finding	Diagnostic possibilities
Blood		
Fasting glucose (N: 60 to 100 mg/100 mL)	Elevated	Diabetes mellitus with autonomic neuropathy and postural hypotension

Fasting glucose	Low ⎫	Hypoglycemic epi-
Glucose tolerance test	Abnormal ⎭	sodes

Procedure	*To detect*
ECG	Complete AV block with Stokes-Adams attacks
Long-term electro-cardiographic monitoring	Arrhythmias responsible for the syncopal episodes
His bundle electro-gram*	Transient AV block; sinus node dysfunction
Echocardiography*	Idiopathic hypertrophic subaortic stenosis; left atrial myxoma
EEG	Epilepsy vs. syncope

* If appropriate.

USEFUL REMINDERS AND DIAGNOSTIC CLUES

Misleading Factor

Complete heart block may be transient; by the time a patient with Stokes-Adams syndrome reaches the hospital, normal atrioventricular conduction may have been restored.

Diagnostic Considerations

Vasodepressor syncope is the most frequent cause of transient loss of consciousness.

In Stokes-Adams syndrome 4 to 8 s of asystole produces coma in the erect position, and 12 to 15 s is required in recumbency; if cardiac standstill is more than 12 s the patient may exhibit a few clonic jerks.

Hysteria almost never begins for the first time in patients over 20 to 25 years old; the diagnosis of hysterical faintings in the middle-aged or elderly is risky.

In case of	*Suspect*
Recurrent syncopes in	
• Young adults	Vasodepressor syncope; epilepsy; hypoglycemia; postural hypotension; hysteria
• Middle-aged and elderly	Complete heart block; aortic stenosis; arrhythmia; pulmonary emboli; postural hypotension; cerebral arterial disease; cough and micturition syncope
Fainting episodes in a young woman showing little concern about them	Hysteria
Unexplained syncope with acute respiratory distress	Pulmonary embolism

SELECTED BIBLIOGRAPHY

Adams RD, Victor M: Faintness and syncope, in *Principles of Neurology,* pp 231–240, New York: McGraw-Hill, 1977

Lee JE, Killip III T, Plum F: Episodic unconsciousness, in Barondess JA (ed), *Diagnostic Approaches to Presenting Syndromes,* pp 133–166, Baltimore: Williams & Wilkins, 1971

Noble RJ: The patient with syncope. JAMA 237:1372–1376, 1976

Weissler AM, Warren JV: Syncope and shock, in Hurst JW (ed), *The Heart,* 3d ed, pp 570–580, New York: McGraw-Hill, 1974

36
Vertigo

DEFINITIONS AND PATHOPHYSIOLOGY

Vertigo sense of "turning" either of one's body or of the surroundings; the term should be restricted to an illusion of movement.

Pseudovertigo (*giddiness*) sensation of uncertainty, light-headedness, without a feeling of rotation or impulsion.

Impulses from the retinas, the labyrinths, the proprioceptors of joints and muscles maintain balanced posture and awareness of the body's position in relation to its surroundings. The cerebellum, the vestibular nuclei, the oculomotor nucleus and the red nucleus in the brainstem, and certain ganglionic centers in the basal ganglia integrate these sensory data and provide for postural adjustment and locomotion.

Generally the problem of vertigo resolves itself into deciding whether it has its origin in the labyrinth, in the vestibular division of the eighth cranial nerve, or in the vestibular nuclei and their immediate connections with other structures in the brainstem. Labyrinthine lesions are the usual causes of paroxysmal vertigo (Ménière's disease, vestibular neuronitis). Vertigo of acoustic nerve origin (acoustic neuroma) is usually mild and intermittent. The association of vertigo with auditory signs and symptoms indicates an aural or eighth nerve lesion. In vertigo of brainstem origin, auditory function is nearly always spared, since the vestibular and cochlear fibers separate upon entering the medulla and pons. Central causes of vertigo are associated with signs of involvement of other structures within the brain.

Giddiness (pseudovertigo) is frequently of circulatory or psychologic origin.

ETIOLOGY

Vertigo

Otologic
  Ménière's disease; Bárány's positional vertigo; vestibular neuronitis

Tumors of middle and inner ear; cholesteatoma
Motion sickness
Ototoxic drugs
Otitis media; labyrinthitis; impacted cerumen
Neurologic
  Cerebellopontine angle tumor (acoustic neuroma)
  Brainstem tumors; cerebellar tumors
  Degenerative and demyelinating diseases; multiple sclerosis
  Vascular: vertebrobasilar insufficiency
  Infectious conditions: brain abscess; aseptic meningoencephalitis
  Convulsive disorders
  Migraine-like syndromes
  Cervical origin: neck trauma; upper cervical sensory root irritation
  Ocular disturbances; ocular muscle paralysis

Pseudovertigo   (without sensation of motion)
Psychogenic: tension-anxiety states; hyperventilation syndrome; introspective persons
Systemic:
  Cardiac diseases; paroxysmal atrial fibrillation
  Hypertension; postural dizziness (unstable vasomotor reflexes)
  Hyperactive carotid reflex
  Anemia; emphysema; posttraumatic

Iatrogenic Causes of Vertigo or Giddiness

Antihypertensive drugs (particularly guanethidine)
Dilantin (toxic doses)
Gentamycin, streptomycin, kanamycin

Minocycline
Neomycin
Quinine
Salicylates (large doses)

QUESTIONNAIRE

Possible *meaning of response*

1 Character of the complaint

1.1 During your dizzy spell, do you feel

• *a rotating sensation?* • *a rotation of your surroundings?* • *a sensation of lateral pulsion when walking?*	True vertigo: a rotational sensation and a feeling of impulsion are particularly characteristic of vertigo

2   *Mode of onset and chronology*

2.1 How long have you had dizzy spells?

Acute process: lesion of middle ear; basilar insufficiency

2.2 Do you have
• repeated episodes of vertigo?

Acute and recurrent peripheral vestibulopathy; chronicity: Ménière's disease; positional vertigo of Bárány

If single attack: acute etiology, inflammation or infection of middle ear; vestibular neuronitis

• persistent dizziness?

Chronic suppurative otitis with labyrinthine fistula

2.3 How long does an episode of dizziness last?
• a few seconds?

Almost always related to a change of position: anoxia of labyrinth due to vascular insufficiency (?)

• from minutes to hours?

Labyrinthine disease; Ménière's disease

• from hours to days?

Vestibular neuronitis; Ménière's disease

• for days to weeks?

Chronic suppurative otitis with labyrinthine fistula; acoustic neuroma; toxic labyrinthitis; brainstem origin

2.4 Is the onset of your dizzy spell
• *abrupt?*

Usually in true vertigo; labyrinthitis

• gradual?

Pseudovertigo

3 *Intensity of the complaint*

3.1 Is your attack of vertigo

•usually mild? Acoustic neuroma

• severe? Ménière's disease

3.2 Does your dizziness pro- Acoustic neuroma
gress gradually in in-
tensity?

4 *Precipitating or aggravating factors*

4.1 Do you have dizziness

• only on change of position? Benign positional vertigo (for a
on rolling over in bed? few seconds)

• *on abrupt arising from a* Postural dizziness (without a
recumbent or sitting position? feeling of rotation or impulse):
may occur in normal persons or
in individuals in poor physical
condition, in many elderly persons, in persons convalescing
from debilitating illness

• on standing? Postural dizziness with orthostatic hypotension

• on sudden head move- Benign positional vertigo; other
ments? on stooping over? vestibular disorders in which
vertigo is present at other times;
vascular insufficiency, vertebral-
basilar involvement

5 *Accompanying symptoms*

5.1 Is your dizzy spell
accompanied by

• nausea? vomiting? head-
aches?

• *a need to keep the head im-* Usually in true vertigo of laby-
mobile? rinthine origin (also in vertigo
of acoustic neuroma)

• *disturbances of balance?*

- a feeling of unsteadiness? light-headedness?
- choking? tingling around the mouth, in the fingers?
- sweating? anxiety?
- *a decreased hearing? tinnitus?*

Giddiness: pseudovertigo

Hyperventilation: in depressed or anxious patients

Disease of the ear or of the auditory nerve and its central connections; labyrinthine vertigo; Ménière's disease; acoustic neuroma (vestibular neuronitis: no tinnitus or deafness)

5.1a Do you sometimes fall to the ground, without loss of consciousness?

May occur in abrupt and severe attack of vertigo

5.2 Do you have
- double vision?
- difficulty swallowing? loss of strength? numbness?
- a decreased hearing, tinnitus, present for months before the vertigo?
- disturbances of gait?

Multiple sclerosis
Brainstem origin of vertigo

Ménière's disease; acoustic neuroma

Acoustic nerve origin; labyrinthine origin

6 *Iatrogenic factors* see Etiology

7 *Personal antecedents pertaining to the vertigo*

7.1 Do you have any of the following conditions:
- a neurologic disease? an ear condition? hypertension? anemia?
- a past cranial trauma?

May be followed by persistent or positional vertigo (traumatic labyrinthine vertigo)

- a recent neck trauma?

Cervicogenic vertigo: the articulations and musculature of the cervical region provide extensive input to the brainstem vestibular system

PHYSICAL SIGNS PERTINENT TO THE COMPLAINT

Finding	**Possible** *significance*
Nystagmus; hearing loss; disturbed balance; unsteadiness of gait; no other neurologic findings	Labyrinthine vertigo (hearing is normal in benign positional vertigo, vestibular neuronitis)
Hearing loss; facial weakness (fifth, sixth, seventh nerves); disturbed balance; ipsilateral ataxia of the limbs; nystagmus	Acoustic neuroma (cerebellopontine angle tumor) (with tinnitus)
Café-au-lait spots; neurofibromas	Unilateral or bilateral acoustic neuromas are common in neurofibromatosis
Nystagmus; involvement of cranial nerves, motor and sensory tracts; dysequilibrium; hearing spared	Central cause of vertigo, brainstem origin (no tinnitus): cerebrovascular disease; multiple sclerosis
Examination of the ear	May reveal: otitis media; perforated tympanic membrane

LABORATORY TESTS PERTAINING TO THE COMPLAINT

Procedure	*Finding*	*Diagnostic possibilities*
Caloric and rotational testing	Abnormal	Vestibular dysfunction: lesion of labyrinth, vestibular nerve, central vestibular connections
Audiometry	Normal	Brainstem lesion
	Abnormal	Lesion of the middle ear, labyrinth, cochlear nerve: Ménière's disease; cerebellopontine angle tumors

Procedure	*To detect*
Skull x-rays and tomograms	Erosion of internal auditory meatus: acoustic neuroma
Cervical spine x-rays	Cervical spondylosis with possible cervicogenic vertigo
EEG, brain scan, computerized tomography*	Intracranial lesions; temporal lobe mass lesions; posterior fossa lesions

* If appropriate.

USEFUL REMINDERS AND DIAGNOSTIC CLUES

Misleading Factors

Equilibrium is deranged in vertigo, but it may be affected by other disorders: loss of joint or muscle sense, cerebellar disease, and motor abnormalities.

Diagnostic Considerations

In vertiginous ataxia (ataxia of gait with vertigo), the coordination of individual movements of the limbs is normal, a point of difference from most instances of cerebellar diseases.

Loss of consciousness as part of a vertiginous attack rarely occurs and usually signifies another category of disorder, such as syncope or seizure.

Vertical nystagmus accompanying vertigo nearly always indicates disease of the brainstem.

When a young person has a severe and protracted attack of vertigo without auditory symptoms, suspect a demyelinative lesion.

Pure vertigo as a manifestation of disease of the brainstem is rare.

If a sense of motion cannot be established, the patient should be described as having dizziness rather than vertigo.

SELECTED BIBLIOGRAPHY

Adams RD, Victor M: Deafness, dizziness, vertigo, and disorders of equilibrium, in *Principles of Neurology*, pp 178–192, New York: McGraw-Hill, 1977

Drachman DA, Hart CW: An approach to the dizzy patient. Neurology 22: 323–334, 1972

Hood NA: Cerebral atherosclerosis, transient ischaemic attacks, Ménière's disease, and disorders of balance. Br Med J 4:398–400, 1975

37
Weakness

DEFINITIONS AND GENERAL CONSIDERATIONS

Weakness   reduction in the maximum force of muscular contraction and in muscular force on repeated contraction.

Motor paralysis   loss of function of voluntary muscles due to interruption of one of the motor pathways from the cerebrum to the muscle fiber. *Paresis* is a lesser, slight degree of paralysis.

Hemiplegia   paralysis of an arm and leg on one side of the body.

Monoplegia   paralysis of all the muscles in one arm or leg.

Paraplegia   paralysis of both legs.

The stimulus for voluntary movement originates in the cerebral cortex. The motor impulse passes from the motor cortex down the corticospinal tract to the anterior horn cell of the spinal cord and thence down the motor nerves to the neuromuscular junction and to the muscle. Muscle tone and movement are also influenced by the effect of the extrapyramidal, cerebellar, and proprioceptive pathways on the anterior horn cells. Motor dysfunction may result from involvement of the upper motor neuron (motor cortex and corticospinal tract), the lower motor neuron (anterior horn cell and motor nerve), the neuromuscular junction, and the muscle fibers. A lesion of the upper motor neuron affects muscle groups diffusely and is associated with spasticity, increased tendon reflexes, clonus, extensor plantar reflex, and no or slight atrophy due to disuse. Lesions of the lower motor neuron may affect individual muscles and are accompanied by marked atrophy, flaccidity, loss of tendon reflexes, and normal plantar reflex, if present; muscular twitchings may be present. Sensory changes are generally absent when the lesion is localized to the anterior horn cell (progressive muscular atrophies) or anterior roots, and are usually present when the lesion is in the peripheral nerves (neuropathies). Weakness may be due to disorders of the neuromuscular junction (myasthenia gravis). It appears that the defect in myasthenia gravis results from partial blockade of nicotinic acetylcholine receptors at the neuromuscular junction by circulating IgG antibodies. Diseases affecting muscle fibers without interfering with their nerve supply (myopathies) also result in weakness with atrophy, flaccidity, and decreased tendon reflexes; sensory loss and fasciculations are absent. In contrast to neuropathies, myopathies are associated with normal nerve conductions; serum enzymes [creatine phosphokinase (CPK), lactic dehydrogenase (LDH), serum glutamic oxalacetic transaminase (SGOT), and aldolase] are usually elevated.

Weakness must be distinguished from fatigue, a subjective sense of loss of energy. The loss of strength of true weakness can generally be demonstrated objectively.

ETIOLOGY

Central nervous system lesions

Vascular; tumor; infection; trauma; demyelinating; hereditary

Anterior horn cells
Poliomyelitis; syringomyelitis; amyotrophic lateral sclerosis; tumor; myelitis; trauma

Neuropathies
Nutritional: alcoholism; malnutrition; pellagra; pernicious anemia; chronic gastrointestinal disease; postgastrectomy conditions
Malignancy: carcinoma of lung; lymphoma; multiple myeloma
Connective-tissue disease: polyarteritis nodosa; systemic lupus erythematosus; rheumatoid arthritis
Metabolic and endocrine disorders: diabetes mellitus; uremia; porphyria; amyloidosis; macroglobulinemia; acromegaly; myxedema
Toxins; heavy metals (lead, arsenic, thallium, mercury); organophosphate compounds; industrial poisons; drugs
Inflammatory states: serum sickness; acute idiopathic polyneuritis (Guillain-Barré syndrome); sarcoidosis
Infections: diphtheria; leprosy; infectious mononucleosis; herpes zoster
Hereditary disorders: progressive hypertrophic polyneuropathy; peroneal muscular atrophy; Refsum's disease
Entrapment neuropathies

Nerve roots
Herniated intervertebral disk; spondylosis

Muscle diseases

Dystrophies: pseudohypertrophic (Duchenne); myotonic; fascio-
scapulohumeral (Landouzy-Dejerine); limb-girdle (Erb); distal
(Gower); myotonic dystrophy (Steinert's disease); ocular dystrophy

Polymyositis, dermatomyositis
Without associated disease
Associated with: connective-tissue disease, systemic lupus erythematosus, scleroderma, rheumatoid arthritis; malignancy; sarcoidosis

Metabolic and endocrine disorders: thyroid myopathy (hyperthyroidism, hypothyroidism); adrenal steroid myopathy (Cushing's
disease, iatrogenic); Addison's disease, hyperparathyroid myopathy; alcoholic myopathy; periodic paralysis; glycogen storage
diseases

Miscellaneous: congenital myopathies; congenital myotonia (Thomsen's disease); myoglobinuria; myositis ossificans; drug-induced

Disorders of neuromuscular transmission

Myasthenia gravis

Carcinomatous myopathy (Eaton-Lambert syndrome)

Episodic kalemic paralyses; familial periodic paralysis

Toxins and chemicals: botulism, anticholesterinase intoxication;
snake venoms; drugs

Iatrogenic Causes of Weakness

Drug-induced polyneuropathies: clioquinol; dimercaprol (BAL); diphenylhydantoin; disulfiram; gold salts; hydralazine; isoniazid;
nitrofurans; vinca alkaloids

Neuromuscular-blocking drugs: curare; decamethonium; kanamycin,
gentamycin, streptomycin; quinine, quinidine; succinylcholine

Drug-induced myopathy: chloroquine; corticosteroids; clofibrate

Drug-induced intracerebral bleeding and stroke: anticoagulants; oral
contraceptives; monoamine oxidase inhibitors associated with
sympathomimetic amines or tricyclic antidepressants

QUESTIONNAIRE

Possible meaning of response

1   Mode of onset and evolution

1.1   When was the weakness
first noted?

• before age 5?	Duchenne's dystrophy
• in adolescence?	Fascioscapulohumeral dystrophy; limb-girdle type
• age 20+?	Distal dystrophy
• after age 35?	In case of muscle diseases: polymyositis; myotonic dystrophy appears early or late

1.2 Has the onset of the weakness been

• sudden? (developing over a period of minutes to hours)	<u>Vascular disorder</u> of spinal cord or brain; upper motor neuron lesion; myelitis; botulism
• acute (days)?	Poliomyelitis; acute idiopathic polyneuritis; porphyria; polyarteritis; periodic paralysis; hyper- or hypokalemia; expanding intracranial lesion
• gradual (weeks to months)?	Muscular dystrophies; chronic polymyositis; brain tumor; disorders of the neuromuscular junction

1.3 Is your weakness

• persistent at all times?	Progressive muscular dystrophy; chronic polymyositis
• variable from day to day?	Myasthenia gravis
• episodic?	Myasthenia gravis; symptomatic myasthenia; familial periodic paralysis; hyper- or hypokalemia; multiple sclerosis

2 Location of the weakness

2.1 Is the weakness

• generalized?	More likely systemic cause: endocrine, metabolic, infectious, drug-induced myopathy; disorder of the motor system unlikely
• localized?	Myopathy of disuse; <u>neuropathy</u>; <u>CNS involvement</u>

2.2 Is the weakness
- *symmetrical?*

Myopathy; <u>polyneuropathy</u> (alcoholic, vitamin B deficiency, nitrofurans, isoniazid therapy, lead, arsenic); acute idiopathic polyneuritis

- *asymmetrical?*

<u>Lesion of central nervous system</u>; multiple sclerosis; poliomyelitis; amyotrophic lateral sclerosis; <u>polyneuropathies</u> (diabetic, polyarteritis nodosa, sarcoidosis); may occur in myasthenia gravis

2.3 Is the weakness
- *proximal?* Myopathy
- *distal?* Neuropathy

2.4 Do you have difficulty in lifting objects? placing packages on high shelves? shaving, brushing your hair?

Proximal weakness of the upper extremities: myopathy

2.5 Do you have difficulty in turning doorknobs, picking up a match, a pin, lighting a cigarette?

Distal weakness of the upper extremities: neuropathy

2.6 Do you have difficulty in walking, ascending and descending stairs, getting out of the bathtub, crossing your knees?

Proximal weakness of the lower limbs: myopathy

2.7 Have you noticed a tendency for your ankles to turn, a flopping of your feet?

Distal weakness of the lower limbs: neuropathy

3 Precipitating or aggravating factors

3.1 Does the weakness occur after
- *a sustained effort?*

Myasthenia gravis

- a violent exercise? ⎫
- a large carbohydrate ⎬ Familial periodic paralysis
  meal? ⎭

4   *Relieving factors*

4.1   *Does rest restore your*   Myasthenia gravis
      muscular strength?

5   *Accompanying symptoms*

5.1   Do you have

- *pain, tenderness, in your*   Peripheral neuropathy (not
  muscles?   prominent in myopathy); may
     occur in inflammatory myop-
     athies (polymyositis); poly-
     arteritis

- *numbness, tingling,* in your   Distal ("stocking-and-glove")
  hands? feet?   sensory loss in peripheral poly-
     neuropathies; sensory changes
     exclude myopathy as the cause
     of weakness

- any impairment in the per-   If dissociated loss of pain and
  ception of pain? tempera-   temperature with preservation of
  ture? touch?   touch: syringomyelia

- twitchings in resting mus-   Fasciculations: amyotrophic
  cles?   lateral sclerosis; benign fascicu-
     lations

- double vision?   Diplopia: myasthenia gravis (in-
     volvement of ocular muscles)

- difficulty swallowing?   Myasthenia gravis: weakness of
  speaking? chewing?   lips, tongue, palate, and pharynx

- pain in your joints?   Inflammatory myopathies; con-
     nective-tissue disease

- low back pain?   Intervertebral disk herniation
     with weakness in lower ex-
     tremity

- a skin rash?   Systemic lupus erythematosus
     (SLE); dermatomyositis;
     scleroderma

- an increase in the size of   Congenital myotonia (without
  some of your muscles?   muscular weakness); calves:

	pseudohypertrophic form of muscular dystrophy
• a reduction in the size of some of your muscles?	Atrophy: myopathy; disease of the lower motor neuron and of muscle; polyneuropathies; debilitating systemic disease; disuse; senility
• no change in the size of your muscles?	Weakness without atrophy: upper motor neuron lesion; disorder of the neuromuscular junction (myasthenia gravis, drugs) or muscle (hypo- and hyperkalemia, hypercalcemia, hypothyroidism)
• heat intolerance?	Thyrotoxicosis
• fever? weight loss?	Underlying systemic condition

6 Iatrogenic factors   see Etiology

7 Environmental factors

7.1 Have you been exposed to toxic products? insecticides? lead fumes?	Peripheral neuropathy

8 Personal antecedents pertaining to the weakness

8.1 Do you have any of the following conditions: diabetes? alcoholism? a thyroid disease?

8.2 Have you recently had an infection? an operation? an immunization?	Acute idiopathic polyneuritis

9 Family medical history pertaining to the weakness

9.1 Are there other members of your family who have weakness?	Myotonic dystrophy: autosomal dominant; familial periodic paralysis: autosomal dominant; porphyria
• only males?	Pseudohypertrophic (Duchenne's) form of muscular dystrophy: sex-linked recessive

PHYSICAL SIGNS PERTINENT TO THE COMPLAINT

Finding	**Possible** *significance*
Individual muscle testing	Objective evaluation of the pattern and degree of weakness
Spasticity; hyperactive tendon reflexes; extensor plantar reflex; no atrophy (or slight atrophy due to disuse); no fasciculations	Upper motor neuron paralysis: lesion of the corticospinal system
Atrophy; flaccidity; decreased or absent tendon reflexes; sensory loss and fasciculations may be present	Lower motor neuron paralysis
Atrophy; flaccidity; decreased tendon reflexes; no sensory loss; no fasciculations	Some diseases of muscle: polymyositis, hyperthyroidism, muscular dystrophy
No atrophy; no alteration in tendon reflexes; no sensory loss	Diseases of the neuromuscular junction or muscle: myasthenia gravis, botulism, potassium or calcium disorders; thyroid myopathies; congenital myotonia
Distribution of weakness: Weakness of individual muscles; marked atrophy	Lower motor neuron paralysis: lesion of one or more peripheral nerves, occasionally of spinal roots
Weakness affecting muscles in groups; no atrophy	Upper motor neuron or supranuclear paralysis
Monoplegia without muscular atrophy	Upper motor neuron lesion; most likely in cerebral cortex; multiple sclerosis; spinal cord tumor
Monoplegia with atrophy • in the upper extremity	Lesion of the lower motor neuron Springomyelia, poliomyelitis, amyotrophic lateral sclerosis; brachial plexus lesion

• in the lower extremity	Lesion of the thoracic or lumbar cord or its roots and nerves
Hemiplegia	Almost always upper motor neuron lesion: involvement of the corticospinal pathways
Paraplegia	Lesion of the corticospinal tracts below the cervical cord; disease of the spinal cord and the spinal roots or of the peripheral nerves
Quadriplegia	Lesion in the cervical segment of the spinal cord
Weakness or sensory loss in a lower extremity; bilateral Babinski sign	Multiple sclerosis ("symptoms in one leg and signs in both")
Symmetrical distal weakness	Polyneuropathy
Symmetrical proximal weakness	Myopathy
Increase in size and weakness of muscles	Pseudohypertrophy: progressive muscular dystrophy
Increased size and strength of muscles	Congenital myotonia
Ptosis; facial weakness; nasal or dysarthric speech; deep-tendon reflexes present; no sensory loss	Myasthenia gravis
Myotonia	Myotonic dystrophy; hyperkalemic periodic paralysis; hypothyroidism
Skin rash; arthritis	Connective-tissue disease with inflammatory myopathy: dermatomyositis, scleroderma, systemic lupus erythematosus
Dry coarse cool skin; delayed relaxation phase of the tendon reflexes	Hypothyroidism with myopathy

LABORATORY TESTS PERTAINING TO THE COMPLAINT

Procedure	Finding	Diagnostic possibilities
Blood CPK, SGOT, LDH, aldolase	Elevated	Myopathies
Potassium	Abnormal	Episodic kalemic paralyses; primary hyperaldosteronism
Thyroid function tests	Abnormal	Thyroid myopathies
Antinuclear antibodies	Positive	SLE
Urine 24-h creatine excretion	Increased	Progressive muscular dystrophy; neurogenic atrophy; reduced muscle mass: polymyositis, hyperthyroidism, etc.
Myoglobin	Positive	Spontaneous myoglobinuria
Nerve conduction velocities	Normal	Spinal cord or muscle diseases (may be normal in alcoholic, diabetic, nutritional, uremic polyneuropathies)
	Slow	Segmental demyelination: neuropathies; idiopathic polyneuritis; entrapment neuropathies

Procedure	*To detect*
Muscle biopsy	Neurogenic vs. myopathic disorders; poly-arteritis; neurogenic atrophy due to lesions of motor nerve cells or peripheral nerves
Electromyography	Short duration, low amplitude, frequently polyphasic potentials: myopathies
	Denervation pattern: loss of motor units, positive waves, fibrillation potentials, prolonged high-amplitude motor unit potentials: neuropathies
	Fasciculations, giant polyphasic potentials: motor neuron diseases
Neostigmine or edrophonium test	Increased muscle strength: myasthenia gravis
EEG, CT scan	Central nervous system lesion
Spine x-rays	Involvement of spinal cord, nerve roots
Chest x-ray	Lung tumor, thymoma, with myasthenic state

USEFUL REMINDERS AND DIAGNOSTIC CLUES

Misleading Factors

Muscle weakness must be distinguished from fatigue. The patient with fatigue feels tired while lying in bed; he is able to drive a car, run to catch a bus, a train, dress, shave, eat. The patient with weakness experiences trouble on exercise or when he begins to move.

Weakness due to muscle dysfunction must be distinguished from limitation of motion due to joint, bursa, tendon, or bone pain, or to contracture.

Diagnostic Considerations

Two-thirds of cerebral vascular accidents are due to arterial thrombosis, 20 percent to intracerebral hemorrhage, 8 percent to subarachnoid hemorrhage, and 5 percent to embolus.

Myasthenic patients have an increased incidence of thymoma (about 10 percent) and hyperthyroidism (3 to 8 percent).

The incidence of malignancy (most often bronchogenic carcinoma) in adults with polymyositis or dermatomyositis is 18 to 24 percent. Muscular weakness, cataract, baldness, gonadal atrophy are present in myotonic dystrophy and absent in congenital myotonia (Thomsen's disease).

SELECTED BIBLIOGRAPHY

Adams RD, Victor M: *Principles of Neurology,* Motor paralysis, pp 25–39; Diseases of the peripheral and cranial nerves; pp 411–463; Diseases of striated muscle, pp 889–967; New York: McGraw-Hill, 1977

Grob D: Weakness, in Barondess JA (ed), *Diagnostic Approaches to Presenting Syndromes,* pp 197–300, Baltimore: Williams & Wilkins, 1971

Osteoarticular System

38
Articular Pain

DEFINITIONS AND GENERAL CONSIDERATIONS

Arthralgia   joint pain in the absence of objective evidence of joint disease.

Arthritis   joint pain with visible or palpable abnormality.

Monoarthritis   affecting one joint.

Polyarthritis   affecting more than one joint.

Joint pain is perceived as diffuse and poorly localized; when severe, it may be felt distally over most of the extremity; it may be referred to another anatomic location. Disorders of the joints are likely to be accompanied by pain on local movements, and the duration of the pain parallels that of the movement. Articular pain may be due to synovial tissue disease or to diseased cartilage and involvement of supporting structures. Inflammatory arthritides (rheumatoid arthritis, systemic lupus erythematosus) are characterized by accumulation of inflammatory cells in the synovial tissue and fluid. Acute inflammation in rheumatoid arthritis is in part caused by the activation of the complement sequence and release of mediators such as prostaglandins. In the seronegative spondylarthritides such as ankylosing spondylitis and Reiter's syndrome, the enthesis (the transitional area of attachment of ligaments to bone) appears to be the primary site of inflammation; the "enthesopathies" are commonly associated with the histocompatibility antigen HL-A-B27. In infectious arthritis, the synovium is most commonly infected by the hematogenous spread of microorganisms from a primary site (skin, respiratory or urinary tract), but occasionally no source can be found. Microorganisms may be introduced directly into the joint by a penetrating wound or intraarticular injection. Rheumatic fever occurs as a delayed sequel to pharyngeal infection with group A hemolytic streptococci. The acute inflammatory lesion in rheumatic fever is attributed to an immunologic mechanism. Microcrystalline synovitis (gout, pseudogout) is characterized by crystal formation within the synovial space, and an accompanying strong inflammatory reaction. Degenerative joint disease (osteoarthritis) is characterized by a chronic low-grade synovial inflammation and the presence in cartilage and supporting structures of alterations induced by continuous wear-and-tear processes; the proteoglycan content of osteoarthritic cartilage is diminished, although its rate of synthesis is increased. Joint pain may be a manifestation of psychologic disorders in anxious or depressed patients (psychogenic rheumatism).

ETIOLOGY

Monoarthritis*

Acute

Infection: gonococcus, pneumococcus, staphylococcus

Crystal-induced: gout, pseudogout

Trauma: tear of ligament or cartilage; meniscus injury; loose bodies

Hemarthrosis: hemophilia

Intermittent hydrarthrosis (knee)

Inflammatory joint disease:
Rheumatoid arthritis
Inflammatory bowel diseases

Subacute and chronic

Degenerative joint disease, osteoarthritis

Rheumatoid arthritis (juvenile form)

Infection: tuberculosis, fungus

Traumatic: tear of ligaments or menisci

Neurogenic arthropathy: tabes, diabetes

Neoplasms

Pigmented villonodular synovitis

* Any form of polyarthritis may present initially with monoarticular involvement.

Polyarthritis

Acute

Infection: bacterial (gonococcus, meningococcus), viral (rubella, hepatitis); subacute bacterial endocarditis

Subacute and chronic

Inflammatory joint disease: rheumatoid arthritis, ankylosing spondylitis, psoriatic arthropathy, Reiter's syndrome

Rheumatic fever
Allergic: serum sickness; drug reaction; Henoch-Schönlein purpura
Connective-tissue disease: systemic lupus erythematosus (SLE), polyarteritis nodosa, scleroderma, dermatomyositis,
Inflammatory joint disease: rheumatoid arthritis, Reiter's syndrome, Behçet's disease
Arthritis of intestinal disease
Microcrystalline: gout, pseudogout
Miscellaneous: sarcoidosis, sickle cell anemia, Whipple's disease, familial Mediterranean fever, neoplasms (lymphoma, leukemia, multiple myeloma)

Connective-tissue disease: systemic lupus erythematosus, polyarteritis, scleroderma, Sjögren's syndrome, mixed connective-tissue disease
Degenerative joint disease: osteoarthritis
Arthritis of intestinal disease
Microcrystalline: gout, pseudogout
Miscellaneous: sarcoidosis, hemophilia, hypertrophic osteoarthropathy, hyperlipoproteinemia, type IV

Iatrogenic Causes of Articular Pain (partial list)

Drug-induced gout   diuretics: chlorothiazides, furosemide, ethacrynic acid; probenecid; sulfinpyrazone; allopurinol; cytotoxic drugs in the therapy of myeloproliferative and lymphoproliferative disorders; low doses of salicylate therapy
Drug-induced polyarteritis nodosa   sulfonamides, penicillin
Drug-induced serum-sickness type of reaction   penicillin, barbiturates, animal serums
Drug-induced SLE and/or positive tests for antinuclear antibodies

Alpha methyldopa
Anticonvulsivants: diphenylhydantoin
Oral contraceptives
Hydralazine
Isoniazid
Levodopa
Penicillin
Phenothiazines
Procainamide
Sulfonamides

Anticoagulant overdosage may produce acute hemarthrosis.
Too rapid withdrawal of corticosteroid therapy may induce arthralgia.

QUESTIONNAIRE

Possible meaning of response

1 Location

1.1   In which joint(s) do you have pain?

• hips and shoulders?

Peripheral joints most frequently affected in ankylosing spondylitis

• sacroiliac joints?
• lumbar spine?

Ankylosing spondylitis; psoriatic arthropathy; Reiter's syndrome; relatively spared in rheumatoid arthritis

• knees and hips?

<u>Osteoarthritis</u>: in weight-bearing joints

• wrists?

Frequently involved in <u>rheumatoid</u> arthritis (RA)

• the small joints of hands or feet?

May be involved in the polyarticular form of gout (with sparing of the great toe)

  • *metacarpophalangeal?*

<u>RA</u> (rarely affected in osteoarthritis)

  • *proximal interphalangeal?*

<u>RA</u>; nontender Bouchard's nodes in osteoarthritis

  • *distal interphalangeal?*

Osteoarthritis (Heberden's nodes); psoriatic arthritis; commonly spared in RA

• a great toe?

Gout (the big toe is involved in 50 to 70 percent of initial attacks)

• any of the above?

Acute rheumatic fever (knees, ankles: commonest); trauma

1.2   How many joints are involved?

• *one?*

<u>Gout</u> (great toe); trauma; bursitis

• *"flitting" from joint to joint, with one or two joints affected at one time?*

Acute rheumatic fever

• *one or a few?*	<u>Osteoarthritis</u>; microcrystalline; infection (gonococcus, others)
• *multiple, more than four joints?*	<u>RA</u>, serum sickness; rheumatic fever; viral arthritis; Reiter's syn drome
• multiple or "all"?	Psychogenic rheumatism

2   *Mode of onset, duration, and evolution*

2.1 How long have you had joint pain?	Less than 6 weeks' duration: microcrystalline, infection, acute rheumatic fever Lasting more than 6 weeks: RA, osteoarthritis
2.2 At what age did the joint condition appear?	
• between 20 to 45?	<u>RA</u>; rheumatic fever is infrequent after age 21
• *in a young man?*	Ankylcsing spondylitis; gout; Reiter's syndrome
• after age 40?	<u>Osteoarthritis</u> (unusual before age 35)
• in older age group?	Carcinomatous arthritis; hypertrophic osteoarthropathy; neurogenic arthropathy; pseudogout
2.3 Was the onset of joint pain	
• *sudden?* (hours to days)	Rheumatic fever; <u>gout</u>; pseudogout; onset of RA may be abrupt
• gradual? (days to weeks to months)	RA; osteoarthritis
2.4 Did the joint involvement	
• appear and stay in one joint?	Gout; infection, gonococcal
• appear simultaneously in several joints?	RA (especially in hands and feet); Reiter's syndrome

2.5 Did the joint condition

- migrate from joint to joint? ⎫
- *tend to leave one joint as a new one was affected?* ⎬

Migratory pattern: common in acute polyarthritis: acute rheumatic fever, serum sickness, gonococcal arthritis, drug sensitivity

- *involve new joints, with persistence of the first affected?*

Additive pattern: RA, Reiter's syndrome

3 *Character*

3.1 Are your joints swollen? tender?

The intensity of joint inflammation is greater in microcrystalline and septic arthritides than in other disorders

3.1a Did the swelling appear

- simultaneously with the pain?

RA: swelling due to synovitis and accumulation of joint fluid

- weeks to months after the pain?

Osteoarthritis: swelling due to proliferative changes in cartilage and bone

3.2 Are your joints painful at rest?

RA; osteoarthritis (advanced stage); infectious arthritis; gout

3.3 Is the joint involvement

- symmetric?

Frequent in RA

- asymmetric?

Osteoarthritis; psoriatic arthritis; Reiter's syndrome

4 *Precipitating or aggravating factors*

4.1 Is the pain in your joints worse

- with movements?

Pain caused by any arthritis

- after prolonged activity?

Osteoarthritis

4.2   Did the joint complaints occur
- *after a trauma?*
- *after a dietary or alcoholic excess?*

Acute attack of <u>gout</u>; <u>trauma</u> may also precipitate **pseudo-gout**

5   *Relieving factors*

5.1   Is the pain in your joints relieved by
- rest?

Osteoarthritis; RA

- aspirin?

Most arthritides; acute rheumatic fever

- *colchicine?*

Gout

5.1*a*   Do salicylates fail to relieve your complaints?

Psychogenic rheumatism (in the absence of physical signs)

6   *Accompanying symptoms*

6.1   Do you have
- *a (generalized) stiffness, most severe in the morning?*

"Gelling" phenomenon: accentuation of the congestion and edema in synovium, joint capsule, and periarticular tissues resulting from inactivity

- persisting for a few minutes?

Osteoarthritis

- *lasting more than 30 min?*
- lasting up to 3 h?

Characteristic of <u>RA</u>

- subsiding with activity?

RA; other polyarthritides

- increased by activity? by weight bearing?

Osteoarthritis

6.1*a*   What part of the day is the most difficult for you?
- the early morning hours?

RA

- the end of the day?

Osteoarthritis

6.2 Do you have

• fever?	Acute rheumatic fever; infection: gonococcal, septic arthritis; gout; connective-tissue disease (fever is absent in osteoarthritis and infrequent in chronic poly-arthritis)
• with chills?	Bacteremia with acute polyar-thritis
• weight loss? fatigue? • pain in your muscles?	Underlying systemic disorder: connective-tissue disease; sub-acute bacterial endocarditis; neoplasm; weight loss may be profound in <u>RA</u> (systemic signs are absent in osteoarthritis)
• skin lesions?	Psoriatic arthritis; SLE; sclero-derma
• chronic diarrhea?	Arthritis associated with ulcera-tive colitis, regional enteritis, Whipple's disease
• difficulty swallowing?	Dermatomyositis; scleroderma
• cough? expectorations? • shortness of breath?	Pulmonary lesions associated with RA, SLE, polymyositis, sar-coidosis, polyarteritis nodosa
• hemoptysis?	Bronchogenic carcinoma with hypertrophic osteoarthropathy
• chest pain?	Pleurisy and pericarditis are common in SLE
• back pain?	Spondylitis is common in pso-riatic arthritis, Reiter's syn-drome, colonic arthritis
• an eye condition?	Episcleritis associated with RA; conjunctivitis in Reiter's syn-drome; keratitis sicca in Sjö-gren's syndrome; anterior uveitis in ankylosing spondylitis
• pain in your fingers when exposed to cold?	Raynaud's phenomenon: SLE, scleroderma, Sjögren's syn-drome; may occur in RA
• pain on urination? • a urethral discharge?	Gonococcal arthritis; Reiter's syndrome

7   *Iatrogenic factors*   see Etiology

8   *Environmental factors*

8.1   Have you ever worked in a coal mine?

Caplan's syndrome: RA with multiple pulmonary nodules on chest x-ray in coal workers

9   *Personal antecedents pertaining to the articular pain*

9.1   Have you ever had x-rays, a biopsy, of your joints? When? With what results?

9.2   Prior to the onset of joint pain, did you have
   • a sore throat?

A group A hemolytic streptococcal infection is usually noted about 2 weeks prior to acute rheumatic fever

   • any injection of serum?

Serum sickness; hepatitis B with arthritis

   • a rubella infection?

Polyarthralgia or polyarthritis synchronous with rubella

   • a rubella vaccination?

Joint involvement begins 2 to 8 weeks after vaccination

   • any sexual contact(s)?

3 to 17 days prior to the arthritis: gonococcal arthritis, more frequent in females (may cause polyarthritis prior to localization to a monoarticular form); Reiter's syndrome

   • an operation? a trauma?

Gout; pseudogout

   • a trauma to the involved area?

Posttraumatic arthritis

9.3   Have you ever had
   • similar attacks in the past?

Gout; pseudogout, Reitor's syndrome (RA is less episodic)

   • an episode of renal colic?

Gouty renal disease

| 9.4 | Do you have a blood ab-normality? | Acute polyarthralgia or poly-arthritis occurs in sickle cell anemia; hemoglobinopathies may be associated with septic arthritis, avascular necrosis of bone |

10 *Family medical history pertaining to the articular pain*

10.1	Is there a family history of	
	• joint pain?	Gout, osteoarthritis of the distal interphalangeal joints (He-berden's nodes), ankylosing spondylitis have a hereditary background
	• psoriasis?	30 percent of patients with pso-riatic arthritis give a family his-tory of psoriasis

PHYSICAL SIGNS PERTINENT TO THE COMPLAINT

Finding	**Possible** *significance*
Joint swelling with	
• fluctuation or bulging	Effusion within the joint space
• a boggy, nonfluctuant feeling	Soft-tissue swelling; synovial thickening: rheumatoid arthritis (RA), gout
• a hard, irregular enlargement	Hypertrophy of cartilage or bone; osteophytes in osteoar-thritis
Periarticular swelling	Disorder of periarticular struc-tures: bursitis, tendonitis, cellu-litis
Direct pressure over the joint elicits	
• pain	Arthritis; inflammatory joint dis-ease
• no pain	Involvement of periarticular tis-sues: bursitis, tendonitis

Swollen joint, with overlying skin

• red and warm

Acute rheumatic fever; RA; other inflammatory joint diseases; gout; pyogenic infection (local heat is absent in chronic inflammation)

• not discolored

Osteoarthritis

Crepitation on motion

Irregularity in the articulating surfaces: granulation tissue in RA; osteophytes and disorganized cartilage in osteoarthritis; may also arise from the soft tissues

Joint deformity

Gross joint destruction or injury; RA (loss of articular cartilage, destruction or weakening of ligaments, tendons, and capsular structures, muscle imbalance); chronic gout; hemophilic arthritis; occasionally: osteoarthritis

• ulnar deviation of the fingers at the metacarpophalangeal joints

Frequently observed deformity in RA

Limitation of motion

Muscle spasm or guarding; effusion distending the capsule; fibrosis of the capsule; fibrous or bony ankylosis; disorder of tendon, muscle, or nerve

Atrophy and weakness of muscles

• adjacent to the affected joints

Primary joint disease (atrophy of skeletal muscles in RA often parallels the severity of the joint disease)

• generalized

Primary muscle disorder; polymyositis

Subcutaneous swellings

- over pressure points, over the extensor surface of the elbows

  Rheumatoid nodules: in 20 percent of patients with RA

- in margin of ear, periarticular areas

  Tophi of gout: in about 50 percent of patients with clinical gout

- nodules at the
  - dorsal margins of the distal interphalangeal joints

    Heberden's nodes in osteoarthritis

  - proximal interphalangeal joints

    Bouchard's nodes in osteoarthritis

Fever

Acute rheumatic fever; connective-tissue disease; juvenile RA (Still's disease); gout; infectious arthritis

Eye:
- keratitis

  Sjögren's syndrome; 15 percent of patients with RA

- anterior uveitis

  Ankylosing spondylitis; sarcoidosis

- conjunctivitis

  Reiter's syndrome

Skin:
- psoriatic lesions; nail lesions

  Psoriatic arthropathy

- butterfly rash of the face

  Systemic lupus erythematosus (SLE)

- violaceous (heliotrope) rash on the eyelids, cheeks, forehead

  Dermatomyositis

- petechiae

  Henoch-Schönlein purpura; SLE; subacute bacterial endocarditis

- various cutaneous manifestations

  Rheumatic fever; Reiter's syndrome; gonococcal arthritis; polyarteritis nodosa, allergic angiitis; dermatomyositis; SLE; scleroderma; rheumatoid arthritis; rubella arthritis; hepatitis-associated arthritis

- mucocutaneous lesions (glans penis, mouth, palms and soles) — Reiter's syndrome
- painful red tender nodules on the legs — Erythema nodosum (see Chap. 40)
- ulcerations of oral mucosae and genitalia — Behçet's syndrome; Stevens-Johnson syndrome

Moon facies; striae	Previous steroid therapy
Splenomegaly	In 5 to 10 percent of patients with RA; Felty's syndrome (with neutropenia)
Lymphadenopathy; splenomegaly	Juvenile RA; SLE
Wheezes; pleural effusion	Pulmonary lesions associated with RA, SLE, sarcoidosis, polyarteritis nodosa
Neurologic abnormalities; loss of proprioception	Neurogenic arthropathy: diabetes mellitus, tabes dorsalis

LABORATORY TESTS PERTAINING TO THE COMPLAINT

Procedure	Finding	Diagnostic possibilities
Blood		
RBCs	Normal	Osteoarthritis
	Normocytic hypochromic anemia	Rheumatoid arthritis (RA)
	Hemolytic anemia	SLE; other connective-tissue diseases
WBCs	Leukocytosis	Infectious arthritis; microcrystalline arthropathy; juvenile RA; RA (occasionally)

	Leukopenia	SLE; Felty's syndrome
ESR	Normal	Osteoarthritis
	Elevated	Not specific: RA; polymyalgia rheumatica
Uric acid	Increased	Gout; hematologic disorders; diuretics; etc.
Rheumatoid factor (latex)	Positive (1:320)	Not specific: RA (75 percent); SLE (20 to 30 percent); infectious diseases; etc.
	Negative	Osteoarthritis; microcrystalline arthropathy; ankylosing spondylitis; Reiter's syndrome; psoriatic arthritis; colonic arthritis
Antinuclear antibodies, lupus erythematosus (LE) cells*	Positive	SLE; RA (10 to 20 percent)
Antistreptolysin O, other streptococcal antibody tests,* C-reactive protein	Abnormal	Acute rheumatic fever
Serum complement* (CH_{50}) (N: 150 to 250 U/mL)	Normal	RA
	Decreased	SLE
HL-A-B27 antigen*	Present	Ankylosing spondylitis; Reiter's syndrome; psoriatic arthritis; colonic arthritis

* If appropriate.

Urine

Urinalysis	Proteinuria	SLE; polyarteritis nodosa; scleroderma; gouty nephropathy; amyloidosis complicating RA
	Pyuria	Gonorrhea; Reiter's syndrome
	RBC casts, cylindruria	Lupus nephritis

Synovial fluid analysis

WBC/mm^3(N: <200)	<2000	Osteoarthritis
	<50,000	Inflammatory effusion: RA, psoriatic arthritis, Reiter's syndrome, ankylosing spondylitis (peripheral joints), acute gout, pseudogout, SLE
	>50,000	Septic arthritis
	Hemorrhagic	Traumatic arthritis; hemophilia
Protein, g/100 mL (N: 1 to 4)	1 to 4.5	Osteoarthritis
	3 to 6	Inflammatory effusion: RA, etc.
Glucose (N: blood glucose level)	Normal	Osteoarthritis
	Reduced	Inflammatory effusion; septic arthritis
	Crystals	Gout; pseudogout

Procedure	*To detect*
Joint x-rays	Juxtaarticular erosions, periarticular osteoporosis: RA
	Marginal sclerosis, bony spurs and bridges: osteoarthritis

Punched-out defects in bone adjacent to joints: chronic gout

Calcification of fibrocartilage and articular hyaline cartilage: pseudogout

Periostitis: hypertrophic osteoarthropathy; Reiter's syndrome

Synovial biopsy* Tuberculosis; sarcoidosis; hemochromatosis; amyloidosis; pigmented villonodular synovitis; synovial tumor; etc.

* If appropriate.

USEFUL REMINDERS AND DIAGNOSTIC CLUES

Misleading Factors

Acute osteomyelitis may produce symptoms very much like those seen in septic arthritis and should be considered in the differential diagnosis of acute joint infection.

Periarticular disease (tendonitis, bursitis) may produce symptoms related to the joint.

Joint pain may occasionally be referred to other sites; in disease of the hip, pain may be felt primarily in the groin, the thigh, or the knee.

Diagnostic Considerations

Joints previously damaged by rheumatoid arthritis, osteoarthritis, or trauma are more liable to infection.

Septic arthritis affects larger joints more frequently.

In rheumatoid arthritis, individual joints once involved usually remain involved, though activity fluctuates.

The monoarticular type of rheumatoid arthritis remains monoarticular in 60 percent of patients; the other 40 percent develop polyarthritis in up to 10 years.

Amyloidosis should be considered in rheumatoid arthritis patients who develop renal insufficiency, especially with a nephrotic syndrome, and in those with unexplained gastrointestinal hemorrhage.

Aortic regurgitation occurs in 3 percent of patients with ankylosing spondylitis.

Arthritides associated with gastrointestinal symptoms Ulcerative colitis, regional enteritis; Whipple's disease; scleroderma; Reiter's syndrome; Behçet's syndrome; necrotizing vasculitis; carcinoma of the bowel; gastrointestinal shunts.

Arthritides associated with pulmonary disease Rheumatoid arthritis; Caplan's syndrome; systemic lupus erythematosus; polymyositis, dermatomyositis; necrotizing vasculitis; sarcoidosis; hypertrophic osteoarthropathy; lung carcinoma; erythema nodosum.
Osteoarthritis is the most common rheumatic disease problem.

SELECTED BIBLIOGRAPHY

Fries JF, Mitchell DM: Joint pain or arthritis. JAMA 235:199–204, 1976
Gilliland BC, Mannik M: Disorders of the joints and connective tissues, in Thorn et al (eds), *Harrison's Principles of Internal Medicine,* 8th ed, pp 2048–2080, New York: McGraw-Hill, 1977
Moskowitz RW: *Clinical Rheumatology: A Problem-oriented Approach to Diagnosis and Management,* Philadelphia: Lea & Febiger, 1975
Shearn M (ed): Rheumatic diseases. Med Clin North Am 61:203–461, 1977

39

Low Back Pain

DEFINITIONS AND GENERAL CONSIDERATIONS

Strain   a minor injury which does not produce gross structural damage.

Local (scleratogenous) pain   caused by any pathologic process which impinges upon or irritates sensory nerve endings in meso-dermal tissues: periosteum, ligaments and fibrous joint capsules, tendons, fascia, muscles. It usually results from low back strain or muscle spasm. The pain thresholds of these structures are vari-able: the periosteum is most sensitive, followed by ligaments and fibrous joint capsules, tendons, fascia, and muscles in that order; bone for the most part is insensitive.

Referred somatic pain   may be projected from the spine into areas related to the lumbar and upper sacral dermatomes (thighs, legs, calves). Decreased sensory and motor function in the lower ex-tremities is never found in association with referred somatic pain.

Referred pain from visceral disease   pain arising in pelvic and ab-dominal viscera may be referred to the spine. The pain of pelvic diseases is referred to the sacral region; lower abdominal diseases are referred to the lumbar region (centering around L2 to L4), and upper abdominal diseases to the lower thoracic spine (T8 to L1 to L2).

Radicular pain   sharp pain radiating from a central position near the spine to some part of the lower extremity and caused by compres-sion and irritation of a spinal root. A space-occupying lesion in the spinal cord or in the intervertebral foramen may be responsible.

It is safe to assume that the patient who complains of low back pain of obscure origin has some type of primary or secondary disease of the spine and its supporting structures or of the abdominal or pelvic viscera.

ETIOLOGY

Mechanical:
  Abnormal posture and strain
  Spondylolisthesis

Congenital: lumbosacral anomaly, spina bifida scoliosis
Trauma: soft tissue; bone; previous surgery
Degenerative: disk lesion; osteoarthritis
Ankylosing spondylitis; Reiter's syndrome; psoriatic arthritis; colonic arthritis
Spinal infections: acute pyogenic; tuberculosis; *Salmonella;* epidural abscess
Generalized and metabolic bone diseases: osteoporosis; osteomalacia; hyperparathyroidism; acromegaly
Neoplastic: primary or metastatic; multiple myeloma
Referred: retroperitoneal structures; pelvic organs; diseases of the colon: colitis, diverticulitis, tumor

QUESTIONNAIRE

Possible *meaning of response*

1   Location and radiation

1.1   Where do you have pain?

1.1*a* Please indicate the site of the pain.	It may be difficult for the patient to localize the pain accurately with words; he may be more specific by pointing to the site of the pain
1.2 Do you have pain • in the midline? (over the lower lumbar area)?	Local back pain: may have its origin in any of the underlying structures
• in one (or both) sacroiliac joint(s)?	Sacroiliac strain; ankylosing spondylitis (in young males)
1.3 *Does the pain radiate down into lower extremity?*	<u>Herniated disk lesion; primary degenerative joint disease</u> of the spine; spondylolisthesis
1.3*a* How far distally does the pain extend?	The extent of radiation in many instances may be used as a rough index of the severity of the lesion

1.3*b* Does the pain radiate into
- *the posterior part of the thigh, the calf, to the heel, sole of the foot?*   L5 to S1 disk and S1 nerve root

- *the posterolateral thigh, lateral calf, and dorsum of the foot? first or second and third toes?*   L4 to L5 disk and L5 nerve root

- the anterior part of the thigh?   L3 to L4 disk and L4 nerve root (rare)

2   Mode of onset and chronology

2.1 How long have you had pain in your back?   At least 3 months (and in men between the ages of 15 and 40 years): ankylosing spondylitis

2.2 Do you have recurring episodes of back pain?   Lumbar disk lesion; recurrent acute <u>strains</u> (any cause of chronic or recurring low back pain can produce an acute attack)

2.3 Was the onset of the pain
- sudden? rapid?   Injury to soft tissue in the lower part of the back

- gradual?   Common onset of lumbar disk lesion; ankylosing spondylitis

2.4 Has the pain
- remained the same?   Stabilized process
- worsened?   Evolutive process
- improved?   In lumbar disk syndrome (chronic stage), when fibrosis of the disk is complete and matured

3   Character and intensity of the pain

3.1 Is the pain
- mild?
- moderate to severe?   An individually variable factor which should be interpreted with caution
- severe, unbearable?

3.2   Does the pain
   • unable you to work? to
     engage in social activi-
     ties?
   • confine you to bed? in-
     terfere with sleep?

   Useful indexes to the degree of
   severity of pain

3.3   Is the back pain
   • dull, aching in character?
     slow in onset, long in
     duration? diffuse?

   Local pain produced by stimuli
   within deep skeletal structures
   (ligaments, fascia, muscles,
   periosteum)

3.4   Is the back pain
   • constant in duration?

   Local (scleratogenous) pain:
   strain; lumbar disk (early stage);
   osteoporosis

   • variable in intensity?

   Lumbar disk lesion (later stage)

   • unremittent, severe, and
     progressive?

   Neoplasm (vertebral tumor); tuberculous infection

   • intermittent, recurrent?

   Ruptured disk causing instability
   of the spine; ankylosing spondylitis

   • throbbing?

   Pain caused by neoplasms

3.5   If a distal radiation is pres-
      ent, is this radiated pain
   • *sharp,* lancinating, intense?
     well localized? rapid in
     onset?

   Radicular type of pain: distortion, stretching, irritation, or
   compression of a spinal nerve
   root

   • dull, aching, steady? deep?
     poorly localized?

   Referred pain from skeletal
   structures

   • mild?

   Spinal cord lesion (associated
   with neurologic abnormalities)

4   *Precipitating or aggravating factors*

4.1   Did the pain accompany or
      follow
   • a <u>trauma</u> to the back?

   The most frequent cause of
   acute low back pain; a vertebral

fracture must be excluded; in the elderly patient: osteoporosis, with collapse or wedging of a vertebra

- a strenuous use of the back, when something "gave way"?
- unaccustomed heavy work?
- a bending forward motion?
- your getting up from bed?

Injury to soft tissue in the lower back: lumbosacral or sacroiliac strain; degenerative disorders (disk, synovial joints)

4.1*a* In case of a trauma prior to the onset of pain, when did it occur?

Persistence of acute symptoms beyond 72 h is highly indicative of some serious underlying process other than mechanical derangement and requires hospitalization

4.2 Did the pain appear spontaneously?

In a considerable proportion of cases of herniated nucleosus pulposus, no trauma is recalled

4.3 Does the pain occur or worsen
  - when moving the trunk?

Local pain; acute strain; lumbar disk lesion (sudden displacement of nuclear material); referred pain from visceral disease is usually unaffected by movement of the spine

  - *when coughing? sneezing? straining?*

Lumbar disk lesion; radicular pain

  - when bending? lifting objects from the floor with the trunk bent?

Lumbar disk syndrome; local pain: traumatic strain

  - when maintaining a particular posture over a period of time?

Postural back pain with inadequate musculature

  - at night?

Ankylosing spondylitis; neoplasms; tuberculous spondylitis; osteomyelitis

  - in the early morning?

Ankylosing spondylitis

4.4   For the female patient with pain in the sacral region: Does the pain appear

- before and/or during the menstruation?

Endometriosis involving the uterosacral ligaments

- when you have been standing for several hours?

Malposition of the uterus; fibroma of the uterus

5   *Relieving factors*

5.1   Is the pain relieved by
- bed rest?

Local pain: traumatic, <u>strain</u>; <u>osteoarthritis</u>

- lying on a firm bed? on the floor?

Lumbar disk lesion (early phase): decrease of the vertebral loading of the spine

- certain positions of the trunk and legs?

Decreasing the tension and pressure of the nerve root: lumbar disk syndrome

- mild activity? "loosening up" in the morning?

May be observed in osteoarthritis

6   *Accompanying symptoms*

6.1   If the pain has appeared immediately after a trauma to the back:
- can you move your legs?

A vertebral fracture must be excluded

- do you have any muscle weakness? loss of sensation in the limbs? urinary incontinence? inability to void?

Vertebral fracture: spinal cord lesion

6.2   If the pain was precipitated by a minor trauma, did you
- feel a "sudden snap" in the lower part of the back?
- experience the sensation of something "tearing," "giving way" in the back?

In lumbar disk lesion: sudden rupture of the defective annulus due to sudden rise in the tension in the nucleus and backward displacement of nuclear material

6.3 In case of chronic and/or recurring low back pain, do you have

- *numbness, tingling of either or both lower extremities?*
- any weakness, wasting of a muscle in a lower extremity?

May accompany pain arising from compression and irritation of nerve roots; space-occupying lesion in the spinal cord or in the intervertebral foramen may be responsible

6.4 Do you have
- fever? a general malaise?

Acute pain in the back may occur in any febrile disorder; infectious lesion of the spine

- any stiffness of your back?
  - increased by exercise?

Local pain; strain; lumbar disk syndrome (in referred pain from visceral disease, there is no stiffness and motion is of full range)

  - especially in the morning?
  - produced by inactivity?
  - relieved by activity?

Ankylosing spondylitis; also in osteoarthritis

- difficulty, burning on urination?
- frequency of urination?

Reiter's syndrome; carcinoma of prostate with metastases to the lower part of the spine

- (female patient) a vaginal discharge?

Gynecologic disease causing low back pain

- pain in other joints?

Occurs in 25 percent of patients with ankylosing spondylitis; osteoarthritis

- conjunctivitis?

Reiter's syndrome with spondylitis

- chronic diarrhea?

Spondylitis may be associated with ulcerative colitis, regional enteritis, Whipple's disease (rarely)

• an increase of weight?	Aggravating factor in traumatic and degenerative disorders of the spine
• a loss of weight?	Neoplasm; tuberculosis of the spine

7   *Environmental factors*

7.1 What is your occupation? What do you do during your leisure time?	Heavy manual workers are liable to degenerative disorders of disks and/or synovial joints; sacroiliac strain is commonly found in occupations where heavy lifting is required (nurses)
7.1*a* Are you suing for compensation for your back pain?	The pain may be exaggerated or prolonged because of psychologic factors, especially when there is the possibility of personal gain (compensation)

8   *Personal antecedents pertaining to the complaint*

8.1   Have you ever had an x-ray of your spine? a myelography? spinal surgery? When? With what results?

PHYSICAL SIGNS PERTINENT TO THE COMPLAINT

Finding	**Possible** *significance*
Muscle spasm and tenderness in involved area	Herniated disk; osteoarthritis; ankylosing spondylitis; lumbosacral strain
Localized tenderness on percussion or pressure over the involved vertebra	Tumor; infection; osteoporosis with vertebral compression
Tenderness on palpation of the sacroiliac joints; paravertebral muscle spasm and tenderness; loss of lumbar lordotic curve	Sacroiliitis: in the early stages of ankylosing spondylitis
Painful lateral compression of the pelvis	Sacroiliac disease: associated with osteoarthritis, ankylosing spondylitis

Difference in midline measurements from sacrum to T12, in flexion and extension less than 7 cm	Diminished lumbar flexion; chronic phase of ankylosing spondylitis
Painful straight-leg-raising maneuver	Disease of lumbosacral joints; herniated lumbar intervertebral disk; lumbosacral roots involvement
Motor, sensory, and reflex changes in the lower extremities (see Chap. 40)	Herniated disk; spinal lesion
Fever; flaccid paraplegia; localized pain with percussion and palpation of the spine	Epidural abscess with compression of the spinal cord
Diminished chest expansion (< 5 cm)	Costovertebral joint involvement in ankylosing spondylitis
Aortic regurgitation murmur	Ankylosing spondylitis: in 3 percent of cases
Iridocyclitis	Ankylosing spondylitis: in 20 to 30 percent of cases
Psoriatic lesions	5 percent of patients with psoriasis and arthritis manifest features identical to those of ankylosing spondylitis
Conjunctivitis; urethritis	Reiter's syndrome with involvement of the spine
Tenderness over the costovertebral angle	Genitourinary disease; adrenal disease; injury to the transverse processes of the first or second lumbar vertebra
Full range motion of the spine; no local signs; no stiffness of the back	Referred pain from visceral disease (colitis, diverticulitis, tumor of the colon, gynecologic disorder)
Abdominal examination Rectal and pelvic examination	May reveal: gastrointestinal, urologic, and gynecologic diseases

LABORATORY TESTS PERTAINING TO THE COMPLAINT

Procedure	Finding	Diagnostic possibilities
Blood ESR	Elevated	Infection of the vertebral column; multiple myeloma; ankylosing spondylitis
	Normal	Osteoarthritis
Serum proteins and electrophoresis	Abnormal	Multiple myeloma; connective-tissue diseases
Alkaline phosphatase	Normal	Osteoporosis; multiple myeloma; hyperparathyroidism
	Elevated	Metastatic carcinoma; Paget's disease
Acid phosphatase	Elevated	Metastatic carcinoma of prostate
HLA-B27 antigen*	Positive	Ankylosing spondylitis; Reiter's disease; enteropathic arthropathy; psoriatic arthritis

Procedure	To detect
Lumbar spine x-rays ⎫ Laminographic films ⎭	Osteophytic overgrowth, spur formation, bridging of vertebrae: osteoarthritis
	Disk narrowing: disk herniation (x-ray may be normal)
	Sacroiliac arthritis, syndesmophytes, "bamboo spine": ankylosing spondylitis
	Bone destruction: neoplasm, tuberculosis, neuropathic disorders
	Collapse, wedging of a vertebra: osteoporosis (nonspecific abnormality)

* If appropriate.

	Vertebral fracture; spondylolisthesis; spondylolysis; Paget's disease
X-ray of other bones and joints	Malignancy; osteoporosis; etc.
Myelography*	Disk herniation (as preparation for surgery); spinal cord tumor
Bone scan	Hot spots: bone destruction associated with malignancy
Barium enema*	Colitis; diverticulitis; tumor of colon
Psychiatric evaluation*	Depression; malingering; compensation hysteria

* If appropriate.

USEFUL REMINDERS AND DIAGNOSTIC CLUES

Diagnostic Considerations

Lumbar disk syndrome

A large group of patients with lumbar disk lesions deny a history of trauma.

The disks most commonly involved in the lumbar spine are the L5 to S1 and the L4 to L5 disks. Disk disease at two levels occurs in 8 to 10 percent of patients, usually at successive levels.

In most patients with sciatica, only one leg is involved, and in subsequent attacks, the sciatica is confined to the same leg.

The fact that there are radiologic changes of the lumbar spine does not mean that these are the cause of the back pain: radiologically speaking, there is no such thing as a normal spine after middle age is passed.

Infection

Tuberculosis and pyogenic osteomyelitis are the most frequent infections of the spine, though brucellosis, typhoid fever, actinomycosis, and blastomycosis are known to occur.

Gynecologic-Urologic

Although gynecologic disorders may manifest themselves by back pain, the pelvis is seldom the site of a disease which causes obscure low back pain.

Low back pain with radiation into one or both thighs is a common phenomenon during the last weeks of pregnancy.

Lesions of the bladder and testes are usually not accompanied by back pain.

When the kidney is the site of disease, the pain is ipsilateral, being felt in the flank or lumbar region.

Tumor

The most common tumors which involve the spine are: metastatic carcinoma (breast, bronchus, prostate, thyroid, hypernephroma, stomach, uterus); multiple myeloma; histiocytic lymphoma.

In case of	*Suspect*
Sudden appearance of obscure lumbar pain in a patient receiving	
• anticoagulants	Retroperitoneal bleeding
• chronic corticosteroid therapy	Osteoporosis with vertebral collapse
Back pain in	
• a postmenopausal female	Osteoporosis; osteoarthritis
• a young man	Ankylosing spondylitis
• an adolescent	Epiphyseal (Scheuermann's) disease of the spine

SELECTED BIBLIOGRAPHY

Adams RD, Victor M: Pain in the back, neck, and extremities, in *Principles of Neurology*, pp 112–133, New York: McGraw-Hill, 1977

De Palma AF, Rothman RH: Salient clinical features of lumbar disc lesions, in *The Intervertebral Disc*, chap 11, pp 181–202, Philadelphia, Saunders, 1970

40
Pain in the Lower Extremities

GENERAL CONSIDERATIONS

Pain in the lower extremities may result from diseases of the skin and of the musculoskeletal, vascular, and nervous systems. Superficial pain (skin and adjacent structures) is well localized and is associated with tenderness and hyperalgesia. The pain from trauma is due to mechanical stimulation of nerve endings. In bacterial infections, rapidly forming edema increases local tissue pressure and causes pain in skin already made hyperalgesic by chemical factors associated with injury. Deep pain originates in fascia, vessels, periosteum, joints, and supporting structures; it is often poorly localized and dull, and may be associated with muscle rigidity and deep tenderness. The pain from ischemia in skeletal muscles (arteriosclerosis) may be produced by the action on sensory nerve endings of metabolites accumulating in the muscles or by changes in the nerves from ischemia. The pain of joint involvement is related to inflammation of the synovial membrane. Pain due to diseases of the peripheral nerves may be associated with areflexia and distal or other sensory impairment. Irritation and compression of nerve roots by a herniated nucleosus pulposus or osteoarthritis can cause pain in the lower extremities. Pain from the deep muscles of the back or from the vertebrae may be the source of pain referred to the extremity. Referred pain is usually well localized.

ETIOLOGY

Skin and soft tissues
Acute trauma to the skin
Cellulitis: bacterial and fungous infections; lymphangitis
Erythema nodosum

Articular and periarticular structures
Arthritis: acute pyogenic arthritis; gout; rheumatoid arthritis; rheumatic fever; osteoarthritis; posttraumatic condition; hypertrophic osteoarthropathy

Bursitis; tendonitis; Baker's (popliteal) cyst

Bone and periosteum
Fracture; osteomyelitis; tumors

Muscles
Acute suppurative myositis; polymyositis, dermatomyositis
Overstrain of untrained muscle fibers
Nocturnal muscle cramp

Arteries and veins
Arterial occlusion: acute: thrombosis, embolism, cholesterol emboli, injury; chronic: arteriosclerosis obliterans, thromboangiitis obliterans
Erythromelalgia
Venous thrombosis: superficial, deep; chronic venous insufficiency; postphlebitic syndrome
Lymphedema

Neurologic
Polyneuropathy; mononeuritis multiplex (polyarteritis, diabetes)
Nerve root compression: herniated nucleus pulposus; spinal cord neoplasm; osteoarthritis
Entrapment neuropathy: meralgia paresthetica
Reflex sympathetic dystrophies: causalgia
Interdigital neuroma; glomus tumor

Iatrogenic Causes of Pain in the Lower Extremities

Oral contraceptives: venous thrombosis
Corticosteroids: avascular necrosis of head of femur; increased liability to septic arthritis
Faulty intramuscular injection: sciatic neuritis
Triamterine: leg cramps
Penicillin, sulfonamides, iodides, bromides, oral contraceptives: erythema nodosum

QUESTIONNAIRE

Possible *meaning of response*

1 Location and radiation of the pain

1.1 Where do you have pain?
  • in a joint?

• a large joint?	Infectious arthritis affects large joints (hips, knees) more frequently
• hip?	<u>Osteoarthritis</u>; ankylosing spondylitis
• knee?	<u>Osteoarthritis</u> (the most common source of major disability in osteoarthritis); <u>loose bodies</u>; juvenile rheumatoid arthritis (monoarticular involvement); tuberculous arthritis; neurogenic, tabes (pain, when present, is mild)
• ankle? foot?	<u>Traumatic</u> injury, sprain (may affect any joint); neurogenic, diabetes (pain, when present, is mild)
• *great toe?*	<u>Gout</u>
• small joints of foot? (metatarsophalangeal, toes)	Rheumatoid arthritis [pseudogout does not affect the small joints of (hands and) feet]
• in an area adjacent to a joint?	Periarticular structure: bursitis, tendonitis
• in thigh? buttock? calf? foot? (nonarticular)	Origin of pain in skin, vessels, nerves, muscle, bone; lumbar spine
• in the calf?	<u>Vascular occlusion</u>, chronic or acute; if sudden onset of severe pain: spontaneous rupture of plantaris tendon
• in both feet?	If acute pain: cholesterol emboli arising from ulcerating plaques in the aorta
• in the foot? toes?	Ischemic rest pain due to chronic arterial occlusion is generally localized to the foot and toes
• along the limb in a linear fashion? crossing over joint and muscle areas?	Lesion of <u>nerve</u> or <u>blood vessel</u>: herniated intervertebral disk; neuropathy; <u>deep-vein thrombosis</u>; arterial occlusion

1.2 Do you have back pain radiating to your limb?	Radicular pain
• *in the lateral region of the thigh, calf? to the dorsum of the foot?*	Lesion of the fifth lumbar root: herniation of disk between the fourth and fifth lumbar vertebrae
• *in the posterior part of the thigh? calf? to the heel and plantar surface of the foot?*	Lesion of the first sacral root: herniation of disk between the fifth lumbar and the first sacral vertebrae
• in the anterior part of the thigh and knee?	Lesions of the fourth and third lumbar roots (rarer)

2   Mode of onset and duration

2.1 How long have you had pain in your limb?	
2.2 Was the onset of pain • acute?	Acute arterial occlusion (thrombosis or embolism); acute infectious process, articular or nonarticular; in calf: spontaneous rupture of plantaris tendon; in both feet: cholesterol emboli arising from ulcerating plaques in the aorta
• gradual?	<u>Chronic arterial occlusion</u>; <u>neuropathy</u>; chronic <u>joint</u> disorder

3   Character and intensity of the pain

3.1 Is your pain • *sharp? shooting?* burning?	Nerve lesions: posterior nerve roots, peripheral neuropathy
• dull? diffuse?	Venous or lymphatic disorders
• aching?	Muscle or joint problems
• throbbing?	Pain arising in the bones
3.2 Is the pain • severe?	Arterial occlusion; osteomyelitis; gout

• mild?	Venous thrombosis; muscle or joint pain is usually not very severe

4 Precipitating or aggravating factors

4.1 In case of articular pain, do you have pain in your joint	
• only with movement?	Hip and knee: osteoarthritis (early stage) Knee: posttraumatic internal joint derangement
• at rest?	Rheumatoid arthritis; osteo-arthritis (advanced stage)
4.1*a* Is the pain induced or made worse upon weight bearing?	Degenerative hip and knee joint disease
4.2 In case of nonarticular pain, is the pain induced or made worse	
• *by sneezing? coughing? straining at stool? bending?* lifting?	Disorders of the vertebral column or of the posterior nerve roots (<u>herniated nucleosus pulposus</u>)
• by elevation of your legs? • by exposure to cold?	Pain of ulceration; ischemic rest pain; <u>chronic arterial occlusion</u>
• by dependency?	<u>Venous obstruction</u>
• by exercise?	Chronic arterial occlusion; osteomyelitis; deep-vein thrombosis
• at night?	<u>Nocturnal muscle cramp</u>; chronic arterial occlusion; involvement of bone
• by prolonged standing?	Chronic venous insufficiency; lymphedema; origin of pain in the lumbar spine or feet
• by movements of the back?	Disorder of the spine or hip
4.3 *Is your pain induced by walking?*	<u>Intermittent claudication</u>: chronic arterial occlusion; also in musculoskeletal disorders

4.3*a*   Where do you have pain
on walking?

• in the calf?

Occlusion of popliteal artery or
higher

• at the arch of the foot?

Occlusion of branches of popliteal artery or higher

• *at the instep?*

Thromboangiitis obliterans

• in the thigh, buttock, and
calf?

Occlusion of common femoral
artery or iliac arteries

• in the thigh and buttock?
• without calf pain?
• with low back pain?

Pseudoclaudication syndrome:
compression of the cauda
equina by protruded lumbar disk
or hypertrophic ridging

4.3*b*   How long are you able to
walk, at an average pace
on level ground, before the
pain appears?

The walking distance required
to produce the pain is usually
fairly constant at any stage of
the chronic arterial occlusion

• half an hour?

Early stage of chronic arterial
occlusion

• between one-half and two
blocks?

Most frequently in chronic arterial occlusion

• 50 to 100 steps?

Advanced stage of the disease

5   *Relieving factors*

5.1   Is the pain relieved by

• elevation of your leg?

Chronic venous insufficiency,
postphlebitic syndrome

• dependency?

(Rest) pain due to chronic arterial occlusion

5.2   In case of pain induced by
walking, is your pain re-
lieved by rest

• *promptly?* (1 to 2 min)

Chronic arterial occlusion with
intermittent claudication

• gradually? Does the pain
persist for longer than 10
min after you have stopped
walking?

Pseudoclaudication syndrome;
degenerative hip and/or knee
joint disease; probably not
chronic arterial occlusion

6　*Accompanying symptoms*

6.1　In case of hip pain, do you have inability to walk? limping?

Osteoarthritis, necrosis of hip; hips may be affected in ankylosing spondylitis

6.2　In case of knee pain, do you have

- a feeling of locking, snapping at times?
- pain on squatting? on running up and down stairs?

Posttraumatic internal joint derangement: involvement of medial meniscus; ligament tear

- concomitant hip pain?

Referred pain from hip

6.2*a*　Is your painful knee swollen? red? hot?

Infection: septic, gonococcal arthritis; microcrystalline arthritis

6.2*b*　Is your swollen knee relatively painless?

Intermittent hydrarthrosis (female preponderance)

6.3　In case of acute nonarticular pain, has the pain been followed by coldness? numbness? tingling? muscle weakness?

Acute arterial occlusion (thrombosis or embolism)

6.4　In case of acute nonarticular pain, is the pain accompanied by

- local swelling? redness?

Cellulitis; lymphangitis; superficial thrombophlebitis

- tender red nodules on the legs?

Erythema nodosum

6.5　Do you have

- fever? chills?

Acute sepsis; septic arthritis; acute osteomyelitis; erythema nodosum; acute suppurative myositis

- *numbness, tingling in the limb?*

Nerve root compression: herniated lumbar intervertebral disk

• skin ulcerations?	Chronic arterial occlusion; multiple sites of vascular occlusion; thromboangiitis obliterans
• swollen legs?	Chronic venous insufficiency
• (male patient) pain on urination?	Gonococcal arthritis or tendonitis
• (female patient) a vaginal discharge?	
• sexual impotence?	With hip, thigh, and buttock claudication: Leriche syndrome: terminal aortic occlusion

7   Iatrogenic factors   see Etiology

8   Personal antecedents pertaining to the pain

8.1   Have you ever had an x-ray of your joints? bones? When? With what results?

8.2   Have you recently had

• a trauma to your limb?	Posttraumatic arthritis; acute attack of gout
	Knee: torn ligament or meniscus; loose bodies
	Hip: avascular necrosis of head of femur
	Infection introduced into the body by the trauma
• an operation? a prolonged immobilization?	Deep-vein thrombosis

8.3   Do you have

• a heart disease? atrial fibrillation?	Acute embolic arterial occlusion
• diabetes?	Neurogenic limb pain; chronic arterial occlusion

8.4   Do you smoke?   Adverse effect on occlusive arterial disease

PHYSICAL SIGNS PERTINENT TO THE COMPLAINT

Finding	Possible *significance*
Local swelling, warmth, erythema; fever	Infectious process: cellulitis, with or without lymphangitis
Swollen, red, warm, tender joint(s)	Acute pyogenic arthritis; post-traumatic; rheumatoid arthritis; microcrystalline arthritis; rheumatic fever
Cold, pallid limb; motor weakness; loss of sensation; absent pulses; no swelling	Acute arterial occlusion: embolism, thrombosis, injury
• with irregular heart rhythm	Atrial fibrillation with arterial embolism
Palpable pulse disappearing with exercise; absent pulse(s); cool limb; extremity becoming pale on elevation; trophic changes in skin and nails; ulceration	Chronic arterial occlusion: atherosclerosis of large and medium-sized arteries
Murmur audible over the aorta and peripheral arteries	Proximal obstruction or stenotic lesion
After a period of elevation of the leg:	
• flushing time >20 s • venous filling time >30 s	Severe arterial obstruction; inadequate collateral circulation
Absent pulses with warm, normally colored extremity	Chronic arterial occlusion with adequate collateral blood flow
Cyanotic mottling of the skin of the feet	Livedo reticularis (with symmetric rest pain in the feet: cholesterol emboli from the aorta)
Tender cords in the path of veins; erythema of the overlying skin; no prominent leg swelling	Superficial-vein thrombosis
Leg edema; tenderness in the calf muscles; calf pain with dorsiflexion of the foot (Homan's sign)	Deep-vein thrombosis

Bone tenderness	Fracture; malignancy
• with fever, chills, local swelling	Osteomyelitis
Warm, tender, red nodules over the tibial areas	Erythema nodosum: associated with streptococcal infection, sarcoidosis, tuberculosis, coccidioidomycosis, ulcerative colitis, regional enteritis, drugs
Palpable, tender temporal artery	Polymyalgia rheumatica (with pain in the limbs)
Absent ankle and knee jerks; sensory impairment; tenderness of deep tissues	Polyneuropathy
Low back and leg pain:	Herniated lumbar intervertebral disk: degenerative disk disease; osteoarthritis, with nerve root compression
• with weakness of the extensors of the big toe and of the foot; difficulty in walking on the heels; no reflex change; sensory deficit in the lateral leg and mediodorsal aspect of the foot	Lesion of the fifth lumbar root
• with diminished to absent ankle reflex, weakness of plantar flexors, difficulty in walking on the toes, sensory deficit in the lateral border and sole of the foot and toes	Lesion of the first sacral root
• with diminished to absent knee jerk, sensory deficit in the anterior part of the thigh and knee	Lesion of the fourth and third lumbar roots (rarer)

LABORATORY TESTS PERTAINING TO THE COMPLAINT

Procedure	To detect
Lumbosacral spine x-rays	Intervertebral disk herniation; primary or metastatic neoplasm

Joint and bone x-rays	Fracture; rheumatoid arthritis; osteoarthritis; gout; pseudogout; osteomyelitis; primary or metastatic tumor
Ultrasonic and/or plethysmographic methods	Thrombosis of the major deep veins of the leg
Radioactive fibrinogen (^{125}I) test	Early calf vein thrombosis
Phlebography	Deep-vein thrombosis
Arteriography	Location and extent of the occlusive involvement in chronic or acute arterial occlusion
Ultrasonic arterial flow detection	Peripheral arterial disease
Myelography	Intervertebral disk herniation; spinal cord tumor
Nerve conduction studies	Neuropathies
Joint fluid analysis*	See Chap. 38
Electromyography*	Lesions of anterior horn cells, muscle, peripheral nerves
Muscle biopsy*	Myopathies vs. neuropathies

* If appropriate.

USEFUL REMINDERS AND DIAGNOSTIC CLUES

Misleading Factors
Pain ascribed to walking may actually be due to standing and may have its source in the lumbar spine or feet.

In meralgia paresthetica (compression of the lateral femoral cutaneous nerve), the pain and numbness in the lateral aspect of the thigh may be confused with sciatica.

Hip pain is frequently referred to the knee and may present as such.

Diagnostic Considerations
A patient with intermittent claudication almost always has objective evidence of impaired circulation.

Intermittent claudication is unilateral at first and may become bilateral at any time.

Nocturnal muscular cramps are not symptoms of arterial disease of any kind; they are more frequent in pregnant women, the middle aged, and the elderly.

The first symptom of deep-vein thrombosis is often pulmonary embolism.

SELECTED BIBLIOGRAPHY

Fairbairn II JF: Approach to the patient with peripheral vascular disease, in Fairbairn II JF, Juergens JL, Spittel, Jr JA: *Peripheral Vascular Diseases,* 4th ed, pp 27–44, Philadelphia: Saunders, 1972

Strandness, Jr DE: Pain in the extremities, in *Harrison's Principles of Internal Medicine,* 8th ed, pp 49–53, New York: McGraw-Hill, 1977

41

Pain in the Neck and Shoulder

DEFINITIONS AND GENERAL CONSIDERATIONS

Local pain   caused by any pathologic process which impinges upon, or irritates, sensory nerve endings in periosteum, synovial membranes, muscles, annulus fibrosus, and ligaments.

Referred pain   produced by stimulation of sensory nerve endings in the structural soft tissues which support the cervical spine and which are part of the cervical disk complex.

Radicular (root) pain   caused by distortion or compression of a spinal root.

Pain arising from the cervical spine is experienced in the neck and back of the head, but may be projected to the shoulder and arm. The pain of herniated nucleosus pulposus is deep and poorly localized to the level of the spine where the disk rupture has occurred. It is usually associated with evidence of neurologic involvement. Nerve roots may also be involved in osteoarthritis of the cervical spine.

Pain of brachial plexus origin (abnormalities of the thoracic outlet) is felt in and around the shoulder, in the supraclavicular region, or between the shoulders; it is associated with neurologic and circulatory abnormalities in the arm.

Shoulder pain resulting from a tear in the rotator cuff or from a calcific tendonitis may radiate into the arm or hand, but is not associated with peripheral sensory, motor, and reflex changes. Apart from acute traumatic lesions, 85 to 90 percent of painful disability of the shoulder is due to nonarticular disorders of tendons, bursas, tendon sheaths, and the musculotendinous cuff.

ETIOLOGY

Neck pain
Fibrositis; chronic cervical muscle spasm
Osteoarthritis: degenerative joint disease of the cervical spine, cervical spondylosis

Herniated intervertebral cervical disk
Juvenile rheumatoid arthritis; ankylosing spondylitis
Tumors: local (hemangioma, osteoid osteoma, neurofibroma, meningioma); metastatic
Whiplash injury
Temporal arteritis

Pain in the shoulder
Local: rotator cuff tear; calcific tendonitis; adhesive capsulitis
Vertebral column: fractures; arthritis; protruded disk
Neurovascular:
  Compression (thoracic outlet) syndromes: cervical rib syndrome, scalenus anticus syndrome, costoclavicular syndrome, hyperabduction syndrome
  Shoulder-hand syndrome: idiopathic; secondary: trauma, cervical osteoarthritis, cervical disk herniation, myocardial infarction, stroke, superior sulcus tumor of the lung, drugs
Peripheral nerves: trauma; tumors; neuritis
Spinal cord: syringomyelia; herpes zoster; tumors
Viscerogenic:
  Thorax: cardiac, aorta, diaphragm, sternal lesions
  Abdomen: gallbladder, diaphragm

Iatrogenic Causes of Shoulder-Hand Syndrome

Barbiturates; ethionamide; isoniazid

QUESTIONNAIRE

Neck Pain

Possible *meaning of response*

1 Location and radiation of the pain

1.1 Where do you have pain?
  • anterior neck pain?

Thyroid; intrathoracic disease with referred pain to the neck: ischemic heart disease

  • in the neck and back of head?

Pain arising from the cervical spine

1.2   Does the pain radiate to
   • the shoulder(s)?
   • the arm(s)?

Cervical nerve root involvement: herniated cervical disk; osteoarthritis

2   *Mode of onset and duration*

2.1   Was the onset of pain
   • abrupt?
   • gradual? (several days)

Herniated cervical disk
Cervical osteoarthritis

2.2   How long have you had pain?
   • hours to days?

Acute cervical strain; whiplash injury

   • weeks to months?

Subacute or chronic process: herniated cervical disk; osteoarthritis; fibrositis

3   *Character and intensity of the pain*

3.1   Is the pain dull? aching?

Pain caused by muscle or joint disorder; chronic cervical muscle spasm

3.2   In case of pain pro- jected to the arm, *is the radiated pain sharp? shooting?*

Pain associated with cervical nerve root lesion; radicular pain of cervical disk disease; coinci- dental involvement of nerve roots in osteoarthritis

4   *Precipitating or aggravating factors*

4.1   Is the pain evoked or enhanced
   • by certain movements or positions of the neck?
   • by hyperextension of the neck?

Cervical nerve root compres- sion: herniated cervical disk, osteoarthritis

   • by activity?

Mechanical pain: disk lesion, osteoarthritis

   • by inactivity?

Fibrositis; chronic cervical muscle spasm

5   *Relieving factors*

5.1   Is your neck pain relieved
   • by rest?

Cervical nerve root compression

   • by movement?

Fibrositis

   • by flexion of the neck?

Cervical nerve root compression

6   *Accompanying symptoms*

6.1   Do you have
   • stiffness, limitation of
     mobility of the neck?

Pain arising from the cervical
spine; osteoarthritis, ruptured
cervical disk, fibrositis

   • numbness, tingling, weakness, in your arm, hand?

Cervical nerve root compression

   • pain and/or swelling in
     other joints?

Juvenile rheumatoid arthritis
(cervical involvement occurs in
50 percent of patients)

   • headaches?

Patients with long-standing
chronic muscle spasm or rheumatoid arthritis of the spine
often develop occipital headaches; meningismus; temporal
arteritis may cause pain in the
occipital and upper cervical
regions

   • fever?

Infection of cervical vertebra;
meningismus

   • episodes of vertigo?
   • visual impairment?

Compression of the vertebral
arteries by degenerative spurs
in the spinal canal may
compromise the blood supply
to the brain

   • a weakness in your legs?
   • disturbance of your gait?
     (ataxia)

Compression of the spinal
cord by cervical disk or by
bony ridges formed in the spinal
canal; primary neurologic
disease: syringomyelia; amyotrophic lateral sclerosis; tumor

7   *Environmental factors*

7.1   What is your profession?

Persons in certain occupations (draftsmen, typists, clerks) are liable to chronic spasm of the posterior cervical muscles (fibrositis)

8   *Personal antecedents pertaining to the neck pain*

8.1   Have you ever had an x-ray of your neck? When? With what results?

8.2   Have you recently sustained

• a trauma to the neck?
• a car accident?

Acute cervical strain; whiplash injury: injury to the ligaments and muscles (the pain may appear 48 to 72 h after the accident)

• *sudden hyperextension of the neck?* diving?

Ruptured cervical disk

Shoulder Pain

1   *Location and radiation*

1.1   Where do you have pain?
• in and around the shoulder?

Tear of the rotator cuff; tendonitis; abnormalities of the thoracic outlet

1.2   Does the pain radiate to the arm?

Thoracic outlet syndrome; may occur in calcific tendonitis

2   *Mode of onset and duration*

2.1   How long have you had pain in your shoulder?
• hours to days?

Acute process: calcific tendonitis, subacromial bursitis

• weeks to months?	Chronic process: <u>adhesive capsulitis</u>; shoulder-hand syndrome

2.2   Was the onset of the pain
   • sudden?   Calcific tendonitis (onset may be subacute)

   • gradual?   Adhesive capsulitis; shoulder-hand syndrome (onset may be acute)

3   Character and intensity of the pain

3.1   Is the pain
   • severe?   <u>Calcific tendonitis</u>

   • interfering with sleep?   Night pain may be prominent in calcific tendonitis

   • constant, dull, aching? }
   • slowly progressive?   } <u>Adhesive capsulitis</u>; also in chronic form of calcific tendonitis; skeletal pain

4   Precipitating or aggravating factors

4.1   Is the pain increased by
   • motion of the shoulder? }
   • rotation? abduction?   }
   • inserting your arm into a } <u>Tear of the tendon cuff</u>; <u>calcific tendonitis</u>; <u>adhesive capsulitis</u>
     coat sleeve?   }

   • certain positions of the }
     arm?   }
   • elevation of the arm above } Thoracic outlet syndrome
     the chest level?   }
   • the performance of certain }
     tasks with arm?   }

5   Accompanying symptoms

5.1   Do you have stiffness,   <u>Adhesive capsulitis</u>
     limitation of mobility,
     wasting of the muscles, of
     the shoulder?

5.2 *Do you have numbness, tingling in the arm? the hand?*	Thoracic outlet syndrome; sensory, or other neurologic changes in the arm indicating disease of the nerve roots, plexus, or peripheral nerves are absent when shoulder pain is due to calcific tendonitis
5.3 Is your hand swollen? painful on motion?	Shoulder-hand syndrome; occasionally thoracic outlet syndrome
5.4 *Do you have pain in your fingers when they are immersed in cold water?*	Unilateral Raynaud's phenomenon may occur in thoracic outlet syndrome; shoulder-hand syndrome

6 *Iatrogenic factors* see Etiology

7 *Personal antecedents pertaining to the pain in the shoulder*

7.1 Have you ever had an x-ray of your shoulder? When? With what results?

7.2 Have you ever had a trauma to your shoulder?	Rotator cuff tears

7.3 Do you have a neurologic disease? rheumatoid arthritis? degenerative arthritis?

PHYSICAL SIGNS PERTINENT TO THE COMPLAINT

Finding	**Possible** *significance*
Tenderness and limitation of motion of the neck	Disease of the ligaments, muscles, or apophyseal joints in the cervical spine; osteoarthritis
Swollen, red, warm, tender joint	Acute pyogenic arthritis, posttraumatic, microcrystalline arthritis
Shoulder pain with	

- loss of radial pulse in bracing and pulling down on shoulders, abducting arm over head, or during Adson's test*
- pallor on elevating the arm

} Thoracic outlet syndrome

- supraclavicular palpable abnormality

Aneurysm of the subclavian artery, cervical rib, tumor, causing the thoracic outlet syndrome

Neck and shoulder pain radiating into the arm, with weakness, deep-tendon reflex, and sensory changes in the arm

Involvement of nerve roots: osteoarthritis of the cervical spine; ruptured cervical disk (see Chap. 42)

Shoulder pain with tenderness and limitation of extension, abduction, rotation; no sensory, motor, and reflex changes

Tear of the rotator cuff; calcific tendonitis; adhesive capsulitis

Shoulder pain with trophic and vasomotor changes of the hand

Shoulder-hand syndrome; thoracic outlet syndrome

* Adson's test: the patient holds a full breath while extending the neck and turning the head toward the affected side.

LABORATORY TESTS PERTAINING TO THE COMPLAINT

Procedure	To detect
Cervical spine x-rays	Osteoarthritis; rheumatoid arthritis; ruptured cervical disk; cervical rib with thoracic outlet syndrome
Shoulder x-rays	Linear calcific deposits: calcific tendonitis
Contrast arthrography*	Rotator cuff tears
Chest x-ray	Thoracic outlet anomalies; superior sulcus (Pancoast's) tumor of the lung

* If appropriate.

ECG	Ischemic heart disease with shoulder-hand syndrome
Joint fluid analysis*	See Chap. 38

* If appropriate.

USEFUL REMINDERS AND DIAGNOSTIC CLUES

Neck Pain

The most common sites of degenerative cervical disk disease are the C5 to C6 interspace (sixth cervical root) and C6 to C7 interspace (seventh cervical root).

Pain in the Neck and Shoulder

In the cervical region, symptoms due to osteoarthritis are far more common than complaints due to a herniated cervical disk.

Pain in the neck extending upward to the suboccipital or post-auricular region, or into the mid- or upper portions of the neck laterally, almost certainly excludes lower cervical nerve root compression.

Shoulder Pain

In the shoulder-hand syndrome, either the shoulder or the hand may be affected first, or the condition may develop in the two simultaneously.

The frequency of the shoulder-hand syndrome following myocardial infarction is decreasing with earlier mobilization of these patients.

A cervical supernumerary rib, usually originating from the seventh cervical vertebra, is often present without clinical symptoms.

Pain in the deltoid area usually reflects intrinsic disease of the shoulder; it is rarely viscerogenic.

Location of referred viscerogenic pain in the shoulder

At the trapezius ridge: diaphragmatic irritation, perforated viscus, pulmonary infarction; pericardial disease

Left pectoral and ulnar regions: myocardial ischemia

Right side of the neck and shoulder: ascending arch of the aorta

Left side of the back and shoulder: transverse or descending portions of the aortic arch

Right scapula: biliary tract disease

SELECTED BIBLIOGRAPHY

Christian CL: The painful shoulder, in Beeson PB, McDermott W (eds), *Textbook of Medicine,* 14th ed, chap 99, pp 161–163, Philadelphia: Saunders, 1975

Moskowitz RW: *Clinical Rheumatology: A Problem-oriented Approach,* chap 15, pp 219–229, Philadelphia: Lea & Febiger, 1975

42
Pain in the Upper Extremities

GENERAL CONSIDERATIONS

Pain in the upper extremities may result from diseases of the skin and of the musculoskeletal, vascular, and nervous systems. Any agent (mechanical, chemical, thermal) causing inflammation, swelling, ischemia, or destruction of pain-sensitive tissues may be painful. Superficial pain (caused by bacterial infection, trauma, burns) is well localized and is associated with tenderness and hyperalgesia. Deep pain arising from vessels, fascia, joints, periosteum, and supporting structures is often poorly localized and dull, and may be accompanied by muscular rigidity and deep tenderness. The pain due to disorders of the joints (acute or chronic process) is usually related to inflammation of the synovial membrane. Pain from ischemic skeletal muscles is due to the action on sensory nerve endings of metabolites accumulating in the muscles or changes in the nerves themselves. Painful intermittent vasospasm in the hands of young female patients, initiated by exposure to cold (Raynaud's phenomenon), is attributed to excessive adrenergic stimulation directed selectively to the vessels of the upper limbs or a defect in basal heat production limiting the ability of these patients to dilate their cutaneous vessels. Pain caused by diseases of the peripheral nerves or by entrapment neuropathy (carpal tunnel syndrome) is usually accompanied by motor, reflex, and other sensory changes. Irritation of the cervical nerve roots (herniated nucleosus pulposus, osteoarthritis) can cause pain in the upper extremities. Pain in the upper limb caused by compression of the neurovascular bundle as it leaves the thorax (thoracic outlet syndrome) is frequently associated with evidence of vascular compression. Pain originating from intrathoracic structures (ischemic heart disease) may radiate to the inner surfaces of the arm.

ETIOLOGY

Skin and soft tissues
Cellulitis: bacterial and fungous infection; lymphangitis
Acute trauma to the skin

Articular and periarticular structures
Arthritis: acute pyogenic arthritis; rheumatoid arthritis; rheumatic
fever; osteoarthritis; gout; posttraumatic; hypertrophic osteo
arthropathy
Bursitis; tendonitis

Bones and periosteum
Osteomyelitis; fractures; tumors

Muscles
Acute suppurative myositis; polymyositis, dermatomyositis

Neurologic
Polyneuropathy, mononeuropathy; carpal tunnel syndrome
Cervical nerve root compression: protruded cervical disk; osteo-
arthritis; spinal cord disorder
Brachial plexus disorders: thoracic outlet syndromes; superior sul-
cus tumor of the lung

Vascular
Raynaud's phenomenon; phlebitis; thromboangiitis obliterans

Iatrogenic Causes of Raynaud's Phenomenon
Propranolol; ergotamine preparations; methysergide

QUESTIONNAIRE

Possible *meaning of response*

1 Location of the pain

1.1 Where do you have pain?
   • in a joint?

Pain resulting from an articular
disorder is perceived as coming
directly from the joint, not from
the bones between the joints

   • elbows? wrists?

Rheumatoid arthritis; septic
arthritis; pseudogout (frequently
symmetric in rheumatoid arthritis)

- *metacarpal phalangeal joints?*
- *proximal interphalangeal joints?*

- *distal interphalangeal joints?*

- *carpometacarpal joint of thumb?*
- in an area adjacent to a joint?
  - at an elbow?
  - at a wrist?

- in the arm? forearm? (nonarticular)

- along the limb in a linear fashion? crossing over joint and muscle areas?

  - *the tip of the shoulder, the anterior upper part of the arm, the radial forearm, the thumb?*
  - *the shoulder blade, pectoral region, posterolateral upper arm, dorsal forearm and elbow, index and middle finger?*
  - the posteromedial part of the arm and forearm?
- *in the first three fingers?*

Rheumatoid arthritis

Rheumatoid arthritis (nontender Bouchard's nodes in osteo-arthritis)
Osteoarthritis (Heberden's nodes; often painless); psoriatic arthritis
Osteoarthritis

Periarticular structures: tendon-itis, bursitis, bone
Epicondylitis (tennis elbow)
Tenosynovitis; tuberculous synovitis
Origin of pain in: skin, muscle, bone, vessels, nerves; pain due to lesions of muscle is usually felt over the muscle belly, not at the areas of insertion near the joints or tendons
Lesion of nerve or blood vessels: nerve root compression; thoracic outlet syndrome; peripheral nerve lesion; referred pain, ischemic heart disease
Fifth to sixth cervical disk disease: involvement of the sixth cervical root

Sixth to seventh cervical disk disease: involvement of the seventh cervical root

Eighth cervical root

Carpal tunnel syndrome: compression of the median nerve at the wrist

• at the ulnar aspect of the hand?	Lesion of the ulnar nerve (commonly at the elbow) **or of** the brachial plexus
• in the entire hand? (and shoulder?)	Shoulder-hand syndrome
• in the fingers? *at the finger tips?*	On exposure to cold: Raynaud's phenomenon or disease

2 Character of pain

2.1 Is the pain
• aching?	Muscle or joint problem
• *shooting? sharp?* burning?	Nerve lesion; cervical root **pain** (protruded cervical disk; <u>cervical spondylosis</u>; cervical intraspinal lesion)
• throbbing?	Pain arising from bone

3 Precipitating or aggravating factors

3.1 In case of articular pain, is the pain
• present only with movements?	Osteoarthritis (early stage)
• present at rest?	Rheumatoid arthritis; osteoarthritis (later stage)
• increased by motion?	Any disorder of the joints

3.2 In case of nonarticular pain, is the pain in your arm induced or made worse
• *by sneezing? coughing?* hyperextension of the neck? when shaving under the chin?	Cervical nerve root pain: protruded cervical disk; <u>cervical spondylosis</u>
• upon rotating the head? • on laterally flexing the neck?	Cervical spine lesion
• on general exertion?	Referred pain, **ischemic heart disease** (inner arm)

• when elevating the arm above the head? bracing the shoulders?	Thoracic outlet syndrome

3.3 If the pain is localized to the first three fingers, does the pain occur
  • at night?
  • when grasping an object for a prolonged time? } Carpal tunnel syndrome (more frequent in women); frequently bilateral

3.4 In case of pain in the fingers, is the pain induced by
  • *exposure to cold?*
  • *an emotional upset?* } Raynaud's phenomenon

4 *Relieving factors*

4.1 In case of nonarticular pain, is the pain relieved by
  • flexion of the neck? Cervical nerve root compression
  • *nitroglycerin?* rest? **Ischemic heart disease** with referred pain

4.2 In case of pain in the fingers, is the pain relieved by heat? Raynaud's phenomenon

5 *Accompanying symptoms*

5.1 In case of articular pain, is the joint swollen? Infectious arthritis (in large joints); microcrystalline (gout, pseudogout); rheumatoid arthritis

5.2 In case of nonarticular pain:
  • Is the involved area swollen? red? Cellulitis, with or without lymphangitis
  • Is the hand swollen? Shoulder-hand syndrome

• Is the arm swollen? discolored?	Occasionally in the thoracic outlet syndrome, with venous occlusion

5.3   Do you have
• fever? chills?	Septic arthritis; acute osteo-myelitis; cellulitis; acute sup-purative myositis
• *numbness, tingling* in the arm?	Nerve root compression syndrome; thoracic outlet syndrome; peripheral neuropathy
• chest pain on exertion?	**Ischemic heart disease** with referred pain in the arm
• bloody expectorations? cough?	Lung tumor with hypertrophic osteoarthropathy; superior sulcus (Pancoast's) tumor involving the brachial plexus

6   Personal antecedents pertaining to the pain

6.1   Have you recently had
• a trauma, an injury to the affected area?	Posttraumatic arthritis or muscular pain; portal of entry for infecting agent: cellulitis, acute suppurative myositis, septic arthritis
• a trauma to the neck? • a "whiplash" injury?	May cause radicular symptoms
• injections into the shoulder muscles? an infectious disease?	May precede acute brachial plexus neuropathy
• a myocardial infarction?	Shoulder-hand syndrome

PHYSICAL SIGNS PERTINENT TO THE COMPLAINT

Finding	*Possible significance*
Local swelling, warmth, erythema; fever	Infectious process; cellulitis with or without lymphangitis
Tender, swollen, red, warm joint(s)	Acute pyogenic arthritis; post-traumatic; microcrystalline; rheumatoid arthritis; rheumatic fever

Weakness and sensory loss in the middle three fingers; tenderness on pressure over the carpal ligament; atrophy of the thenar eminence; positive Tinel's sign*	Carpal tunnel syndrome (may occur in multiple myeloma, amyloidosis)
Bone tenderness	Fracture; malignancy
• with fever, chills, local swelling	Osteomyelitis
Color changes in the fingers brought about by putting the patient's hands into ice water for a few minutes	Raynaud's phenomenon; may occur in: connective-tissue disease, rheumatoid arthritis, thromboangiitis obliterans, dysproteinemia, cryopathies, occupational trauma, thoracic outlet syndrome, drugs
Clubbing	Hypertrophic osteoarthropathy: lung cancer
Palpable tender temporal artery	Polymyalgia rheumatica (with pain in the limbs)
Pain in the arm and the neck:	Osteoarthritis of the cervical spine; ruptured cervical disk, with involvement of cervical nerve roots
• with sensory impairment in the tip of the shoulder, anterior upper part of the arm, radial forearm, thumb; weakness in flexion of the forearm; absent biceps and supinator reflexes; retained biceps reflex	Protruded disk between the fifth and sixth cervical vertebrae: involvement of the sixth cervical root
• with sensory impairment in the second and third fingers; weakness in extension of the forearm and in the hand grip; absent triceps reflex; retained biceps and supinator reflexes	Protruded disk between the sixth and seventh vertebrae: involvement of the seventh cervical root

* Tinel's sign: tingling sensation in the fingers on tapping the median nerve at the wrist.

LABORATORY TESTS PERTAINING TO THE COMPLAINT

Procedure	To detect
Cervical spine x-rays	Osteoarthritis; intervertebral disk herniation; cervical rib with thoracic outlet syndrome
Chest x-ray	Superior sulcus tumor of the lung (Pancoast's syndrome)
Joint and bone x-rays	Rheumatoid arthritis; osteoarthritis; fracture; osteomyelitis; tumor, primary or metastatic; hypertrophic osteoarthropathy
Joint fluid analysis*	See Chap. 38
Nerve conduction studies*	Neuropathies; thoracic outlet syndromes; carpal tunnel syndrome (delayed conduction at the wrist)
Electromyography*	Lesions of anterior horn cells, muscle, peripheral nerves
Muscle biopsy*	Myopathies vs. neuropathies
Angiography,* Venography* Ultrasonic methods*	Location and extent of occlusive vascular involvement
Myelography*	Intervertebral disk herniation; spinal cord tumor

* If appropriate.

USEFUL REMINDERS AND DIAGNOSTIC CLUES

Misleading Factors

Pain in the left arm associated with chest pain does not necessarily indicate the presence of ischemic heart disease; almost any condition capable of causing chest pain may induce radiation to the left arm.

The pain in the carpal tunnel syndrome may extend up the arm; the syndrome may then be mistaken for disease of the shoulder or neck.

Diagnostic Considerations

Recurrent bursitis of shoulder or elbow may be a manifestation of gout.

Clubbing associated with carcinoma of the lung is often painful; clubbing associated with nonneoplastic conditions (chronic pulmonary disease, biliary cirrhosis, ulcerative colitis, regional enteritis, congenital cyanotic heart disease, bacterial endocarditis) is usually asymptomatic.

SELECTED BIBLIOGRAPHY

Moort ME, Tourtelotte CD: Pain in the extremity and back, in Conn HF, Conn RB; *Current Diagnosis 5*, pp 63–70, Philadelphia: Saunders, 1977

Strandness, Jr DE: Pain in the extremities, in *Harrison's Principles of Internal Medicine*, 8th ed, pp 49–53, New York: McGraw-Hill, 1977

Hematologic-Metabolic Disorders

43
Anemia

DEFINITION AND PATHOPHYSIOLOGY

Anemia reduction below normal in the concentration of hemoglobin or red blood cells in the blood.

In normal subjects the erythrocyte is produced by the bone marrow and released to the circulation, where it remains for approximately 120 days. It is then removed by the reticuloendothelial system of the spleen, the liver, and the bone marrow. The major stimulus to erythroid cell production is tissue oxygen deficit. The rate of erythropoiesis is regulated by erythropoietin, a glycoprotein produced by the kidney in response to tissue oxygen requirements. The erythrocyte transports oxygen bound to hemoglobin, which comprises about 95 percent of the dry weight of the red blood cell (RBC). Iron, vitamin B_{12}, and folic acid are necessary for normal erythropoiesis.

Physiologically, anemia may be defined as a reduction in oxygen-carrying capacity of the blood as reflected by its hemoglobin concentration. Anemia may develop as the result of inadequate production of RBCs. This may be due to a decrease in the number of functioning erythroid stem cells (aplastic anemia, marrow fibrosis).

Impaired production of RBCs may also result from abnormal maturation of erythroid cells. A defect in hemoglobin synthesis may be due to iron deficiency, a defect in the synthesis of heme (sideroblastic anemia), or globin (thalassemia). Maturation disorders due to deficiency of vitamin B_{12} or folic acid result in megaloblastic anemias and reflect impaired DNA synthesis involving all replicating tissues.

Anemia may result from excessive destruction of RBCs. A shortening of erythrocyte survival occurs in hemolytic anemias, which may be inherited or acquired. Inherited hemolytic disorders usually result from intrinsic (or intracorpuscular) defects and include hemoglobinopathies (sickle cell anemia), enzymopathies, and membrane defects (hereditary spherocytosis with undue rigidity of the red cells). Acquired hemolytic anemias usually reflect extrinsic (extracorpuscular) defects. In antibody-mediated, idiopathic or secondary, hemolysis (positive Coombs' antiglobulin test), presence of either IgG or complement renders the red cell vulnerable to phagocytosis. Coombs-negative hemolytic anemias may result from mechanical damage to red cells (microangiopathic hemolytic anemia, "heart valve hemolysis"). In anemias of chronic diseases (chronic inflammation, rheumatoid arthritis, malignancy), erythropoietin levels are usually low and a mild hemolytic process is common, with failure of the bone marrow to increase RBC production. The anemia of chronic renal failure is attributed to lack of erythropoietin, hemolysis, and deficient erythropoiesis due to accumulation of toxic metabolites.

Anemia may also appear as the result of acute blood loss. Iron deficiency due to chronic blood loss (from pelvic organs in women and from the gastrointestinal tract in men) is probably the most common form of anemia.

Evaluation of any patient with anemia requires a careful interpretation of a peripheral blood film and of the three erythrocyte indexes:

Mean corpuscular volume (MCV):
$$\frac{\text{Volume of packed red cells/1000 mL blood}}{\text{red cells, millions/mm}^3}$$
normally: $90 \pm 5 \ \mu m^3$/red blood cell

Mean corpuscular hemoglobin concentration (MCHC):
$$\frac{\text{hemoglobin, g/100 mL} \times 100}{\text{packed cell volume, \%}}$$
normally: 34 ± 2 g/100 mL red blood cells

Mean corpuscular hemoglobin (MCH):

$$\frac{\text{hemoglobin, g/1000 mL blood}}{\text{red cell count, millions/mm}^3}$$

normally: 29 ± 2 pg/red blood cell

On the basis of the three erythrocyte indexes, anemias may be classified into normocytic, hypochromic microcytic (MCV: 50 to 80 μm^3; MCH: 12 to 27 pg; MCHC: 24 to 32 g/100 mL), and macrocytic (MCV: 94 to 160 μm^3; MCH: 32 to 50 pg; MCHC: 32 to 36 g/100 mL) anemias.

ETIOLOGY

Anemias Due to Decreased RBC Production

Normocytic normochromic
Primary bone marrow failure: aplastic anemia; myelophthisic anemias (leukemia, lymphoma, other neoplasms, myelofibrosis, granulomas)
Chronic inflammation (rheumatoid arthritis, connective-tissue disorders); uremia; liver disease; endocrine deficiencies: hypothyroidism, Addison's disease, panhypopituitarism, hypogonadism

Microcytic hypochromic anemias
Iron deficiency: deficient heme synthesis
Thalassemias: deficient globin synthesis with mild extravascular hemolysis
Sideroblastic anemias: defect in heme synthesis

Macrocytic (megaloblastic) anemias
Vitamin B_{12} deficiency: pernicious anemia; malabsorption; increased requirements (pregnancy, neoplastic diseases)
Folic acid deficiency: decreased intake (alcoholism, malabsorption); increased requirements (pregnancy, malignancy)
Drug-induced; orotic aciduria; some refractory anemias

Anemias Due to Excessive Destruction of RBCs

Hemolytic anemias   nearly always normochromic normocytic
Intracorpuscular, hereditary:
  Membrane disorders: hereditary spherocytosis (increased MCHC, hyperchromic)

Enzymopathies: glucose-6-phosphate dehydrogenase (G-6-PD), pyruvate kinase, hexokinase, other enzymes, deficiency
Hemoglobinopathies: sickle cell anemia; hemoglobin C disease; etc.
Intracorpuscular, acquired:
Membrane disorder: paroxysmal nocturnal hemoglobinuria
Extracorpuscular, acquired:
Immune mechanisms
With warm-reacting antibodies
Isoimmune: transfusion reactions
Autoimmune: chronic lymphocytic leukemia, lymphoma, SLE, carcinoma; drug-related
With cold antibodies
Idiopathic
Secondary: *Mycoplasma pneumoniae,* infectious mononucleosis, neoplasms, paroxysmal cold hemoglobinuria
Mechanical disruption: cardiac valve prothesis, microangiopathic hemolytic anemia, march hemoglobinuria
Acquired membrane alteration: drugs, poisons; liver failure (spur-cell anemia); kidney failure; infectious agents (malaria, septicemia)

Blood Loss

Acute: normocytic if recent loss
Chronic: microcytic hypochromic; lesions in GI tract or uterus

Iatrogenic Causes of Anemia (partial list)

Megaloblastic anemia folic acid antagonists (methotrexate, amethopterine); diphenylhydantoin; barbiturates; oral contraceptives

Immune hemolytic anemia alpha methyldopa; cephalosporins; levodopa; penicillin; quinidine; sulfonamides

Hemolytic anemia, glucose-6-phosphate dehydrogenase deficiency nitrofurans; phenylhydrazine; sulfonamides; sulfones

Sideroblastic anemia chloramphenicol; isoniazid, cycloserine; nitrogen mustard, melphalan, azathioprine

Aplastic anemia analgesics; antimetabolites, alkylating and anti-mitotic agents; carbamazepine (Tegretol); chloramphenicol; gold compounds; phenylbutazone; (ionizing radiation)

(Peptic ulceration and hemorrhage: anticoagulants; corticosteroids; indomethacin; phenylbutazone; salicylates)

QUESTONNAIRE

Possible *meaning of response*

1 Mode of onset and duration

1.1 How long have you been aware that you have anemia?

Since birth: thalassemia, other hemoglobinopathies
At late middle-age or elderly: pernicious anemia
Any age: iron deficiency; folate deficiency

1.1*a* Do you know the most recent date at which a blood examination indicated that you had no anemia?

Will help to date the onset of anemia

Anemia of recent onset: acquired disease

Rapidly appearing anemia: bleeding or hemolysis

Gradually developing anemia: marrow failure

Chronic anemia or recurrent episodes of anemia: hereditary disease; chronic or episodic bleeding

1.2 How was your anemia detected?

• at a routine checkup examination?

Anemia may be initially asymptomatic if insidious in onset

• because you were sick?

2 Accompanying symptoms

2.1 Do you have

• dizziness or faintness upon arising from a sitting or recumbent position?

Rapidly developing anemia

• palpitations?	Tachycardia; cardiac adjustment to anemia; when hemoglobin is less than 7.5 g/100 mL, cardiac output usually increases because of increased heart rate and stroke volume
• shortness of breath on exertion?	Decrease in hemoglobin prevents maximum O_2 flow to tissues, with decreased exercise tolerance
• fatigue?	May be produced by <u>iron deficiency</u> without any anemia at all
• chest pain on exertion? • pain in the calves when walking?	Angina pectoris Intermittent claudication } may become manifest in anemic patients with underlying organ disease
• headaches? vertigo? • roaring in the ears? }	Cerebral hypoxia due to marked anemia
• a humming sound in your head?	Rapid blood flow through cranial arteries indicating significant anemia
• black, tarry stools? • blood on your stools? }	**Gastrointestinal bleeding:** the most common cause of chronic iron deficiency in men
• diarrhea?	Neoplasm of the colon and rectum underlying the anemia; malabsorption: <u>folic acid</u> or vitamin B_{12} deficiency
• constipation alternating with episodes of diarrhea?	Neoplasm of colon and rectum
• *a semisolid stool in the morning immediately upon arising?*	Achlorhydria, in pernicious anemia
• *epigastric pain? relieved by eating? antacids?*	<u>Peptic ulcer</u> with chronic blood loss
• burning sensations of the tongue?	Pernicious anemia; iron-deficiency anemia
• sores around the angles of the mouth?	Iron-deficiency anemia

- painful ulcers in your mouth?
- a sore throat?
- difficulty swallowing?

Aplastic anemia with neutropenia and infection of oral mucosa

Dysphagia in chronic iron-deficiency anemia (Plummer-Vinson syndrome); mucosal ulcerations in aplastic anemia

- loss of appetite? vomiting?
- abdominal discomfort?

Underlying or associated gastrointestinal disease

- episodic abdominal pain?

Acute hemolysis; painful vasoocclusive episodes, in sickle cell anemia; gallstones (develop frequently in patients with chronic hemolytic disorders)

- difficulty walking? unsteadiness of gait?
- numbness, tingling ("pins-and-needles") in the hands, toes?

Vitamin B_{12} deficiency with subacute combined degeneration: ataxia, loss of position sense, paresthesias

- jaundice?

Congenital or acquired hemolytic anemia; pernicious anemia

- a weight loss?

Carcinoma; leukemia; lymphoma

- fever?

Infection; leukemia; lymphoma or other neoplasm; connective-tissue disease; infection complicating aplastic anemia

- chills?

Accompany severe hemolytic process

- a bleeding tendency?

The disorder producing the anemia is not confined to the RBCs (aplastic anemia with pancytopenia); presence of additional disturbance of the other marrow elements or of the liver; the anemia itself may be due to the blood loss resulting from a disorder of hemostasis

• bone pains?	Congenital hemolytic anemias (sickle cell anemia): infarction of bone and bone marrow; malignancies
• bone tenderness?	Myeloid metaplasia; leukemia; multiple myeloma
• an abnormal color of your urine?	Blood or hemoglobin: may signify urinary tract disease or hematologic problem; hematuria: in sickle cell trait; hemoglobinuria: intravascular hemolysis (bilirubin does not occur in the urine in uncomplicated hemolytic anemia)
• *darkly discolored urine in the morning, clearing during day?*	Paroxysmal nocturnal hemoglobinuria

2.2 For the female patient: What is the frequency, the duration of your periods?

2.2*a* How many pads per day, per period, do you use?

<u>Increased menstrual blood loss</u> is the single most common cause of iron deficiency in temperate countries

2.2*b* Do you have vaginal bleeding between your periods?

Menstrual disorders (menorrhagia, irregularity of flow) are common in, and may aggravate, <u>iron-deficiency anemia</u>

3 *Iatrogenic factors* see Etiology

4 *Environmental factors*

4.1 What is
• your daily diet?

Inadequate diet may produce nutritional <u>folate deficiency</u>

• your alcohol intake?

<u>Alcoholism</u> associated with folate deficiency, sideroblastic anemia

4.1*a* Do you follow any particular diet?

Identifies individuals who follow "fad" diets, any type of unusual diet, who exclude important foods from their diet

4.2 What is (were) your present (past) occupation(s)

(Drugs and) chemicals may produce hemolytic or aplastic anemia

4.2*a* Do you often use cleaning fluids? insecticides? any paints? hair dyes? deodorants? depilatories?

May produce blood dyscrasias (may be overlooked by the patient)

4.3 Have you ever lived in, or traveled to, tropical countries? Vietnam?

Endemic areas of malaria

5 *Personal antecedents pertaining to the anemia*

5.1 Have you ever had past examinations of your blood? stools? bone marrow? x-rays of your stomach? bowel? When? With what results?

5.2 Do you have any of the following conditions:

• a peptic ulcer?

Iron-deficiency anemia due to chronic blood loss

• past surgery on the stomach? the intestine?

Iron-deficiency anemia following subtotal gastrectomy: iron malabsorption, persistent bleeding; megaloblastic anemia after partial or total gastrectomy, anastomoses, ileal resection

• chronic leg ulcers?

Sickle cell anemia; rarely in hereditary spherocytosis and other long-standing hemolytic anemias

• gallstones?

Bilirubin stones in congenital hemolytic anemias: increased excretion of bile pigment through the hepatobiliary system

• a chronic liver condition?	Megaloblastic anemia is observed in about 20 percent of patients with <u>alcoholic cirrhosis</u>
• a thyroid condition?	Anemia of hypothyroidism:(?) decreased erythropoietin production
• a chronic infection?	May cause impaired iron metabolism
• a chronic condition of the joints?	Connective-tissue disease; leukemia; rheumatoid arthritis with impaired iron metabolism; sickle cell disorders
• a chronic renal disease?	Anemia of chronic renal insufficiency: normocytic normochromic

6 *Family medical history pertaining to the anemia*

6.1 Are there any members of your family who have • anemia? jaundice? gallstones? • a splenectomy?	Helps establishing the presence of a hereditary type of anemia; pernicious anemia; sickle cell trait (in about 8 percent of American blacks); G-6-PD deficiency (about 10 percent of American blacks); thalassemia (in persons of Mediterranean ancestry)

PHYSICAL SIGNS PERTINENT TO THE COMPLAINT

Finding	**Possible** *significance*
Pallor of the skin and mucous membranes	The most evident sign of anemia; skin color is affected by the thickness of the epidermis, pigmentation, blood flow, fluid content of the subcutaneous tissues
Sallow color of the skin	Chronic anemia due to iron deficiency
Lemon-yellow pallor	Pernicious anemia: combination of pallor of anemia and low-grade icterus from hemolysis

Pallor; cold, clammy skin; **clinical shock**	Acute hemorrhage: blood loss of 2000 mL
• systolic blood pressure <100 mmHg	Blood volume probably less than 70 percent of normal
• pulse rate of 100 or more beats per minute	Blood volume probably less than 80 percent of normal
Pallor of the palmar creases	Hemoglobin below 7 g/100 mL
Pallor with mild icterus	Hemolytic anemia
Marked pallor with petechiae or ecchymoses	Acute leukemia; aplastic anemia
Fever	Infection; malignancy; lymphoma; collagen tissue disease
Lymphadenopathy	Lymphoma; leukemia; infection; metastatic carcinoma
Tachycardia; systolic murmur (most marked at the pulmonic area)	Increased cardiac output; hemoglobin less than 7.5 g/100 mL
Heart murmur; fever; splenomegaly	Subacute bacterial endocarditis with anemia
Sternal tenderness	Leukemia; multiple myeloma
Splenomegaly	Infectious disease; hemolytic anemia; connective-tissue disease; neoplastic disorder
Enlargement of the malar bones ("Chipmunk" facies); frontal bossing	Congenital hemolytic anemias with expansion of red marrow within the maxillary bones
Nail changes: brittleness, longitudinal ridging, flattening (spooning: koilonychia, rare)	Chronic iron-deficiency anemia
Smooth tongue	Glossitis: pernicious anemia; iron-deficiency anemia
Chronic leg ulcers	Sickle cell anemia; rarely in other hemolytic anemias

In the lower legs: weakness, incoordination, loss of position sense, abnormal tendon reflexes; unsteady gait	Degeneration of the dorsal and lateral columns of the spinal cord in vitamin B_{12} deficiency
Rectal and pelvic examination	May reveal: tumor or infection causing anemia
Optic fundi: hemorrhages, exudates	May occur in severe anemia; aplastic anemia; pernicious anemia; leukemia

LABORATORY TESTS PERTAINING TO THE COMPLAINT

Procedure	Finding	Diagnostic possibilities
Blood Blood smear	Poikilocytosis	Disordered erythropoiesis: iron-deficiency anemia; thalassemia
	Spherocytes	Hereditary spherocytosis
	Teardrops	Myelophthistic anemia; myeloid metaplasia
	Target cells	Sickle cell disease; thalassemia; liver disease
	RBC fragmentation	Microangiopathic hemolysis; cardiac mechanical hemolysis; disseminated intravascular coagulation
	Punctate basophilia	Disorders of hemoglobin synthesis: thalassemia

Reticulocytes (N: 0.5 to 2.0 percent of RBCs)	Normal or decreased	Bone marrow failure; iron deficiency; vitamin B_{12} deficiency; folic acid deficiency; uremia; chronic inflammation
	Increased	Hemolysis; response to acute blood loss; recovery from suppression of erythropoiesis
Iron (N: 75 to 175 μg/100 mL)	Iron decreased IBC increased	Iron-deficiency anemia
Iron-binding capacity (IBC) (N: 250 to 410 μg/100 mL)	Iron and IBC decreased	Infections; malignancy; uremia; chronic illnesses
	Iron increased, IBC normal	Aplastic anemia
	Iron increased IBC decreased	Thalassemia; hemolysis
Haptoglobin (N: 40 to 170 mg/100 mL)	Decreased	Hemolysis
Sickle cell preparation	Positive	Sickle cell anemia
Hemoglobin electrophoresis	Abnormal	Hemoglobinopathies (C, D, etc.)
Coombs' test	Positive	Immunohemolytic anemia
Erythrocyte enzyme assays	Abnormal	Red cell enzymes deficiencies
Unconjugated bilirubin (N: 0.2 to 0.7 mg/100 mL)	Increased	Hemolysis
Lactate dehydrogenase	Increased	Hemolysis

WBCs	Hypersegmented neutrophils	Vitamin B_{12} deficiency; folic acid deficiency
	Leukopenia	Vitamin B_{12} and folic acid deficiency; aplastic anemia
	Immature	Leukemia
Leukocytic alkaline phosphatase	Increased	Myeloid metaplasia
	Decreased	Paroxysmal nocturnal hemoglobinuria (PNH)

Urine

Hemosiderin	Positive	Hemoglobinuria: PNH

Stools

Occult bood	Positive	Chronic blood loss

Procedure	*To detect*
Bone marrow examination (indicated in any unexplained anemia)	
Smears	Aleukemic leukemia; multiple myeloma; lymphoma; maturation defect: megaloblastic anemia; bone marrow failure; metastatic lesions
Bone marrow biopsy	Tumor cells; granulomas; fibrosis

USEFUL REMINDERS AND DIAGNOSTIC CLUES

Misleading Factors

An extracellular fluid deficit may mask an underlying anemia.
If the anemia has been insidious in onset and cardiopulmonary disease is absent, the hematocrit may be 25 mL/100 mL or less, and

the hemoglobin concentration 8 g/100 mL or lower, before the patient has significant symptoms.

Vitamin B_{12}–deficient patients who are eating large amounts of folate-containing green vegetables may present with advanced neurologic symptoms and near-normal hemoglobin.

About 40 percent of women with excessive menstrual blood loss considered their periods to be "moderate" or even "scanty."

Diagnostic Considerations

Iron deficiency is the most common cause of anemia and is usually due to blood loss.

In the United States, about 50 percent of pregnant women, 20 percent of adult women, and 3 percent of adult men are deficient in iron.

Pica, a compulsive eating of anything, may appear in iron-deficiency anemia.

Blood donation of 3 pt a year doubles the amount of iron that must be absorbed.

Intestinal malabsorption may be associated with either or both vitamin B_{12} or folate deficiency, but folate deficiency is the more common, because folate stores are adequate for only 6 months, whereas vitamin B_{12} stores are sufficient for 3 to 10 years after deprivation.

Patients with sickle cell anemia have a predisposition to *Salmonella* osteomyelitis.

Anemia should never be thought of as a diagnosis in itself, but rather as a manifestation of an underlying disorder.

SELECTED BIBLIOGRAPHY

Williams WJ: Approach to the patient, in Williams WJ, Beutler E, Erslev AJ, Rundles RW (eds), *Hematology*, 2d ed, pp 3–9, New York: McGraw-Hill, 1977

Wintrobe MM: The approach to the patient with anemia, in Wintrobe MM, *Clinical Hematology*, 7th ed, pp 529–565, Philadelphia: Lea & Febiger, 1974

44
Bleeding Tendency

DEFINITIONS AND PATHOPHYSIOLOGY

Hemostasis the process which spontaneously arrests the flow of blood from vessels carrying blood under pressure.

Primary hemostasis the formation of the platelet plugs that seal gaps in the damaged vasculature.

Coagulation orderly sequence of enzymatic reactions which lead to the conversion of a soluble protein, fibrinogen, into an insoluble fibrous substance, fibrin.

The hemostatic mechanism involves the blood vessels, the platelets, and the plasma coagulation factors. Any vascular injury provokes a reflex vasoconstriction which slows blood flow to the injured area. Platelets adhere to the exposed collagen fibers and connective tissue in the injured vessel wall. Adenosine diphosphate released from the adherent platelets causes other platelets to aggregate, and a platelet plug is formed at the site of trauma. Contact of blood with exposed collagen fibers activates the intrinsic coagulation system. Activated factor XII, in the presence of prekallikrein and Fitzgerald factor, activates factor XI. Factor IX is then activated and, in the presence of platelet factor 3 and factor VIII, activates factor X. Activated factor X, in the presence of factor V, calcium, and phospholipids, activates prothrombin (factor II) to thrombin. Thrombin converts fibrinogen (factor I) to fibrin. In addition, tissue factor (thromboplastin) released from the injured endothelium activates the extrinsic coagulation mechanism: activated factor VII activates factor X, which in turn catalyzes the conversion of prothrombin to thrombin. The coagulation mechanism is balanced by the fibrinolytic system and various inhibitors.

A bleeding tendency may be caused by vascular abnormalities, platelet disorders, and plasma coagulation factor abnormalities (coagulopathies). Vascular defects are common, but they seldom lead to serious bleeding. Platelet disorders may be due to altered function or number of the platelets. Qualitative platelet disorders (defective adhesion, aggregation, or release reaction) may be inherited or acquired. Quantitative platelet disorders include thrombocytopenia and thrombocythemia. Thrombocytopenia is the most common serious bleeding disorder involving platelets. In idiopathic thrombocytopenic purpura, platelets are coated with an abnormal protein which sensitizes platelets for sequestration by the spleen and liver. Coagulopathies may be primary (congenital) or secondary to some underlying disease. The congenital disorders are often familial and almost always involve a single coagulation factor. The defect may be due to a total lack of the molecule (e.g., afibrinogenemia) or, more often, to a defective function of the molecule (e.g., hemophilia). Secondary or acquired coagulopathies are far more common than the inherited disorders. They usually involve multiple coagulation factors. Liver diseases and vitamin K deficiency are major causes of lack of production or defective synthesis of coagulation factors. Disseminated intravascular coagulation, another common problem, results from pathologic activation of the hemostatic mechanism within the circulation because of introduction of foreign material into the bloodstream (endo- and exotoxins, red cell products in transfusion reactions, tissue factors from neoplasms, trauma, surgery, burns, amniotic fluid).

Precise diagnosis of a bleeding tendency requires specialized laboratory evaluation.

ETIOLOGY

Vascular Abnormalities (nonthrombocytopenic purpuras)

Simple purpura; senile purpura
Dysproteinemias: macroglobulinemia; multiple myeloma; cryoglobulinemia
Allergic: Henoch-Schönlein purpura; drugs
Hereditary hemorrhagic telangiectasia
Hereditary connective-tissue disorders: Ehlers-Danlos syndrome, Marfan's syndrome
Miscellaneous: infections; scurvy; Cushing's syndrome

Platelet Abnormalities

Thrombocytopenia
Decreased production
  Reduced megakaryocytes: marrow failure: acquired, congenital; marrow injury: drugs, chemicals, radiation; marrow infiltration: leukemia, lymphoma, carcinoma; thrombopoietin deficiency

Normal or increased megakaryocytes: vitamin B_{12}, folic acid deficiency; hereditary: Wiskott-Aldrich syndrome; May-Hegglin anomaly
Increased destruction
  Immune thrombocytopenia: idiopathic thrombocytopenic purpura, systemic lupus erythematosus (SLE), drugs, posttransfusion purpura
  Nonimmunologic: increased consumption: disseminated intravascular coagulation, thrombotic thrombocytopenia purpura, hemolytic-uremic syndrome; acute infections; prosthetic heart valves
Sequestration: splenomegaly
Intravascular dilution: massive transfusion; loss by hemorrhage

Thrombocythemia
Essential
Polycythemia vera; chronic myelogenous leukemia

Qualitative platelet defects
Congenital or acquired: defective adhesion; defective primary aggregation (thrombosthenia); defective platelet release reaction; uremia, dysproteinemia

Coagulation Defects

Congenital
Hemophilia: A (factor VIII deficiency) and B (factor IX deficiency): X chromosome-linked recessive traits
von Willebrand's disease: autosomal dominant
Deficiency of each of the following factors: I (fibrinogen), II (prothrombin), V, VII, X, XIII, XII (Hageman: asymptomatic)

Acquired
Vitamin K deficiency: obstructive jaundice, hepatocellular disease, intestinal malabsorption, drugs, nutritional
Disseminated intravascular coagulation: shock, infections, burns, amniotic fluid embolism, retained dead fetus, neoplasms
Fibrinolytic states: administration of streptokinase, urokinase; (?)primary
Circulating anticoagulants

Iatrogenic Causes of Bleeding Tendencies (partial list)

Vascular abnormalities atropine; corticosteroids; iodides; penicillin; phenacetin; quinine; sulfonamides

Thrombocytopenia
Suppression of platelet production: myelosuppressive drugs; thiazides; estrogenic hormones
Immunologic platelet destruction: digitoxin; diphenylhydantoin; gold salts; methyldopa; quinidine, quinine; rifampin; Sedormid; sedatives; stibophen; sulfonamides

Abnormal platelet function (impaired release reaction) aspirin; clofibrate; dipyridamole; indomethacin; phenylbutazone; dextran; sulfinpyrazone

Impaired coagulation heparin; oral anticoagulants

QUESTIONNAIRE

Possible *meaning of response*

1 Mode of onset and duration
1.1 When did the bleeding symptoms appear?
- at birth?

Large cephalohematomas: more common in acquired bleeding disorders: hemorrhagic disease of the newborn; may occur in hemophilia

- from the umbilical stump?
- following circumcision?

Hemorrhagic disease of the newborn; hypofibrinogenemia; factor XIII deficiency; uncommon in the other hereditary coagulation disorders

- *until you began to walk?*
- in childhood?

Hereditary bleeding disorders, hemophilia; hemarthroses in hemophilia do not develop until 3 to 4 years of age; idiopathic thrombocytopenic purpura (ITP)

- in adolescence?
- during military service?

Hereditary bleeding disorder, if mild, may manifest itself in adolescence

• during adulthood?

Acquired bleeding disorder; <u>pur-</u><u>puric syndrome</u>; hereditary hemorrhagic telangiectasia: usually symptomatic in early adulthood or middle age

1.2 In case of bleeding of recent onset, did it appear

• abruptly?

<u>Acute disseminated intravascu-</u><u>lar coagulation</u> (DIC); acute ITP; allergic purpura; intoxication

• chronically?

Chronic DIC; circulating anticoagulants

2 *Location of bleeding*

2.1 *Do you have small superficial bruises?*

Skin (and mucosal surfaces) involved in platelet or vascular disorder with purpuric syndrome

2.2 Do you bleed
• under the skin?
• *into muscles?*
• *into joints?*

Subcutaneous and deep hematomas and hemarthroses are characteristic of hereditary coagulation disorders, most commonly hemophilia A or hemophilia B

2.3 Do you bruise easily and bleed into the muscles?

von Willebrand's disease; DIC

2.4 Do you bleed from the gums? the nose? Is there blood in your urine? Have you ever vomited blood? passed black, tarry stools?

Spontaneous bleeding from bodily orifices may complicate any significant hemorrhagic diathesis; however an underlying local lesion may be responsible

2.4*a* Do your gums bleed easily when you brush your teeth?

Localized gum disorder or severe platelet deficiency; scurvy

3 *Severity of bleeding*

3.1 Do you have
• single, localized bleeding spots on the skin?

Vascular malformation: hereditary hemorrhagic telangiectasia; areas of vasculitis: allergic purpura

• multiple, small generalized bleeding spots?
• larger areas of discoloration?

Petechiae: any of the platelet or vascular disorders
Ecchymoses: coagulation defect (also in vascular or platelet disorder); DIC; bruises larger than the palm of the hand, especially if spontaneous, are suggestive of a hemostatic disorder

3.2 For the female patient: What is the duration of your periods?

3.2a How many pads per day, per period, do you use?

3.2b Do you have vaginal bleeding between your periods?

If the duration of the periods exceeds 7 days and/or if the patient uses more than 4 pads per day or 12 pads per period: menometrorrhagia: usually due to gynecologic disorders; however may be the sole complaint in women with thrombocytopenia, von Willebrand's disease, or other rare autosomally inherited coagulation disorders

4 Precipitating or aggravating factors

4.1 Does your bleeding appear

• *spontaneously?*
• without perceptible trauma?

Petechiae and/or ecchymoses due to platelet or vascular disorder usually appear spontaneously; may occur in hereditary coagulation disorder, when trauma is so slight as to go unnoticed by the patient; hemarthroses (in hereditary coagulation disorder) often develop without significant trauma

• *following a trauma?*

Bleeding in coagulation disorders (also in purpuric syndromes)

4.1*a* Is the bleeding after a
      trauma
      • *delayed? persistent?*   Coagulation disorder, with
                          normal platelet plug formation

      • immediate? shortlived?   Purpuric (vascular or platelet)
                          syndrome

4.2 Do you bleed from   If persistent, profuse bleeding:
      superficial minor cuts?   disorder of platelet or vessel
      scratches? razor nicks?   (inadequacy of primary
                          hemostasis); seldom in patient
                          with coagulation disorder

4.3 Do you bruise or bleed   Significant: suggests a hemo-
      under the skin (hema-   static disorder
      toma) at the sites of in-
      jections? immunizations?

5 *Relieving factors*

5.1 In case of external bleed-
      ing, does local pressure
      stop the bleeding
      • promptly?   Purpuric syndrome: vascular or
                          platelet defect
      • slowly? not at all?   Coagulation disorder

6 *Accompanying symptoms*

6.1 Do you have
      • fever? chills? fatigue?   Underlying disorder; leukemia
                          with thrombocytopenia

      • *pain, swelling in your joints?* Hemarthroses in <u>hemophilia;</u>
                          SLE with circulating anti-
                          coagulants

      • pain in the joints and the   Allergic (Henoch-Schönlein)
      abdomen?   purpura
      • pain in the bones?   Multiple myeloma with vascular
                          purpura, platelet dysfunction,
                          or coagulation factor ab-
                          normality

• chronic diarrhea?	Malabsorption with vitamin K deficiency
• jaundice?	Biliary tract obstruction with deficiencies of the vitamin K–dependent coagulation factors: II, VII, IX, X; liver disease with lack of production of coagulation factors

6.2   *Is the healing of wounds slow? protracted?*
  • with abnormal scar formation?

Factor XIII deficiency; hereditary afibrinogenemia; dysfibrino-genemias

7   *Iatrogenic factors*   see Etiology

7.1   Do you take
  • aspirin?

Inhibits the platelet release reaction; may provoke bleeding in a patient with a bleeding tendency

  • anticoagulants with any other drugs?

Some drugs may potentiate the anticoagulant effects of coumarins

8   *Environmental factors*

8.1   Do you think that you are exposed to any chemical agents?

8.1a   Do you have any hobbies?

Possible <u>toxic</u> action of chemical(s) on bone marrow with thrombocytopenia

9   *Personal antecedents pertaining to the bleeding tendency*

9.1   Have you ever bled following a trauma? an accident? tooth extraction? surgery? (tonsillectomy? circumcision?)

9.1a   *Was the bleeding out of proportion to the extent of the injury?*

Characteristic of a hemostatic defect

9.1*b* Did the bleeding persist for days or weeks?	If bleeding after a dental procedure persists for 3 days or more: hemorrhagic diathesis
9.1*c* Was the onset of bleeding • immediate? (following trauma) • delayed, developing several hours or even days after injury?	Usually in platelet or vascular disorder Common in hereditary coagulation disorders: temporary hemostatic efficacy of the platelet thrombus
9.1*d* Did you have to receive blood transfusions?	A rough guide to the severity of the postsurgical or posttraumatic bleeding
9.2 *Have you ever had a major trauma, surgery, and/or multiple tooth extraction without abnormal bleeding?*	Evidence against a hereditary hemorrhagic disorder; present bleeding is <u>acquired</u>
9.3 In case of prior pregnancy, was there any severe bleeding during delivery?	von Willebrand's disease; thrombocytopenia; DIC; hereditary deficiency of factor II, V, VII, or X (autosomal recessive; rare)
9.4 Do you have • a liver disease?	<u>Cirrhosis</u> with deficiency of vitamin K–dependent coagulation factors: II, VII, IX, X; deficiency of fibrinogen and factor V; fibrinogenolysis
• a renal disease?	Platelet dysfunction
9.5 Have you ever had • acute episodes of abdominal pain?	In hemophilia: **retroperitoneal hemorrhage;** bleeding into the psoas sheath may mimic appendicitis; **hemorrhage into the bowel** may be confused with intestinal obstruction; allergic purpura

- an intracranial hemorrhage?
  - spontaneously?

    The most serious complication of ITP (in 1 percent or less of the patients); usually subarachnoid

  - following a minor trauma?

    May occur in coagulation disorders: subdural, epidural, or intracerebral

10 Family medical history pertaining to the bleeding tendency

10.1 *Are there any members of your family who have bleeding tendency?*

Hereditary coagulation disorder (sex-linked or autosomal dominant); hereditary hemorrhagic telangiectasia

- one of your parents?

  Excludes hemophilia A or B in the patient

- maternal uncles?
- male siblings?

  Hemophilia A and B: X-linked recessive inheritance

10.2 Are (were) your parents related?

An autosomal recessive disease may emerge when both asymptomatic parents are heterozygotes: most likely to occur with consanguinity

PHYSICAL SIGNS PERTINENT TO THE COMPLAINT

Finding
Small capillary hemorrhages

Possible *significance*

- not blanching on pressure

  Purpuric lesions: hemorrhages into the skin

- blanching on pressure

  Lesions of hereditary hemorrhagic telangiectasia, where the blood is within the capillary dilatation

- *about 1 mm in diameter, not blanching on pressure*

  Petechiae: abnormality in the vessels or the platelets

• about 1 mm to 1 cm, not blanching on pressure	Purpura: coalescence of multiple petechiae: vascular or platelet disorder
• around hair follicles	Scurvy (on thighs and buttocks)
Superficial ecchymoses	Coagulation disorder; may accompany petechiae
Deep dissecting hematoma	Coagulation disorder
Purpura and periarticular swelling	Henoch-Schönlein purpura
Purpura and splenomegaly	Thrombocytopenia due to hypersplenism: liver disease with portal hypertension; congestive splenomegaly (very rare in ITP)
Purpura with anemia; lymphadenopathy; fever	Acquired bleeding disorder; leukemia
Purpura with neurologic abnormalities, fever	Thrombotic thrombocytopenic purpura
Hemorrhage into synovial joints	Hemarthroses: virtually diagnostic of a severe hereditary coagulation disorder: hemophilia A or B; rare in acquired coagulation disorders or in purpuric syndromes
Joint deformities; ankyloses	Repeated hemarthroses: hemophilia A or B
Jaundice	Impaired hepatic synthesis of coagulation proteins; biliary tract obstruction with impaired absorption of vitamin K and deficiency of factors II, VII, IX, X
Purpura, ecchymoses; bleeding from venipuncture wounds, from skin suture sites; multiple bleeding sites	Disseminated intravascular coagulation (DIC)

Abnormal scar formation	Hereditary afibrinogenemia; dysfibrinogenemia; factor XIII deficiency
Funduscopic examination: small retinal hemorrhages	Common in thrombocytopenic and other purpuric disorders; rare in hereditary coagulation disorders

LABORATORY TESTS PERTAINING TO THE COMPLAINT

Procedure	Finding	Diagnostic possibilities
Bleeding time (Ivy method, N: <7 min)	Prolonged	Vascular or platelet defect: thrombocytopenia; thrombasthenia; platelet release defects; von Willebrand's disease
Platelet count (N: 150,000 to 400,000 per cubic millimeter)	Normal	Thrombasthenia; platelet release defects; von Willebrand's disease; coagulopathies
	Decreased	Thrombocytopenias; DIC
Clot retraction (N: apparent in 60 min)	Normal	Platelet release defects; von Willebrand's disease
	Deficient	Thrombocytopenia; thrombasthenia
Prothrombin time (N: 11 to 14 s)	Normal	Deficiency of factors VIII, IX, XI, XII, or XIII; thrombocytopenia; von Willebrand's disease

	Prolonged	Abnormality of extrinsic and common pathway coagulation systems: deficiency of factors VII, II, V, or X; vitamin K deficiency; DIC; hypofibrinogenemia; dysfibrinogenemia; heparin or coumarin effect; liver failure
Activated partial thromboplastin time (N: 35 to 45 s)	Normal	Deficiency of factors VII or XIII; thrombocytopenia
	Prolonged	Abnormality of intrinsic and common pathway coagulation systems: deficiency of factors XII, VIII, IX, XI, II, V, or X; DIC; von Willebrand's disease; vitamin K deficiency; heparin or coumarin effect; liver failure; hypofibrinogenemia; dysfibrinogenemia
Thrombin time (N: 15 to 21 s)	Normal	Deficiency of factors XII, XI, VIII, IX, VII, II, V, or X
	Prolonged	DIC; dysfibrinogenemia; liver failure; presence of heparin; hypofibrinogenemia
Fibrinogen (N: 200 to 400 mg/100 mL)	Decreased	DIC; liver failure; hypofibrinogenemia

Fibrin degrada- tion products	Positive	DIC; primary fibrinolysis
Fibrin monomers ⎫ (protamine test) ⎭	Positive Negative	DIC Primary fibrinolysis
Platelet aggregation	Abnormal	Thrombasthenia; platelet release defects; von Wille- brand's disease (in response to ristocetin)

USEFUL REMINDERS AND DIAGNOSTIC CLUES

Misleading Factors

Approximately 30 percent of patients with hereditary coagulation disorders give a negative family history. The family history is usually negative in the autosomal recessive traits.

Hemarthrosis in hemophilia A or B may develop without discoloration or other external evidence of bleeding, and the patient may attribute the symptoms to arthritis rather than to bleeding.

Diagnostic Considerations

Vessels and platelets

Most disorders of vessels and platelets are acquired.

Spontaneous bleeding rarely occurs in patients whose platelet concentrations are greater than 50,000 per cubic millimeter.

The development of thrombocytopenia in an adult should arouse suspicion of a chemical etiologic agent.

Bruising with normal platelet count is a frequent complaint and occurs often in apparently normal people, especially in women; small bruises have little significance; large bruises (more than 6 cm in diameter) may be significant.

Coagulation disorders

Classic hemophilia (factor VIII deficiency) comprises approximately 80 percent of the hereditary coagulation disorders.

Bleeding manifestations usually are less severe in the acquired forms than in the hereditary forms of bleeding disorders.

In a patient with hemophilia A	*Suggest a factor VIII level of*
Spontaneous serious bleeding, with frequent hemarthroses	0 to 2 percent of normal
Serious bleeding from minor injury, with infrequent hemarthroses	2 to 5 percent of normal
No spontaneous bleeding, some bleeding only after minor trauma, and severe bleeding after surgical operations	5 to 25 percent of normal
Moderate bleeding after major trauma	25 to 50 percent of normal

Hemoptysis is rarely due to a hemorrhagic disorder.
Bleeding from the gastrointestinal or genitourinary tract in a patient with a hemorrhagic diathesis should be ascribed to an organic lesion until proved otherwise.

SELECTED BIBLIOGRAPHY

Lewis JH, Spero JA, and Hasiba U: *Coagulopathies,* Disease-a-Month, Chicago: Year Book, June 1977

Nossel HL: Bleeding, in Thorn GW et al (eds), *Harrison's Principles of Internal Medicine,* 8th ed, pp 294–301, New York: McGraw-Hill, 1977

Weiss HJ: Platelet physiology and abnormalities of platelet function. N Engl J Med 293:531–541, 580–588, 1975

Wintrobe MM: The diagnostic approach to the bleeding disorders, in Wintrobe MM, *Clinical Hematology,* 7th ed, pp 1043–1070, Philadelphia: Lea & Febiger 1974

45
Fever of Unknown Origin

DEFINITION AND GENERAL CONSIDERATIONS

Fever of unknown origin (FUO) an illness of at least 3 weeks' duration, with temperature exceeding 101°F (38.3°C) on several occasions, and no established diagnosis after 1 week of hospital investigation.

The average normal oral temperature is 98.6°F (37.0°C), the axillary temperature 97.6°F (36.5°C), and the rectal or vaginal temperature 99.6°F (37.5°C). There is a normal diurnal variation in body temperature, the lowest oral reading being in the early morning, and the highest [99°F (37.2°C) or more] between 6 P.M. and 10 P.M. The febrile patterns of most diseases tend to follow this normal diurnal temperature variation. An oral temperature above 99°F (37.2°C) in a subject at bedrest should be regarded as indicating a disease.

Fever probably results from disturbance of cerebral thermoregulation produced by product(s) of tissue injury. Gram-negative bacterial endotoxins can produce fever by stimulating certain cells, principally neutrophils and mononuclear macrophages, to synthesize and release endogenous pyrogens into the circulation. These humoral factors act on the thermoregulatory centers of the central nervous system to produce fever. Fever following exposure to viruses, bacteria, antigens, antigen-antibody complexes, and sterile inflammatory reactions, is also mediated through the production of endogenous pyrogens.

ETIOLOGY

Infections (40 percent)
Tuberculosis (miliary)
Subacute infective endocarditis
Miscellaneous rare infections: brucellosis, chronic meningococcemia, gonococcemia, toxoplasmosis, cytomegalovirus infection, disseminated mycoses; psittacosis
Localized pyogenic infections

Hepatic infections: liver abscess; cholangitis
Other visceral infections: pancreatic, tuboovarian abscesses; empyema of gallbladder; pericholecystic abscess; osteomyelitis
Intraperitoneal infections: subhepatic, subphrenic, paracolic, appendiceal, pelvic and other abscesses; diverticulitis
Urinary tract: pyelonephritis; renal carbuncle; perinephric abscess; prostatic abscess

Neoplasms (*20 percent*)
Hypernephroma; carcinoma of the gastrointestinal tract; tumor of the pancreas; hepatic carcinoma; carcinoma of the lung and pleura; atrial myxoma; lymphoma, leukemia

Connective-tissue disease (*15 percent*)
Rheumatoid arthritis; systemic lupus erythematosus; polyarteritis nodosa; Wegener's granulomatosis; rheumatic fever; polymyositis; temporal arteritis

Less common causes (*25 percent*)
Granulomatous disease, other than that due to known infectious agents: sarcoidosis; granulomatous hepatitis
Inflammatory bowel disease: regional enteritis, ulcerative colitis, Whipple's disease
Pulmonary embolization; pelvic thrombophlebitis
Drug fever
Hepatic cirrhosis with active hepatocellular necrosis
Miscellaneous: familial Mediterranean fever; porphyria; gout; hyperthyroidism
Factitious fever; habitual hyperthermia

Undiagnosed (*5 to 8 percent*)

Iatrogenic Causes of Fever (partial list)

Antibiotics	Hydralazine	PAS
Antihistamines	Iodides	Procainamide
Arsenicals	Isoniazid	Propylthiouracil
Atropine	Laxatives (phenol-	Quinidine
Barbiturates	phthalein)	Sulfonamides
Hydantoins	Methyldopa	Thiazides

QUESTIONNAIRE

Possible *meaning of response*

1 *Mode of onset and duration*

1.1 How long have you had fever?

• for years?

Habitual hyperthermia (in young women); factitious fever

1.1*a* How was your fever discovered?

The perception of fever by patients varies enormously

2 *Pattern of fever*

2.1 At what site do you measure your temperature?

• oral?

Normal average temperature: 98.6°F (37.0°C)

• axillary?

Normal average temperature: 97.6°F (36.5°C)

• rectal?

Normal average temperature: 99.6°F (37.5°C)

2.2 What are the average, the maximum readings?

Low-grade fever: disseminated fungal infection; above 105°F: urinary tract infection caused by gram-negative bacilli, meningococcemia; tuberculosis; malaria; excessively high fever, greater than 106°F: factitious fever (in adults)

2.3 At what time of the day do you have fever?

In most patients with fever higher levels of temperature usually occur in the evening

2.4 Is your temperature always above 100°F?

• with little or no variations throughout the day?

Sustained fever: typhoid fever, endocarditis, drug fever

• with greater than one degree variation during the day? (but with temperature remaining above normal)

Remittent fever: accentuation of the normal diurnal temperature pattern; this type of fever is seen in most cases and is not characteristic

2.5 Does your temperature drop to normal at least once in a day?	Intermittent fever (hectic fever when the variations in temperature are very large): pyogenic infection; abscesses; lymphomas; miliary tuberculosis; gram-negative bacteremia
2.6 Do you have fever for prolonged periods with periods of normal temperature?	Relapsing or recurrent fever: malaria; relapsing fever (Southwest United States, Texas); rat-bite fever; localized pyogenic (biliary, GU, GI, respiratory) infections (rare); Hodgkin's disease ("Pel-Ebstein fever"); drug reaction; inflammatory bowel disease; familial Mediterranean fever

3 Precipitating or aggravating factors

3.1 Prior to the onset of the fever did you • have a boil? • have a tooth extracted? • have any genitourinary procedure?	<u>Bacteremia</u>; subacute bacterial <u>endocarditis</u>
3.1*a* Do you habitually squeeze pimples, pull hair?	An insignificant skin puncture may be the starting point of a septicemia

4 Accompanying symptoms

4.1 Do you have • shaking chills?	Repeated chills in infectious diseases: bacteremia, pyogenic abscess, bacterial endocarditis (especially staphylococcal), pylephlebitis, pelvic thrombophlebitis, intermittent biliary duct obstruction, malaria, pyelonephritis, rat-bite fever, brucellosis; drug reaction; neoplasms; collagen disorders; intermittent administration of antipyretics

• excessive sweats?	A common response to infection, marking the falling, or defervescent, phase of fever
• during the night?	Miliary tuberculosis
• a loss of weight?	<u>Neoplasm</u>; <u>tuberculosis</u>; if weight unchanged despite fever of long duration: factitious fever, habitual hyperthermia (usually in young, psychoneurotic women)
• chest discomfort?	Repeated small pulmonary emboli
• trouble breathing?	Miliary tuberculosis; pulmonary emboli (pulmonary sarcoidosis is usually a nonfebrile disease)
• headaches?	Temporal arteritis (polymyalgia rheumatica); typhoid fever; brucellosis
• pain in your joints?	<u>Connective-tissue disease</u>; rheumatic fever; sarcoidosis; drug fever; bronchogenic tumor; familial Mediterranean fever
• pain in the muscles?	Polyarteritis; polymyalgia rheumatica; trichinosis; brucellosis
• pain in the chest?	Multiple pulmonary emboli; familial Mediterranean fever
• pain in the abdomen?	Cholangitis with intermittent biliary fever; biliary obstruction due to stone; perinephric abscess; hypernephroma; gynecologic infection; familial Mediterranean fever
• pain in the back?	Osteomyelitis of a vertebra; perinephric abscess
• pain in a bone?	Osteomyelitis
• a sore throat?	Infectious mononucleosis; retropharyngeal abscess; streptococcal tonsillitis followed by rheumatic fever

• frequent, or painful urination?	Urinary tract infection
• altered bowel habits? diarrhea?	Regional enteritis; ulcerative colitis; typhoid fever; schistoso-miasis; amebiasis
• a skin rash?	Meningococcal infection; sarcoidosis; polyarteritis; lymphoma; rheumatic fever; Rocky Mountain spotted fever
• swollen glands?	Lymphoma; leukemia; drug fever; sarcoidosis

5   *Iatrogenic factors*   see Etiology

5.1 Did you recently receive any antibiotics	
• before the onset of your fever?	Drug fever
• after the onset of your fever?	May modify the clinical picture; may mask subacute bacterial endocarditis

6   *Environmental factors*

6.1 Have you recently been exposed to a person with tuberculosis?	Tuberculosis remains the most prominent cause of FUO
6.2 Have you traveled in last 6 months to a tropical area?	Amebic liver abscess; malaria: Asia, Africa, some areas of South and Central America; schistosomiasis: Caribbean islands, Africa, Far East
6.3 Where do you live?	Southwest United States: coc-cidioidomycosis; Western United States: tick-borne re-lapsing fever; Mississippi River Valley: histoplasmosis
6.4 What is your profession?	In farmers, veterinarians, slaughterhouse workers: brucel-losis; contact with various plastics: polymer-fume fever; medical and paramedical per-sonnel: factitious fever

6.5 Do you have any contact with domestic or wild animals? birds?	Brucellosis; rat-bite fever; birds, pigeons: psittacosis
6.5a Have you had a tick bite within the last 2 weeks?	Rocky Mountain spotted fever
6.6 Did you ever ingest	
• unpasteurized milk? cheese?	Brucellosis
• poorly cooked pork?	Trichinosis
6.7 Do you use narcotics?	In intravenous drug users: bacterial endocarditis, frequently on the tricuspid valve; malaria

7 *Personal antecedents pertaining to the FUO*

7.1 Have you ever had a tuberculin skin test? tuberculosis?

7.2 Do you have any of the following conditions:

• a valvular heart disease?	Subacute bacterial endocarditis; rheumatic fever; atrial myxoma
• rheumatic fever during childhood?	Valvular disease with subacute bacterial endocarditis
• a recent operation?	Postoperative abscess

8 *Family medical history pertaining to the FUO*

8.1 Does anyone else in your family have fever?	Tuberculosis; exposure to a common etiologic agent; familial Mediterranean fever

PHYSICAL SIGNS PERTINENT TO THE COMPLAINT

Finding	*Possible significance*
Tachycardia	The heart rate normally increases about 9 to 10 beats per degree of fever (Fahrenheit)

Relative bradycardia	Typhoid, paratyphoid fever; psittacosis; heart disease with AV block; factitious fever
Skin: • petechiae (also in conjunctivas) • splinter hemorrhages (nails)	Subacute bacterial endocarditis
• rash	Meningococcal infection; sarcoidosis; polyarteritis; lymphoma; rheumatic fever; Rocky Mountain spotted fever
• nodules	Metastatic malignancy
Heart murmur	Subacute bacterial endocarditis; atrial myxoma
Lymphadenopathy	Malignancy; lymphoma; leukemia; sarcoidosis; drug fever
Splenomegaly	Lymphoma; leukemia; infection; subacute bacterial endocarditis
Hepatosplenomegaly	Lymphoma; leukemia; chronic infection; cirrhosis
Hepatomegaly without splenomegaly	Liver abscess; metastatic cancer
Abdominal mass	Neoplastic disease; hypernephroma; intraabdominal abscess
Palpation of the navel	Intraabdominal neoplasms may metastasize early to the navel
Arthritis	Connective-tissue disease; rheumatic fever; subacute bacterial endocarditis
Sternal tenderness	Chronic granulocytic leukemia; acute leukemia; **metastatic** tumor; multiple myeloma
Bone tenderness	Osteomyelitis; metastatic tumor
Inflamed, tender temporal artery	Polymyalgia rheumatica

Abnormal testicles

Teratoma; tuberculosis

Rectal and pelvic examination

May reveal: masses, abscesses, perirectal abscess; pelvic thrombophlebitis

Funduscopic examination:
• choroidal tubercles
• flame-shaped hemorrhages

Miliary tuberculosis
Subacute bacterial endocarditis

LABORATORY TESTS PERTAINING TO THE COMPLAINT

Procedures

Blood
Complete blood cell count, erythrocyte sedimentation rate, biochemical screening

Serologic tests: antistreptolysin O titers, antinuclear antibodies, latex fixation tests; febrile agglutinins

Blood smears for: abnormal morphology, parasites, LE cells

Cultures of: blood (aerobically and anaerobically), urine, bone marrow, other body fluids

Skin tests
Tuberculin, histoplasmin, coccidioidin, etc.

Stool
Occult blood tests; ova, parasites, culture

Procedure	*To detect*
Chest x-ray	Pulmonary tuberculosis
IV pyelogram	Tumor; intrarenal or perinephric abscess
Bone x-rays	Osteomyelitis; primary or metastatic tumor
GI barium studies	Colonic tumor; diverticulitis
Upper GI x-rays	Regional enteritis; Whipple's disease
IV cholangiogram Endoscopic retrograde cholangiopancreatography	Biliary tract disorder

Lymphangiograms	Abdominal or retroperitoneal lymphomas
Liver scan	Right upper quadrant disorder
Lung scan	Pulmonary emboli
Simultaneous liver and lung scans	Subphrenic abscess
Bone scans	Osseous metastases
Biopsy of:	
Liver	Primary or metastatic tumor; granulomas, tuberculosis, histoplasmosis, sarcoidosis; lymphoma; etc.
Lymph node	Lymphomas; metastatic cancer; tuberculosis; mycotic infection
Bone marrow	Metastatic carcinoma; granulomas; leukemias
Muscle	Polyarteritis nodosa; dermatomyositis; sarcoidosis; trichinosis
Temporal artery Accessible masses	Polymyalgia rheumatica
Abdominal aortography and selective arteriography	Tumor of the kidneys, pancreas, liver; retroperitoneal mass lesions
Cardiac angiogram Echocardiogram }	Atrial myxoma
Peritoneoscopy	Tuberculous peritonitis; peritoneal carcinomatosis; cholecystitis; pelvic inflammatory disease

USEFUL REMINDERS AND DIAGNOSTIC CLUES

Misleading Factor

Factitious fever is usually of long duration, lacks the normal diurnal variation, is excessively high (above 106 to 107°F in adults), and is associated with normal pulse and respiratory rates.

Diagnostic Considerations

Tuberculosis

The sites in which tuberculosis is most likely to be present with no manifestations other than fever are the liver, pericardium, peritoneum, abdominal and hilar lymph nodes, and female genital tract, as well as the disseminated (military) form of the infection.

The fever in disseminated tuberculosis is usually intermittent and well tolerated by the patient, who often is unaware of its presence despite peaks to 103 to 105°F.

Increased susceptibility to tuberculosis occurs in adolescence, senescence, malnutrition, postgastrectomy state, diabetes mellitus, pregnancy, silicosis, uremia, lymphomas, sarcoidosis, immunosuppressive therapy, corticosteroid therapy, live virus vaccination.

Endocarditis

In the patient with FUO who has had a variety of sequential illnesses (influenza, stroke, urinary tract infection, arthritis), suspect subacute bacterial endocarditis.

Bacterial endocarditis is uncommon in patients with pure mitral stenosis, so that fever in these patients is more likely related to multiple pulmonary emboli or pneumonia.

The absence of a detectable cardiac murmur does not exclude the possibility of bacterial endocarditis. A cardiac murmur is often not present when infection involves the right side of the heart or when it involves the mural endocardium overlying a myocardial infarction.

Patients with atrial myxoma may have a pattern of illness with fever and embolic manifestations simulating bacterial endocarditis.

Miscellaneous

Amebic abscesses of the liver occur mostly in men, are frequently solitary, commonest in the right lobe, and often associated with right pleural effusion. Pyogenic abscesses of the liver have no sex predilection, are frequently multiple, and involve both hepatic lobes.

There is an increased incidence of *Salmonella* infections in: thalassemia, sickle cell disease, leukemia, cirrhosis of the liver, neoplastic disease, and after spenectomy.

Postoperative fever is usually related to the surgical procedure, not to some unrelated disease.

A drug well tolerated for many years may abruptly induce a reaction, including fever.

In a patient past middle age, even low-grade fever should be regarded as a probable indication of organic disease.

The majority of obscure fevers ultimately prove to be an atypical manifestation of commoner diseases rather than of exotic illnesses.

SELECTED BIBLIOGRAPHY

Jacoby GA, Swartz MN: Fever of undetermined origin. N Engl J Med 289:1407–1410, 1973

Petersdorf RG, Beeson PB: Fever of unexplained origin: Report of 100 cases. Medicine (Baltimore) 40:1–30, 1961

Vickery DM, Quinnell RK: Fever of unknown origin: An algorithmic approach. JAMA 238:2183–2188, 1977

46
Glycosuria

DEFINITIONS AND PATHOPHYSIOLOGY

Glycosuria   a condition in which glucose is excreted in the urine.
Melituria   a condition in which any type of sugar is excreted in the urine.

The concentration of glucose in the renal glomerular filtrate equals that in plasma water. Glucose is reabsorbed in the proximal convoluted tubules. When arterial blood glucose levels reach 150 to 180 mg/100 mL, the amount of glucose presented to the tubules usually exceeds the transfer maximum for glucose (normally: 300 to 350 mg/min) and glucose appears in the urine. The blood glucose concentration which results in glycosuria is called the *renal threshold.* Some patients with glycosuria have a low renal threshold (idiopathic renal glycosuria, pregnancy, chronic renal disease). Usually the presence of glucose in the urine is associated with hyperglycemia and diabetes mellitus.

The principal determinants of the blood glucose level are the dietary intake of glucose, the rate of entry of glucose into the cells of muscles, adipose tissue, and other organs, and the regulatory activity of the liver, which takes up glucose and stores it as glycogen (glycogenesis) when the blood glucose is high, and discharges glucose into the circulation through glycogenolysis (breakdown of glycogen) when the blood glucose is low. The overall control of glucose homeostasis is affected by the action of numerous hormones. When carbohydrate is fed, the increase of blood glucose concentration provokes increased secretion of insulin. Insulin acts to decrease blood sugar by stimulating hepatic glycogenesis and decreasing hepatic gluconeogenesis (conversion of nonglucose molecules to glucose). In addition, insulin increases the entry of glucose into muscles and adipose tissue, and stimulates the synthesis of protein from amino acids and the synthesis of lipids from fatty acids. Many of the effects of insulin in muscle and in adipose tissue are attributed to an insulin-induced alteration in the cell plasma membrane. Carbohydrate metabolism is also regulated by other hormones. Glucagon stimulates hepatic glycogenolysis, thereby increasing blood glucose concentration, and increases gluconeogenesis in the liver; epinephrine favors glycogenolysis in liver and muscles and decreases the uptake of glucose by tissues; glucocorticoids increase gluconeogenesis, with resulting hyperglycemic effect; growth hormone increases hepatic glucose output and decreases glucose uptake into some tissues.

Insulin deficiency, either absolute or relative, causes diabetes mellitus. In the absence of insulin, the entry of glucose into various peripheral tissues is decreased (decreased peripheral utilization), and liberation of glucose into the circulation from the liver is increased (due in part to hypersecretion of glucagon). Decreased peripheral utilization with inadequate removal of ingested glucose, and increased hepatic glucogenesis result in hyperglycemia and glycosuria. In addition, lipolysis and protein catabolism are increased, with resulting increased ketogenesis and protein deficiency. Nondiabetic meliturias with normal glycemia have no relation to diabetes mellitus and are due to various rare metabolic defects.

ETIOLOGY

Glycosuric Meliturias (positive glucose oxidase urine test)

Usually associated with hyperglycemia
Diabetes mellitus
Destruction of the islets of Langerhans: pancreatitis, acute or chronic; carcinoma; surgery; hemochromatosis; cystic fibrosis
Endocrinopathies: hyperadrenocorticism; pheochromocytoma; functioning beta-cell or alpha-cell tumor; hyperthyroidism; acromegaly
Nervous system diseases: hypothalamic damage; brain tumors; brain trauma; cerebral hemorrhage
Gastrointestinal disease: severe hepatic disease; postgastrectomy syndrome; glycogen storage diseases
Miscellaneous: obesity; uremia; infections; poststarvation feeding; burns; postmyocardial infarction; drugs

Not associated with hyperglycemia
Renal glycosuria: idiopathic, pregnancy, chronic renal disease
Fanconi's syndrome
Chemical agents: heavy metal salts, carbon monoxide, phlorhizin

Nonglycosuric Meliturias

Pentosurias; fructosurias (essential, hereditary fructose intolerance); galactosuria; heptosuria; disaccharidurias (lactosuria, maltosuria, sucrosuria)

Iatrogenic Causes of Glycosuria

Oral contraceptives; corticosteroids; thiazides, furosemide, diazoxide

Drug-induced false-positive copper-reduction type tests
Antibiotics: penicillin, cephalosporins, isoniazid, PAS, tetracyclines, chloramphenicol; ascorbic acid; chloral hydrate; L-dopa; salicylates; certain x-ray contrast media

QUESTIONNAIRE

1 Mode of onset and duration

Possible *meaning of response*

1.1 At what age were you found to have sugar in your urine?

Approximately ten times as many cases of diabetes are diagnosed in people over the age of 45 as in those under 45

• under 20 years of age?

Juvenile-onset type

• over 40 years of age?

Maturity-onset type

1.2 Under which circumstances was diabetes discovered?

• during a routine examination?

Patients with the milder maturity-onset type of diabetes may be asymptomatic

• because you had any complaints?

Younger subjects have commonly rapid onset of symptomatic hyperglycemia; older age groups have more commonly milder, more stable diabetes appearing more slowly; polydipsia, polyuria, peripheral vascular insufficiency, paresthesias (diabetic neuropathy), vulvar pruritus, furunculosis may be the first manifestations of maturity-onset diabetes

1.2*a* How long have you had these complaints?

2 *Precipitating or aggravating factors*

2.1 In case of rapid (days to weeks) development of symptoms, did you have, prior to the appearance of your complaints
  - an acute infection? a trauma?
  - an operation? a pregnancy?
  - an emotional upset?

Explosive onset of diabetes may be related to stresses which simultaneously increase the need for insulin and decrease the ability to secrete it

2.2 What is your usual weight?

Obesity precipitates diabetes among those predisposed to it

3 *Accompanying symptoms*

3.1 Do you
  - *urinate more than usual?*

Acute or subacute onset of diabetes: polyuria: excretion of the osmotically active glucose molecules provokes an osmotic diuresis

  - ingest more fluids than usual because of *increased thirst?*

Polydipsia: the dehydrating osmotic diuresis activates the mechanisms regulating water intake

  - have an increased appetite?

Polyphagia: (?) decreased activity of the hypothalamic satiety center (due to deficient glucose utilization in its cells) with unopposed activity of the feeding center

3.1*a* Do you have
- a loss of weight?
- a loss of strength?

In diabetes, increased protein catabolism and diminished protein synthesis lead to protein depletion and wasting

- frequent skin infections?
- boils?

Diabetics are liable to bacterial infections: sugar-rich body fluids are favorable culture media for microorganisms, protein depletion is associated with poor resistance to infection

- pruritus?

Diabetes may provoke generalized pruritus without apparent cause (not frequent)

- for the female patient: vulvar pruritus?

Associated with bacterial and *Candida albicans* infections of vulva and vagina

3.2 Do you have, several hours after a starchy meal, episodes of sweating, hunger, palpitation, confusion, weakness?

Iatrogenic hypoglycemia or postprandial hypoglycemia, an uncommon mode of presentation of diabetes

3.3 Do you have headaches? drowsiness? loss of appetite? nausea? vomiting?

Early phase of ketoacidosis
Digestive complaints may also result from delayed gastric emptying (diabetic autonomic neuropathy)

3.4 Do you have
- pain in your calves when walking?
  - disappearing when you stop walking?

Complications of diabetes:

Peripheral occlusive arterial disease, primarily due to premature atherosclerosis

- chest pain on exertion?

Atherosclerotic coronary heart disease

- leg ulcers?

Atherosclerosis in the smaller arteries is more common in diabetics than in nondiabetics

• numbness, tingling, burning in your feet? hands?	Due either to vascular narrowing or to an associated neuropathy ("glove-and-stocking" pattern)
• weakness in an arm, a leg?	Diabetic motor neuropathy
• severe pain in a leg? • loss of movement of an eye? • double vision?	Mononeuropathy multiplex The third and sixth cranial nerves may be involved unilaterally
• a decreased vision?	Diabetic retinopathy; microaneurysms, exudates, and hemorrhages, retinitis proliferans
• episodes of • pain in the flank? • fever? chills? • pain on urination?	Recurrent urinary tract infections Dysuria, in urinary tract infection
• nocturnal diarrhea? • urinary retention?	Autonomic neuropathy
• sexual impotence?	Perhaps the most common symptom of diabetic autonomic neuropathy

4 Iatrogenic factors see Etiology

5 Personal antecedents pertaining to the glycosuria

5.1 How do you control your disease?

5.1a Are you treated with:

• diet? • insulin?: type? number of units? • oral hypoglycemic agents? specify	Extensive education and emotional support of the patient are vital in the proper management of diabetic patients
5.1b How do you adapt your medication and diet to the results of urine tests?	
5.2 How do you adapt to your diabetes?	

5.3 Have you ever had episodes of unconsciousness?   **Hypoglycemia; ketoacidotic coma; hyperglycemic hyperosmolar nonketotic coma; lactic acidosis**

5.4 Do you have any of the following conditions:

- recurrent episodes of abdominal pain? attacks of pancreatitis?
- a past operation on your pancreas?

Diabetes has been reported in 13 percent of the patients with chronic pancreatitis without pancreatic calcinosis and in 45 percent of those with it

- a heart disease?   Ischemic heart disease
- a kidney disease?   Glomerulosclerosis
- urinary tract infections?   Pyelonephritis
- a high blood pressure?   Hypertensive vascular disease frequently complicates diabetes

5.5 For female patients: Has a transitory glycosuria (or hyperglycemia) been detected during one of your pregnancies?   Heralds the future development of permanent diabetes in the mother

5.5*a* What was the birth weight of your children?   The likelihood of large babies (more than 10 lb) is greater in diabetes mellitus

6 *Family medical history pertaining to the glycosuria*

6.1 Are there any other members of your family who have sugar in their urine?   A positive family history increases the frequency two to four times; renal glycosuria (very rare); Fanconi's syndrome, hereditary form

PHYSICAL SIGNS PERTINENT TO THE COMPLAINT

Finding   **Possible** *significance*

Obesity   Diabetes is four times more common in obese than in lean adults

Cellulitis; furunculosis; gingival abscesses   Diabetics are predisposed to staphylococcal and streptococcal soft-tissue infections

Clusters of raised papules (over buttocks and extremities)	Eruptive xanthomatosis with hyperlipidemia
Peripheral vascular insufficiency Gangrene of feet	Premature atherosclerosis of diabetes; ischemic gangrene is seventy-fold more frequent in diabetics
Symmetrical stocking type of anesthesia; decreased vibratory sensation; decreased to absent deep-tendon reflexes in the legs	Peripheral diabetic neuropathy with segmental demyelinization (appearing after 8 to 12 years of overt diabetes)
Orthostatic hypotension	Autonomic diabetic neuropathy
Strabismus; pupil reaction maintained	Lesion of the third cranial nerve [due to a small vascular infarction within the nutrient vessels of the nerve(?)]
Senile cataract	Tends to appear at an earlier chronologic age in diabetics
Round moon facies; truncal obesity; buffalo hump; purple striae	Cushing's syndrome
Skin pigmentation; hepatomegaly; cardiac failure	Hemochromatosis
Funduscopic examination: diabetic retinopathy (microaneurysms, hemorrhages, waxy exudates)	The cause of one-sixth of all cases of acquired blindness; observed in two-thirds of patients with diabetes for 15 years

LABORATORY TESTS PERTAINING TO THE COMPLAINT

Procedure	Finding	Diagnostic possibilities
Blood		
Fasting glucose (N: 60 to 100 mg/100 mL)	>100 mg/100 mL	Diabetes mellitus

Oral glucose tolerance test (100 g glucose) (OGTT)

½ h	>170 mg/100 mL	Diabetes mellitus; OGTT affected by age, diet, pregnancy, physical activity, liver disease, myocardial infarction, stroke, endocrinopathies, fever, infection, uremia, drugs (diuretics, corticosteroids, oral contraceptives)
1 h	>170 mg/100 mL	
2 h	>120 mg/100 mL	
3 h	>110 mg/100 mL	
Triglycerides, cholesterol	Elevated	Poorly controlled diabetes

Urine

Glycosuria (1–2 h after a heavy carbohydrate meal)	Positive	Diabetes mellitus; renal glycosuria
Ketones	Positive	Uncontrolled diabetes

Procedure	*To detect*
ECG	Coronary artery disease

USEFUL REMINDERS AND DIAGNOSTIC CLUES

Misleading Factors

A false-positive glucose oxidase enzyme test may result from unclean glassware (certain cleansers and detergents).

With heavy proteinuria, hexosamines may be transported with protein into the urine and glucose may be liberated, producing a minimal glycosuria (less than 100 mg/100 mL).

Diagnostic Considerations

Paper or stick test materials are prepared with glucose oxidase enzyme (Clinistix, Tes-Tape): glucose is the only sugar which produces a positive glucose oxidase test.

Copper reduction types of test (Clinitest) detect any sugar having a keto group. The only sugar appearing abnormally in the urine that has no keto group and thus cannot reduce copper or other oxidizing agents is sucrose.

The incidence of diabetes in females is approximately 25 percent higher than in males.

Sexual impotence in the diabetic male has been partly overshadowed in the past, mainly because of poor history taking; it has recently been reported in as many as 60 percent of patients within 5 years of diagnosis of diabetes.

There is an increased association of carcinoma of the pancreas with diabetes mellitus.

Only 2 percent of patients with acute pancreatitis develop permanent diabetes.

The glucose tolerance test is abnormal in 25 to 50 percent of patients with carcinoma of pancreas and is a more frequent abnormality than frank glycosuria or fasting hyperglycemia.

In case of	*Suspect*
Diabetes in a patient with	
Mandibular prognathism	Acromegaly
Centripetal obesity and muscular atrophy	Cushing's syndrome
Onset of unstable diabetes in an elderly nonobese patient (with no family history of diabetes)	Pancreatic carcinoma
Development of unstable insulin-requiring diabetes in a previously stable non-insulin-dependent diabetic	

SELECTED BIBLIOGRAPHY

Cahill GF, Jr: Diabetes mellitus, in Beeson PB, McDermott W, *Textbook of Medicine*, 14th ed, chap 806, pp 1599–1619, Philadelphia: Saunders, 1975

Knowles Jr HC: Evaluation of a positive urinary sugar test. JAMA 234:961–963, 1975

Podolsky S (ed): Symposium on diabetes mellitus. Med Clin North Am 62:625–869, 1978

Steinke J, Soeldner JS: Diabetes mellitus, in Thorn GW et al (eds), *Harrison's Principles of Internal Medicine*, 8th ed, pp 563–583, New York: McGraw-Hill, 1977

47

Masses in the Neck

GENERAL CONSIDERATIONS

Masses in the neck are generally due to enlargement of the thyroid, the cervical lymph nodes, or the salivary glands.

Enlargement of the thyroid gland (goiter) may be generalized or focal. Generalized enlargements (with the right lobe tending to enlarge more than the left) are associated with normal, increased, or decreased hormone secretion, depending upon the underlying disturbance. Focal enlargement of the thyroid is usually due to neoplastic (benign or malignant) transformation.

Lymph node enlargement (lymphadenopathy) may be due to an increase in the number and size of lymphoid follicles with proliferation of lymphocytes or reticuloendothelial cells. A lymph node can also be infiltrated by cells normally not present in it (leukemia, metastatic carcinoma cells, polymorphonuclear cells).

Enlargement of the salivary glands may result from inflammatory swelling associated with infection (mumps) or the presence of a stone in a salivary duct, granulomatous inflammatory changes (as in sarcoidosis), or lymphocytic infiltration (as in Sjögren's syndrome).

ETIOLOGY

Enlargement of the thyroid
Goiter associated with hypothyroidism
    Iodine deficiency: endemic, sporadic
    Iodine excess
    Heritable biosynthetic defect in hormonogenesis
    Multinodular colloid goiter
    Chronic thyroiditis (Hashimoto's disease)
    Drug-induced condition
Goiter associated with hyperthyroidism
    Graves' disease; T3-toxicosis
    Toxic multinodular goiter
    Jod-Basedow's phenomenon

Goiter associated with euthyroidism
  Iodine deficiency: endemic, sporadic
  Autoimmune thyroid disease
  Drug-induced condition
  Acute thyroiditis
  Neoplasms: benign, malignant

Enlargement of cervical lymph nodes
Neoplastic
  Lymphomas; leukemias
  Metastatic neoplasms: nasopharynx, oral cavity, pharynx, thyroid,
    lung, breast, kidney
Nonneoplastic
  Infections:
    Acute: bacterial, rickettsial, viral; oropharyngeal or dental infec-
      tions
    Chronic: tuberculosis, syphilis, toxoplasmosis, fungus
  Connective-tissue diseases: systemic lupus erythematosus, derma-
    tomyositis, rheumatoid arthritis
  Hypersensitivity states: serum sickness, drug reactions (hydantoin)
    sarcoidosis

Enlargement of the salivary glands
Infection: bacterial, viral (mumps)
Calculus in a salivary duct
Tumors; lymphoma
Sarcoidosis; Sjögren's syndrome; Mikulicz's disease
Malnutrition: liver cirrhosis, chronic alcoholism
Advanced uremia
Drug-induced condition

Miscellaneous
Congenital abnormalities: branchial cleft cyst, thyroglossal duct
  cyst, dermoid cyst
Benign tumors: lipomas, fibromas, neurofibromas
Abscess

Iatrogenic Causes of Masses in the Neck

Goiter with or without thyroid dysfunction
Amiodarone
Aniline derivatives

Antipyrine
Cobalt

Iodides
Lithium carbonate
Mercaptoimidazole
PAS
Phenylbutazone

Resorcinol
Salicylamide
Sulfonamides
Derivatives of thiourea

Lymph node enlargement
Allopurinol
Antileprosy agents
Antithyroid agents

Hydantoin derivatives
Isoniazid
Phenylbutazone

Parotid enlargement
Guanethidine; iodine; isoproterenol; mercurialism; phenylbutazone;
  vincristine

QUESTIONNAIRE

Medial Mass

Possible *meaning of response*
Usually the thyroid gland

1 Mode of onset and evolution

1.1 How long have you known
      that you have a swelling in
      your neck?

May be difficult to determine exactly when onset is insidious

1.2 Was the onset of the swell-
      ing
      • acute? (hours to days)

Hemorrhage into thyroid; pyogenic thyroiditis

      • subacute? (days to weeks)

Subacute thyroiditis; thyroid
carcinoma

      • gradual, insidious? (months
        to years)

Nontoxic goiter; hypothyroidism;
Graves' disease; thyroid ade-
nomas

1.3 If the swelling has been
      present for years, has its
      volume

      • remained unchanged?

Nontoxic goiter

      • recently increased?

• gradually and without tenderness?	Thyroid carcinoma
• rapidly, with local pain?	Hemorrhage into a nodule; thyroiditis

2 *Accompanying symptoms*

2.1 *Do you have intolerance to heat?* Do you • sleep with fewer blankets? • kick off the covers while asleep? • find hot weather intolerable?	Hyperthyroidism

2.1a Do you have

• excessive sweating?	Adrenergic overactivity
• irritability? anxiety? emotional instability?	Increased nervousness predominates in younger subjects with hyperthyroidism
• palpitations?	Sinusal tachycardia, atrial fibrillation of hyperthyroidism (cardiovascular symptoms of hyperthyroidism predominate in older subjects)
• Have friends observed that your eyes were prominent?	Proptosis of hyperthyroidism

2.2 *Do you have intolerance to cold?* Do you sleep with more blankets on the bed?	Hypothyroidism

2.3 Do you have

• *frequent loose bowel movements?*	Hyperthyroidism (hyperdefecation); medullary carcinoma of thyroid
• constipation?	Hypothyroidism
• a gain in weight?	Hypothyroidism
• a loss of weight?	Hyperthyroidism
• an increased appetite?	Hyperthyroidism

• a decreased appetite?	Hypothyroidism; thyroid carcinoma
• pain (and/or stiffness) in your muscles?	Myopathy of hypothyroidism
• difficulty in climbing stairs? • a wasting of some of your muscles?	Myopathy in Graves' disease (proximal) (myopathic symptoms predominate in older subjects with hyperthyroidism)
• fatigue?	Hypo- as well as hyperthyroidism
• swollen legs?	Congestive heart failure or pretibial myxedema of Graves' disease
• oligomenorrhea or amenorrhea?	Commoner than menorrhagia in hyperthyroidism
• menorrhagia?	Frequent in younger women with hypothyroidism
• a deeper voice?	Hypothyroidism
• hoarseness?	Compression of the recurrent laryngeal nerve: suggests thyroid carcinoma (extension beyond the capsule of the gland); rare in simple goiter
• any difficulty in • breathing?	Compression and displacement of the trachea by the enlarged thyroid
• swallowing?	Compression and displacement of the esophagus by a massively enlarged thyroid; also in carcinoma; chronic thyroiditis
• hearing?	Hypothyroidism; defect of thyroid hormone synthesis with congenital deafness
• excessive sleepiness?	Hypothyroidism
2.4 In case of acute or subacute, and painful swelling, *does the pain in the swelling radiate to lower jaws? the ears?*	Subacute (de Quervain's) thyroiditis

2.4*a* Prior to the appearance of the swelling, did you have fever? malaise? a sore throat?

Subacute thyroiditis frequently occurs 2 to 3 weeks after viral upper respiratory infection

2.5 Have you noticed a swelling at another site in your neck?

Local metastasis of a thyroid carcinoma

3 Iatrogenic factors see Etiology

4 Environmental factors

4.1 Are there any other people with a goiter in the area where you are living?

Endemic goiter

5 Personal antecedents pertaining to the complaint

5.1 Have you ever had previous thyroid tests? radioactive uptake? scan? When? With what results?

5.2 Did you have x-ray therapy to the head or neck during your childhood? Why?

Associated with a high incidence of thyroid carcinoma in later life

5.3 Do you have any of the following conditions:
a thyroid condition? thyroid surgery? a cardiac disease? an eye disease?

6 Family medical history pertaining to the complaint

6.1 Does someone in your family have a thyroid condition? a goiter?

Familial predisposition to Graves' disease, Hashimoto's disease, myxedema, congenital defects of thyroid hormone synthesis, medullary carcinoma of the thyroid

Lateral Masses

Usually cervical lymph nodes: metastatic carcinoma, lymphomas, leukemias, infections

1   Mode of onset and duration

1.1   When did you notice the swelling for the first time?

Patients with neoplastic nodes have a longer history (months) than patients with infectious or inflammatory adenopathy (days)

1.2   Have you noticed
- only one lump? several lumps?
  - on one side of the neck?

Unilateral cervical mass: <u>metastasis</u> from (an undetected) nasopharyngeal tumor; <u>lymphoma</u>, Hodgkin's disease; infection; parotitis

  - on both sides of the neck?

Bilateral cervical adenopathy prominent in: tuberculosis, coccidioidomycosis, infectious mononucleosis, toxoplasmosis, sarcoidosis; <u>lymphomas</u>; <u>leukemias</u>; bilateral parotid enlargement (mumps, sarcoidosis)

1.3   Has the onset of the mass(es) been
- sudden?

Nonneoplastic: acute infection; hypersensitivity states

- gradual?

Neoplastic; tuberculosis; fungus

2   Precipitating or aggravating factors

2.1   If the onset has been sudden, have you recently had
- a dental abscess? a sore throat?

Oropharyngeal or dental <u>infections</u> can cause cervical adenopathy

- a sore throat with a skin rash?

Infectious mononucleosis

3   Accompanying symptoms

3.1   If the onset was sudden, was it associated with

- fever?
- local pain, redness, heat? } Acute infection; parotitis

3.2 If the swelling has progressed slowly, is it
- tender?

  Acute infection (may occur in tuberculosis); acute leukemia

- painless?

  Lymphoma; metastasis; chronic lymphocytic leukemia; chronic infections, tuberculosis; sarcoidosis

3.3 Do you have
- a blockage in one of your nostrils?
- frequent bleeding from the nose?
- increased pain in a sinus? } Metastatic lymph nodes from primary oral, nasal, or pharynx cancer
- a sore in your mouth?
- hoarseness?
- difficulty swallowing?
- fever? a weight loss?
- a decrease of appetite? } Neoplasm
- easy bruising?

  Leukemia with thrombocytopenia

4 *Iatrogenic factors*   see Etiology

5 *Environmental factors*

5.1 Do you have any pets? cats? dogs?   Implicated in toxoplasmosis

5.2 Have you been exposed
- to someone with mumps?
- to a venereal sexual contact?

  Lymphadenopathy associated with extragenital initial lesion of syphilis

6 *Personal antecedents pertaining to the complaint*

6.1 Do you have any of the following conditions: tuberculosis? a venereal disease? recurrent infections? recurrent sore throats? dental problems?

PHYSICAL SIGNS PERTINENT TO THE COMPLAINT

Finding	**Possible** *significance*
Medial masses:	
Enlarged thyroid; systolic thyroid bruit; fine tremor; warm moist thin skin; tachycardia; wide pulse pressure; stare; lid lag; lid retraction	Hyperthyroidism
Proptosis; chemosis; ophthalmoplegia	Ophthalmopathy of Graves' disease
Raised thickened area on legs or feet	Pretibial myxedema in Graves' disease
Thyroid palpable (or absent); somnolent patient; dry, sparse hair; dry, thickened, cool skin; periorbital puffiness; macroglossia; enlarged heart; bradycardia; prolonged tendon reflex relaxation time	Hypothyroidism
Solitary thyroid nodule	Toxic or nontoxic adenoma; malignancy
Enlarged, firm, irregular thyroid	Multinodular goiter (usually euthyroid); single nodules; Hashimoto's thyroiditis
Hard, fixed gland, or nodules	Malignancy
Fever; enlarged, tender thyroid	Acute or subacute thyroiditis
Mass in the thyroid; Marfanoid habitus	Medullary carcinoma of the thyroid (often with associated pheochromocytoma)
Proximal muscular weakness and atrophy	Chronic thyrotoxic myopathy; may occur in overt or masked hyperthyroidism
Stridor; dyspnea	Tracheal obstruction: massively enlarged thyroid; simple (nontoxic) goiter; retrosternal goiter; carcinoma

Lateral masses:

Tender soft nodes (matted together); inflamed overlying skin — Acute infectious lymphadenopathy

Firm, rubbery, nontender, discrete movable nodes — Lymphadenomatous nodes; chronic infection

Very hard, fixed nodes — Carcinomatous nodes

Sinus tract — Tuberculosis; aspergillosis; actinomycosis

Location of lymphadenopathy:

• occipital — Infection (origin in the scalp); malignancy unlikely

• posterior auricular — Rubella; uncommon in lymphoma

• anterior auricular — Infection of eyelid and conjunctiva; may occur in lymphoma

• anterior cervical — Infection of the oral cavity and pharynx

• posterior cervical; submental — Scalp infection; tuberculosis; infections of dental origin

• unilateral cervical mass — Malignancy: metastatic tumor; Hodgkin's disease; histiocytic or lymphocytic lymphoma

• bilateral cervical — Tuberculosis; coccidioidomycosis; infectious mononucleosis; toxoplasmosis; sarcoidosis; lymphoma; leukemia

• supraclavicular fossae — Metastases from intrathoracic or intraabdominal malignancy; inflammatory process unlikely

• generalized — Chronic lymphocytic leukemia; non-Hodgkin's lymphoma; histiocytoses (uncommon in nonhematologic malignancies); infectious mononucleosis; cytomegalovirus infection; histoplasmosis; toxoplasmosis; tuberculosis; brucellosis; infectious hepatitis

Asymmetric cervical lymphadenopathy	Hodgkin's disease; histiocytic lymphoma
Symmetric cervical lymphadenopathy	Leukemia; lymphocytic lymphoma
Salivary gland enlargement; uveitis; facial nerve palsy	Heerfordt's syndrome: sarcoidosis
Nasopharyngeal examination	May reveal a primary tumor with cervical metastases
Dental caries; pharyngitis	Possible infectious origin of cervical lymphadenopathy

Adenopathy with

• splenomegaly	Infectious mononucleosis; connective-tissue disease; sarcoidosis; neoplastic (lymphoma, leukemia, chronic granulocytic leukemia)
• hepatomegaly	Malignancy; hepatitis
• a skin rash	Viral infection
• ecchymoses; petechiae	Bleeding tendency: leukemia, lymphoma
• fever	Infectious process; neoplasm

LABORATORY TESTS PERTAINING TO THE COMPLAINT

Procedure	Finding	Diagnostic possibilities
Serum T4 concentration (N: 4 to 11 μg/100 mL)	Elevated	Hyperthyroidism; increased thyroxine-binding globulin (TBG)
	Decreased	Hypothyroidism; decreased TBG
Serum T3 concentration (N: 80 to 160 ng/100 mL)	Elevated	Hyperthyroidism; T3-toxicosis
	Decreased	Hypothyroidism

Resin-T3 uptake (RT3U) (N: 25 to 35 percent)	Elevated	Hyperthyroidism; decreased binding
	Decreased	Hypothyroidism; increased binding
T4-RT3 index	Elevated	Hyperthyroidism
	Decreased	Hypothyroidism
Serum cholesterol	Elevated	Hypothyroidism of thyroidal origin
	Decreased	Hyperthyroidism
TSH assay (N: <5 μU/mL)	Increased	Hypothyroidism of thyroidal origin
	Undetectable	Pituitary or hypothalamic hypothyroidism; thyrotoxicosis
TRH stimulation test	Subnormal or no response	Pituitary hypothyroidism; thyrotoxicosis
	Supranormal response	Primary (thyroidal) hypothyroidism
Thyroid radioactive iodine uptake (RAIU)	Elevated	Hyperthyroidism; iodine deficiency
	Normal	May occur in: thyroiditis; multinodular goiter; T3-toxicosis
Thyroid suppression test	Normal	Excludes the presence of hyperthyroidism
	Abnormal	Hyperthyroidism; also in: autonomous hyperfunctioning adenoma; after treatment of hyperthyroidism in Graves' disease

| Antithyroglobulin antibodies | Positive | Hashimoto's disease; primary thyroprivic hypothyroidism; Graves' disease |

Procedure	*To detect*
Thyroid scan	Areas of increased or decreased function within the thyroid; retrosternal goiter; ectopic thyroid tissue; functioning metastases of thyroid carcinoma
Thyroid ultrasonography	Thyroid cysts vs. solid nodules
X-rays of chest, paranasal sinuses, trachea, with barium swallow	Tumor of lung, sinuses; pulmonary tuberculosis; deviation or compression of trachea; retrosternal goiter; extrinsic pressure on esophagus
Biopsy of lymph node or accessible mass	Lymphoma; tumor; granulomas, tuberculosis, etc.

USEFUL REMINDERS AND DIAGNOSTIC CLUES

Misleading Factor

Benign hypertrophy of both masseter muscles may be confused with painless parotid swelling.

Diagnostic Considerations

Thyroid metastases often present a lump in the neck as the first sign of thyroid cancer.

Any patient with an unexplained neuromuscular disorder should be investigated for underlying hyperthyroidism.

In anxiety of emotional origin, the skin of the extremities is usually cold and clammy; in anxiety occurring in hyperthyroidism, the skin is usually warm and moist.

Enlargement of lymph nodes in the posterior auricular and supraclavicular areas must always be considered pathologic.

A nonthyroid neck mass in an adult patient should be considered neoplastic until proved otherwise.

In case of	*Suspect*
Hypothyroidism with a small heart	Pituitary hypothyroidism
Unexplained cardiac failure or arrhythmias (especially atrial in origin)	Hyperthyroidism

SELECTED BIBLIOGRAPHY

Burrow GN (ed): Current concepts of thyroid disease. Med Clin North Am 59:1043–1277, 1975

Ingbar SH, Woeber KA: Diseases of the thyroid, in Thorn GW et al (eds), *Harrison's Principles of Internal Medicine,* 8th ed, pp 501–519, New York: McGraw-Hill, 1977

Weinstein IM: Lymphadenopathy and splenomegaly, in Williams WJ, Beutler E, Erslev AJ, Rundles RW, *Hematology,* 2d ed, pp 950–956, New York: McGraw-Hill, 1977

48
Obesity

DEFINITIONS AND GENERAL CONSIDERATIONS

Ideal weight weight associated with lowest mortality according to insurance company data. Ideal weight approximates that at age 20 to 25.

Obesity adiposity in excess of that consistent with good health. A person is considered obese if his or her weight exceeds by 9 to 10 kg the ideal weight; obesity requires the presence of excessive amounts of fat.

Indices used to express obesity

Ponderal index: height/$\sqrt[3]{\text{weight}}$ (height in inches, weight in pounds)

Body mass index: weight/height^2 × 100

Skin-fold thickness (subscapular or triceps): correlates rather well with total body fat. Obesity is diagnosed when the triceps skinfold thickness is greater than 20 mm in men or 30 mm in women between the ages of 20 and 50.

Obesity occurs when the caloric intake exceeds the energy requirements of the body for physical activity and growth. Caloric intake is controlled by a satiety center in the hypothalamic ventromedial nucleus (destruction of this center causes overeating and obesity) and a feeding center in the lateral hypothalamus area (destruction of this center causes anorexia and lack of eating). A disturbance of the appetite-controlling mechanisms permitting the assimilation of more food than is needed may lead to obesity. Pituitary, thyroid, adrenal, and sex hormones influence the regulation of fat deposition.

Obesity due to hypothalamic or endocrine disorders is rare. In most cases of obesity various developmental, psychologic, socioeconomic factors play critical roles. There is no evidence that obese patients have an intrinsic abnormality of energy expenditure or a greater efficacy in their ability to digest, absorb, and utilize food. Individuals who develop obesity in early or late childhood have an increased number of adipocytes with variable degrees of enlargement of fat cells (hyperplastic hypertrophic obesity), whereas in those who develop obesity in adult years, the adipocytes are increased in size but not in number (normocellular hyperplastic obesity).

ETIOLOGY

Increased caloric intake
Psychologic, social, cultural factors
Iatrogenic (e.g., intensive ulcer regimen)
Hypothalamic damage

Decreased energy expenditure
Diminished physical activity
Increased metabolic efficiency(?)

Endocrine
Cushing's syndrome; hypothyroidism; diabetes mellitus; insulinoma, hyperinsulinism; hypogonadism

Genetic
Unusual syndromes associated with obesity: Prader-Labhart-Willi syndrome; hyperostosis frontalis interna; others

Iatrogenic Causes of Obesity

Anabolics; oral contraceptives; glucocorticoids; insulin excess; phenothiazine drugs and other tranquilizers; ulcer regimens (milk, cream)

QUESTIONNAIRE

	Possible *meaning of response*
1 Mode of onset and chronology	
1.1 At what age did obesity appear?	
• during childhood?	Hypercellular obesity
• during adulthood?	Normocellular hyperplastic obesity
1.2 Do you know your weight at birth?	Generally normal in both types of obesity

1.3 Do you know your weight
- during childhood?

Heavy children usually become heavy adults

- *at age 25?*

Desirable weight approximates that at age 25

- during military service? at marriage? at age 40?

If thin or of average weight until age 20 or 40: adult-onset obesity, associated with environmental factors

1.3*a* For female patients: What was your weight before your first pregnancy? after each pregnancy?

There exists a relationship between parity and obesity

1.4 Do you have serial photographs of yourself?

The patient with Cushing's syndrome is sometimes unrecognizable in his earlier photographs, whereas the appearance of the obese patient has not changed much during adult life

2 Severity of obesity

2.1 What has been your

- highest weight?
- lowest weight?

Variations possibly related to stressful events in patient's life history

2.2 Is your weight still increasing?

When weight is more than 20 percent above normal, medical complications become likely (e.g., skin infections, osteoarthritis, diabetes mellitus; hypertension)

3 Location of obesity

In the female, obesity is more pronounced in the lower part of the trunk and extremities; in the male, it is frequently more pronounced in the upper part of the trunk, often sparing the extremities

3.1   Is the obesity
- distributed both on the trunk and on the extremities?

Hypercellular (early or late childhood-onset) obesity

- confined to the trunk?

Acquired hyperplastic (adult-onset) obesity

- *distributed over the back of the neck, trunk and face?*

Cushing's disease

4   *Precipitating or aggravating factors*

4.1   How many meals a day do you eat?

May reveal peculiar eating habits, usually with high carbohydrate and low protein intake

4.2   What did you eat for
- breakfast today?
- lunch today?
- supper last night?

The questions about the patient's diet must be specific; the major caloric intake of the very obese subject usually occurs during late afternoon and evening

4.3   Do you skip breakfast? lunch? supper?

Frequent in teenagers or in obese patients on a self-reducing diet; prevalence of obesity is inversely proportional to meal frequency

4.4   Do you eat between meals?

Many obese patients do not regard a midmeal or bedtime snack as food and do not report it as part of their daily food intake

4.5   How much and/or how many times a day do you eat any of the following items:

- sugar and starches:
  - bread?

Gives an estimate of the total ingested foods with respect to both type and amount; the amounts of sugar and starch foods, and of fats, readily show the main sources of calories
Carbohydrate yields 4 kcal/g
1 slice = 80 kcal

- potatoes?
- fruit?
- candy bars? crackers? pie? cake? ice cream?
- fats:
  - butter? margarine? gravy? mayonnaise? nuts? peanuts? fried foods? sauces?
- proteins:
  - meat? fish? poultry? milk? cheese? eggs?
- side dishes of: rice? spaghetti? potatoes?

1 apple = 100 kcal

Pure fat yields 9 kcal/g
1 pat butter = 90 kcal

Protein gives 4 kcal/g
3 oz meat = 90 kcal
1 egg = 75 kcal
Spaghetti (1 serving) = 400 kcal

4.6 How many times a day (a week) do you eat any of the following snack foods?
- whole milk? (white)

- chocolate milk shake?
- tea?
  - with sugar?
- Coca-cola?
- ice cream? (vanilla)
- ice milk? (vanilla)
- popcorn?
- potato chips?
- plain gelatine dessert?
  - with whipped cream?
- plain doughnut?

"Snack foods" have usually a high-calorie, low-protein content

8 oz = 161 kcal (skim milk, 8 oz = 81 kcal)
8 oz = 421 kcal
8 oz = 2 kcal
1 tsp (level) = 18 kcal
8 oz = 104 kcal
4 oz = 145 kcal
4 oz = 102 kcal
1 cup = 54 kcal
5 = 54 kcal
1 cup = 130 kcal
1 tbsp = 182 kcal
1 = 125 kcal

4.7 What is your intake of beer? alcohol? wine? a day? a week?

Use and abuse of alcohol contribute to obesity; alcohol has significant caloric value: 1 glass beer = 114 kcal; 1 martini = 24 oz beer = ± 200 kcal

4.8   How many meals a day do you eat at home? in restaurants? on your job?

Economic considerations frequently lead to low-protein, high-carbohydrate and high-fat meals

4.9   Do you often attend meetings? celebrations? cocktail parties?

Social contributing factors: calorie-rich refreshments

4.10   Do you have any psychologic problems?

Weight gain with emotional stress is a common characteristic of obese patients

4.10*a*   *When you are confronted with worry or psychologic stress, does your food intake increase?*

Frequent in the juvenile obese group

4.10*b*   Do you have many days of unplanned leisure?

May lead to excessive eating and drinking to "have something to do"

4.11   Did you recently stop smoking?

May contribute to weight increase

5   *Ameliorating factors*

5.1   Do you lose weight on a strict diet?

5.1*a*   Do you regain weight when you discontinue the diet?

Probably psychologic basis for the obesity problem; patients with adult-onset obesity are more amenable to treatment than patients with lifelong obesity

6   *Accompanying symptoms*

Hypercellular early-onset obesity tends to be associated with fewer metabolic disorders (hyperlipemia, diabetes mellitus, hypertension) than the hyperplastic adult-onset obesity

6.1   Do you have
• headaches? a (partial) loss of vision?

Pituitary tumor (chromophobe adenoma); compression of hypothalamus

- fatigability? easy bruising? purple striations on your skin?
- muscular weakness?

Cushing's syndrome (with centripetal obesity)

- intolerance to cold? constipation?

Hypothyroidism

- episodes of hunger? sweating? palpitations? trembling?

Hypoglycemia leading to frequent feedings with resulting obesity

  - after a prolonged fast?
  - 1 to 2 h after eating?

Insulinoma
"Reactive" hypoglycemia

- pain in your knees? hips? spine?

Osteoarthritis: mechanical complication of obesity

- skin lesions? axillae? perineal region? under the breasts?

Moist folds with fungal lesions

- *somnolence?*

Severe obesity with "Pickwickian" syndrome; extreme adiposity of thoracic and abdominal wall can interfere with the mechanics of ventilation and result in alveolar hypoventilation leading to carbon dioxide retention

6.2 For female patients: Do you have absent or scanty menstruations?

Oligomenorrhea or amenorrhea is frequently observed in obesity; Cushing's syndrome

7 *Iatrogenic factors*   see Etiology

8 *Environmental factors*

8.1 What is your present profession? What were your past professions?

Sedentary work contributes to obesity; patients who have previously been physically active may fail to reduce their caloric intake when they suddenly change to a sedentary occupation

8.2   What is your daily activity pattern?

Decreased activity rather than increased food intake is recognized in many obese subjects

8.2*a*   Do you engage in active sports?

The obese adult patient may continue previous alimentary habits despite less physical activity

8.3   What is (was) your relationship with your parents? school? friends? society?

A cause for overeating may be found in a maladjustment problem

8.4   Does your obesity cause you any problem: personal? psychologic? professional? social? sexual?

Obesity makes the satisfaction of social and sexual desires less likely; it may also be a symptom of psychologic maladjustment

8.5   Do you have any reason—social, economic, medical—for undertaking a weight reduction program? Do you want to lose weight?

Motivation is the single most important factor in weight reduction

9   *Personal antecedents pertaining to the obesity*

9.1   Have you ever attempted to lose weight
  • by adhering to a diet?
  • by increased exercise?
  • by group therapy?
  • with Weight Watchers?
  • with medications? specify

A high percentage of persons in the juvenile obese group show poor response to therapy

9.1*a*   Have you ever had any depression after a weight-reducing treatment?

Severe psychologic reaction to treatment may occur in juvenile type of obesity, in obese patients whose increased food intake was a manifestation of anxiety or depression

9.2 Do you have

• diabetes?	Obesity both predisposes to and accompanies diabetes mellitus (diabetes is four times more common in obese than in lean adults); hyperglycemia may reflect a diminished sensitivity of peripheral tissues to insulin; also in Cushing's syndrome
• an elevated blood pressure? • high cholesterol?	Hypertension and hyperlipemia are more common in obese than in lean adults
• a thyroid condition? depression? anxiety?	

10 *Family medical history pertaining to the obesity*

10.1 Do you know the weight of your

• parents? siblings?	Obesity occurs more frequently in near relatives of the juvenile obese than in those of the adult obese (environmental factor?)
• twin, if any?	If obese: genetic factor(?); the variability in body weight between identical twins is much less than that observed in fraternal twins
10.2 Is there any member of your family who has (had) obesity? diabetes? hyperlipemia?	Genetic and/or environmental influences

PHYSICAL SIGNS PERTINENT TO THE COMPLAINT

Finding

Osteoarthritis; flat feet; varicose veins; intertriginous dermatitis; ventral hernias

Possible *significance*

Mechanical trauma of excessive body weight

Hypertension	More common among the obese (due in part to increased cardiac output and stroke volume); Cushing's syndrome
Rounded plethoric facies; truncal obesity; "buffalo hump"	Cushing's syndrome
Purple striae over abdomen, shoulders, hips, elsewhere	Cushing's syndrome; also observed with rapid weight gain
Nonviolaceous striae over breasts, abdomen, upper arms, hips, thighs	Frequently observed in obese adolescents with normal adrenal function
Dry, coarse, cool skin; prolonged tendon reflex relaxation time	Hypothyroidism (the weight gain in hypothyroidism is usually only moderate)
In a female patient: hirsutism	Stein-Leventhal syndrome (with polycystic ovaries, infertility)

LABORATORY TESTS PERTAINING TO THE COMPLAINT

Procedure	To detect
Blood	
Glucose tolerance test	Diabetes mellitus
Thyroid function tests*	Myxedema
Cortisol diurnal variation*	Absence in Cushing's syndrome
Arterial blood gases* Pulmonary function tests*	Elevated P_{CO_2}, depressed P_{O_2}, reduced lung volumes in hypoventilation associated with obesity (Pickwickian syndrome)
Skull films*	Cushing's disease; acromegaly
Psychologic evaluation*	Psychologic problems, depression, anxiety, associated with obesity

* If appropriate.

USEFUL REMINDERS AND DIAGNOSTIC CLUES

Misleading Factors

Weight gain in excess of 1 kg/day almost invariably implies excess fluid retention (edema).

Obese patients notoriously underestimate the calories they consume.

Obese patients who state that they do not eat much frequently refer to the bulk of intake rather than the caloric value.

Diagnostic Considerations

Endocrine abnormalities are an unusual cause of obesity.

Patients with Cushing's syndrome are not extremely obese, rarely weighing more than 225 lb.

Obesity of arms or legs is against the diagnosis of Cushing's syndrome.

Some 30 percent of men and 40 percent of women are 20 lb or more above ideal weight.

SELECTED BIBLIOGRAPHY

Albrink MJ: Obesity, in Beeson PB, McDermott W, *Textbook of Medicine,* 14th ed, pp 1375–1386, Philadelphia: Saunders, 1975

Guggenheim FG: Basic considerations in the treatment of obesity. Med Clin North Am 61:781–796, 1977

Mann GV: The influence of obesity on health. N Engl J Med 291:178–185, 226–232, 1974

Thorn GW, Cahill Jr GF: Gain in weight. Obesity, in Thorn GW et al, *Harrison's Principles of Internal Medicine,* 8th ed, pp 228–233, New York: McGraw-Hill, 1977

49
Weight Loss and/or Anorexia

DEFINITIONS AND GENERAL CONSIDERATIONS

Anorexia loss of the desire to eat.
Sitophobia fear of eating because of subsequent or associated discomfort.

Anorexia is common in patients with gastrointestinal, extraintestinal, and psychologic disorders and therefore is an important but nonspecific symptom. Anorexia may be due to toxic products released by microorganisms, breakdown products of tumor tissue, or retention of metabolic end products in late-stage renal and hepatic disease. Anorexia with decreased food intake results in undernutrition and weight loss. Anorexia nervosa, a chronic illness principally affecting young girls after puberty, is characterized by a neurotic fear of becoming obese, extreme aversion to food, and a marked weight loss; it reflects a severe psychologic disturbance. Weight loss with normal appetite and adequate caloric intake may occur because of increased caloric utilization (increased tissue catabolism of hyperthyroidism or febrile states), decreased intestinal absorption, or abnormal loss of calories (diabetes mellitus with glycosuria, fistulas).

ETIOLOGY

Weight loss with anorexia
Psychologic difficulties: depression; anxiety; anorexia nervosa
Gastrointestinal disorders: gastric carcinoma; malabsorption syndrome; regional enteritis; ulcerative colitis; carcinoma of the colon; chronic liver disease, cirrhosis; carcinoma of the pancreas
Extraintestinal disorders: severe congestive heart failure; chronic pulmonary insufficiency; uremia; endocrinopathies (Addison's disease, hyperparathyroidism, hypercalcemia, hypokalemia); chronic infections, tuberculosis; hematologic diseases (leukemia, myelofibrosis); neoplasms; intoxication (alcohol; lead; excessive smoking); thiamine deficiency

Weight loss without anorexia or with increased appetite
Endocrine and metabolic disorders: hyperthyroidism; diabetes mellitus; pheochromocytoma; carcinoid syndrome
Gastrointestinal disorders; painful lesions of mouth and pharynx; obstructive lesion in esophagus; postgastrectomy syndromes; partial intestinal obstruction; intestinal resection; draining fistulas
Severe food allergies; intestinal parasites
Intracranial disease; neuromuscular disorders with dysphagia
Anxiety
Drugs: thyroid

Iatrogenic Causes of Anorexia

Any medication, particularly:

Amphetamines	Digitalis	Propranolol
Broad-spectrum	Fenfluramine	Salicylates
oral antibiotics	Methylphenidate	(X-ray treatment)
Antimetabolic drugs	(Ritaline)	
Codeine	Morphine	

QUESTIONNAIRE

Possible meaning of response

1 Mode of onset and duration

1.1 How long have you been losing weight?

1.2 How many pounds have you lost?

The magnitude of weight loss reflects either the seriousness or the duration of the underlying disorder; profound loss in anorexia nervosa

1.3 Are you still losing weight?

Underlying process still present

1.4 What was your
• average weight?
• maximum weight?
• minimum weight?

Comparison with prior measurements documents the reliability of the patient's history concerning the importance and duration of weight loss

• *weight at age 25?*

Has proved to be a useful standard for comparison

2 *Precipitating or aggravating factors*

2.1 Please describe your present daily intake at breakfast, at lunch, at dinner

May reveal nutritional deficiencies (in <u>alcoholics</u>, <u>addicts</u>, <u>elderly</u> or <u>poor</u> people)

2.1*a* Please describe your daily diet at your previous normal weight

2.2 Do you avoid eating certain foods?

Food faddism or aversion to certain foods may produce malnutrition

2.2*a* What happens if you eat them?

Allergy to certain foods may produce abdominal discomfort and result in avoidance of these foods

2.2*b* Do you observe
• a reducing diet?
• a therapeutic diet?

May initiate or perpetuate weight loss, or inadvertently cause malnutrition

2.3 Do you have
• any dental problems?

Ill-fitting dentures, or lack of dentures, may interfere with mastication, resulting in a decreased intake of food

• painful lesions in your mouth?

May be caused by vitamin B group or C deficiencies; oral candidiasis

2.4 What is your daily consumption of
• alcohol?

Alcoholics often drink instead of eating; alcohol produces anorexia

• cigarettes?

Smoking dulls the sense of taste

3 *Accompanying symptoms*

3.1 Do you eat less than usual
- *because eating produces abdominal discomfort?*

Sitophobia: anxiety, dumping syndrome following gastrectomy, carcinoma of stomach or pancreas, aerophagic magenblase, partial obstructing intestinal lesion, regional enteritis

- because of a loss of appetite?

Anorexia

3.1a In case of anorexia, is the loss of appetite
- constant?

Organic disease

- intermittent?

Anorexia nervosa

3.2 *Has your appetite remained the same, or increased?*

Thyrotoxicosis; diabetes mellitus

3.2a Do you have
- heat intolerance?
- palpitations?

Thyrotoxicosis

3.2b Do you drink, urinate, more than usual?

Polydipsia, polyuria: diabetes mellitus, chronic renal disease, diabetes insipidus, disorders associated with hypercalcemia or hypokalemia

3.3 Do you have
- a change in your bowel habits?

Gastrointestinal carcinoma

- chronic diarrhea?

Malabsorption syndrome; regional enteritis; ulcerative colitis

- constipation?

Tumor of bowel; anorexia nervosa

- black, tarry stools?

Melena: gastrointestinal carcinoma

- pain in the abdomen?

Neoplasm; pancreatic carcinoma

• difficulty swallowing?	Obstructive esophageal lesion; neuromuscular disorders impairing swallowing and resulting in an insufficient caloric intake
• nausea? vomiting?	Uremia; anorexia nervosa; increased intracranial pressure (brain tumor)
• fever?	Tuberculosis; chronic infection; fever by itself can cause weight loss

3.4   Do you feel depressed? anxious?

3.4*a*   Has any recent familial or professional change occurred in your life?

Functional origin of anorexia and weight loss

4   *Iatrogenic factors*   see Etiology

5   *Environmental factors*

5.1   Where do you usually eat?

Unfavorable environmental factors may adversely influence appetite

5.1*a*   For the single male patient: Who prepares your meals?

Adequate food may be made unpalatable because of the way it is prepared or served

6   *Personal antecedents pertaining to the weight loss*

6.1   Have you ever had a chest x-ray? an x-ray of your stomach? intestine? When? With what results?

6.2   Have you ever had any GI surgery?

Some weight loss is common after subtotal gastrectomy; it may be due to fear of eating because of the dumping syndrome, reduced caloric intake because of early satiety, or mild steatorrhea following surgery
In case of intestinal resection: decreased absorptive surface

6.3 Do you have any of the following conditions: diabetes? a thyroid condition? a renal disease? a cardiac condition? a liver disease? chronic bronchitis? emphysema? tuberculosis?

PHYSICAL SIGNS PERTINENT TO THE COMPLAINT

Finding	**Possible** *significance*
Fever	Chronic infection; tuberculosis
Enlarged thyroid; tremor; warm, moist skin; tachycardia	Thyrotoxicosis
Lymphadenopathy; splenomegaly	Malignancy: leukemia; lymphoma
Abnormal abdominal examination	Malignancy; gastrointestinal obstruction
Hepatomegaly	Cirrhosis; chronic hepatitis
Hypotension; hypothermia; dry skin; lanugo-type hair; retained breast tissue, and pubic and axillary hair	Anorexia nervosa
Examination of mouth and pharynx	May reveal local causes of decreased intake of food: lack of dentures, ulcerations of tongue or oral mucosa; candidiasis
Neurologic abnormalities	Neuromuscular disorders may interfere with mastication: stroke, brainstem lesions, amyotrophic lateral sclerosis, muscular dystrophy

LABORATORY TESTS PERTAINING TO THE COMPLAINT

Procedure	*To detect*
Blood RBCs; WBCs	Anemia; leukemia
Erythrocyte sedimentation rate	Not specific: infection; malignancy; connective-tissue diseases; etc.

BUN, creatinine	Chronic renal failure
Fasting glucose	Uncontrolled diabetes mellitus
Electrolytes	Endocrinopathies: Addison's disease; hypercalcemia; hypokalemia
Protein electrophoresis	Hypoproteinemic states; connective-tissue disease; multiple myeloma
Thyroid function tests	Thyrotoxicosis

Urine

Urinalysis	Chronic renal failure; diabetes mellitus
Culture	Urinary tract infection

Stool

Occult blood tests	Gastrointestinal tumor
Ova, parasites	Parasitic diseases
Fat	Malabsorption syndromes
Skin tests	Tuberculosis; histoplasmosis; etc.
Sputum examination	Tuberculosis; tumor; etc.
Chest x-ray	Tuberculosis; bronchogenic carcinoma; etc.

Complete GI series; IV pyelography; bone x-rays; radioisotope scanning procedures; tissue biopsy

Psychologic evaluation*	Anxiety; depression; anorexia nervosa

* If appropriate.

USEFUL REMINDERS AND DIAGNOSTIC CLUES

Misleading Factors

Anorexia without weight loss or with an actual gain in weight may be due to an accumulation of edema (ascites in cirrhosis or pancreatic carcinoma), which may mask the overall weight loss.

A clue to the presence of ascites may be gained from a history of changing abdominal girth.

If poor appetite and diminished food intake are accompanied by weight gain, a detailed dietary history often establishes that caloric consumption is excessive.

The patient who complains of thinness or of being underweight may actually have normal weight.

Diagnostic Considerations

Anorexia precedes amenorrhea in anorexia nervosa, whereas the amenorrhea may occur months or years before the anorexia of anterior pituitary deficiency.

Despite a loss of weight, patients with anorexia nervosa retain a good tolerance for physical activity and are typically indifferent to their disease.

Patients with panhypopituitarism have a normal weight or mild obesity.

Caloric allowances (at a mean environmental temperature of 20°C, assuming average physical activity):

	25 years	*45 years*	*65 years*
Men	725 + 31 W*	650 + 28 W	550 + 23.5 W
Women	525 + 27 W	475 + 24.5 W	400 + 20.5 W

* W = weight in kilograms.

SELECTED BIBLIOGRAPHY

Krehl WA: The evaluation of nutritional status. Med Clin North Am 48:1129–1140, 1964

Thorn GW: Loss of weight, in *Harrison's Principles of Internal Medicine*, 8th ed, pp 227–228, New York: McGraw-Hill, 1977

PART THREE

Obtaining General Information

50
Evolution of the Illness

1   Have you ever had the same complaints before? When?

1.1   Were you in good health during the symptom-free period(s)?

1.2   How long has it been since you were perfectly well?

2   Do you know someone (relative, friend, acquaintance) who has the same complaint as you?

3   Have you visited other physicians since the beginning of your trouble? Name(s)? When?

3.1   Have they ordered blood tests? x-rays? other examinations? Date of tests? Results?

3.2   What was their diagnosis?

3.3   Did they give you any treatment? When? Result? Any side effect(s)?

4   Did you take any medication for your trouble? On your own? Prescribed by a physician? Which ones? Dosage? Results? Any side effects?

5   Has your trouble caused you
- to stop working?
- to stay in bed?

For how long?

6   Is your trouble getting worse? Better? Spontaneously? Due to treatment? Since when?

6.1   Has your illness remained stationary since its beginning?

7   Do you suspect any factors which could possibly be playing a role in your illness?

8   What illness do you think you are suffering from?

8.1   What do you think is causing your trouble?

9   What prompted you to consult a physician at this time?

51
Personal Past Medical History

1   Have you ever been sick before? What did you have? When?

1.1   What were the symptoms of the illness?

1.2   What kind of treatment did you receive?

1.3   Do you have any aftereffects of the illness? Of the treatment?

2   Have you ever been confined to bed at home? Why? When?

2.1   For how long? For more than 2 weeks?

2.2   Did you call for a physician?

2.3   What was his diagnosis? Treatment?

2.4   What were the results of the treatment?

3   Have you ever been hospitalized? When? Where? For how long?

3.1   What was the diagnosis made by the physicians?

3.2   What kind of treatment did you receive?

3.3   What were the results of the treatment?

4   Have you ever been operated on? Why? When? Where? Name of hospital, city, state? Surname of surgeon(s)?

4.1   What kind of operation was it?

4.2   What was the result of the operation? Any aftereffects?

5   Have you ever had an accident? When?

5.1   Under which circumstances?

5.2   Was it followed by a period of unconsciousness?

5.3   Did you have any fractures?

5.4   Were you hospitalized?

5.5   What was the treatment given?

5.6   Did it necessitate blood transfusion(s)?

5.7   Do you have any aftereffects?

5.8   Are you currently seeking compensation for your injury?

6   For the female patient:

6.1   Have you ever had any miscarriages? abortions? stillbirths? curettages? cesarian deliveries?

6.2   Have you ever used contraceptives?

7   Were you a full-term baby?

7.1   Were you delivered spontaneously (normally)? With forceps?

7.2   Did you have any abnormalities at birth?

7.3   How was the health of your mother during pregnancy?

8   Did you have during your childhood: Chickenpox? Measles? German measles? Scarlet fever? Mumps? Pertussis? Diphtheria? Rheumatic fever?

8.1   Were you excused from participating in sports in school? Why?

9   Allergic disorders: Have you ever had migraine? Asthma? Allergy? Hives? Hay fever? Eczema?

9.1   Are you allergic to any foods? Animals? Feathers? Paints? Soaps? Ointments? Hair discolorants? Chemical products? Drugs?

9.1a Are you allergic to aspirin? Penicillin? Other antibiotics? Sulfonamides? Sedatives? Laxatives? Others?

9.2   Are there any drugs which have adversely affected you?

9.2a What happened when you took these drugs?

9.3   Have you ever received injections of immune serums, antitoxins? Why? Without any side effects?

10   Have you ever received blood transfusions? Why? When? Any side effects?

10.1 Do you know your blood group?

11   Have you been immunized against poliomyelitis? Tetanus?

Smallpox? Rubella? Diphtheria? Measles? Tuberculosis (BCG)? Influenza? Typhoid?

11.1   Date of last active immunization?

12   Have you ever lived in, or traveled to, foreign countries? Where? When? Were you ever sick while there?

13   Have you ever been treated for a venereal disease? Diagnosis? When? Treatment received? For how long? With what results?

14   Have you ever been treated for nervous exhaustion? When? At home? Hospitalized? Treatment received? With what results?

15   Have you ever had to stop working because of health problems? When? How often? For how long? Why?

16   Have you ever had a medical examination for life insurance? Employment purposes? Military service? When? With what results? Date of last thorough medical examination?

16.1   Have you ever been turned down because of health problems?

17   When did you last consult a physician? Why?

17.1   Did he prescribe any treatment?

18   Have you ever had any blood tests done? Urine tests? Pap smears? ECG? X-rays? Isotopic examinations? Eye (ocular fundus) examinations? EEG? Endoscopic examinations?

18.1   When were these tests performed? Why? Results?

18.2   Do you possess any report of these tests?

52

Family Medical History

1   Is your mother still living? Age?

1.1   Is she in good health?

1.1*a* If not: What disease is she suffering from?

1.2   If deceased: Age at death? Cause of death?

2   Is your father still living? Age?

2.1   Is he in good health?

2.1*a* If not: What disease is he suffering from?

2.2   If deceased: Age at death? Cause of death?

3   Are your grandparents still living?

3.1   If so: Which ones? Age? State of health?

3.2   If deceased: Age at death? Cause of death?

4   Do you have any brothers? Sisters? Twins? Age?

4.1   State of health? Diseases, if any?

4.2   If deceased: Age at death? Cause of death?

5   Is your wife (husband) in good health? Age?

5.1   If not: What disease is she (he) suffering from?

5.2   If deceased: Age at death? Cause of death?

6   If any children: Age and state of health?

7   Do you know of any diseases running in your family?

8   Have any of your relatives suffered from:

Diabetes?	Coronary artery	High cholesterol?
Arterial hyper- tension?	disease? Stroke?	Gout? Obesity?

Tuberculosis?
Allergy?
Asthma?
Hay fever?
Renal disease?

Anemia?
Bleeding tendency?
Cancer?
Goiter?
Arthritis?

Migraine?
Depression?
Mental disease?
Epilepsy?

8.1   Have any of your relatives committed suicide?

53
Review of Systems

1 General information

1.1 Have you recently noticed any change in weight? How many pounds? Since when?

1.2 Do you have fever?

1.3 Do you feel tired?

2 Head

2.1 Do you have headache or pain anywhere in the head?

3 Eyes

3.1 Do you need glasses to see things at a distance? to read?

3.2 Do you ever see double?

3.3 Do you ever see halos about light?

3.4 Do you have any blurring, loss of vision? Recent? Old?

3.5 Are your eyes often red or inflamed?

3.6 Does light hurt your eyes?

3.7 Do you have a cataract?

3.8 Have you recently noticed any swelling about the eyes?

4 Ears

4.1 Do you have difficulty hearing? Congenital? Following an infection? With increasing age?

4.2 Do you have any earaches?

4.3 Do you have any ear discharge?

4.4 Do you have constant buzzing in your ears?

5   *Nose*

5.1   Do you have nasal obstruction when you do not have a cold?

5.2   Does your nose run constantly?

5.3   Do you have sinus trouble?

5.4   Do you ever have excessive bleeding from the nose?

5.5   Can you smell coffee, flowers, perfume, as usual?

6   *Mouth*

6.1   Do you have any problems with your teeth?

6.2   Do you wear dentures? Do they fit comfortably? Can you chew well with them?

6.3   Do you have bleeding gums?

6.4   Do you have any sore swellings on your gums?

6.5   Do you have any pain or burning of the tongue or mouth?

6.6   Has your sense of taste changed lately?

7   *Throat*

7.1   Do you have frequent or severe sore throats?

7.2   Has your voice become hoarse lately?

8   *Neck*

8.1   Do you have pain, stiffness in the neck?

8.2   Does twisting your neck cause pain?

8.3   Have you noticed a swelling or lumps in your neck?

9   *Breasts* (female patient)

9.1   Do you have any bleeding, discharge from the nipples?

9.2   Have you felt any lump, or tenderness, in the breasts?

10   *Respiratory system*

10.1   Are you troubled by constant coughing?

10.2   Are you troubled by expectorations? Amount? Character?

10.3   Have you ever coughed up blood?

10.4   Do you have shortness of breath?

10.5   Do you ever have wheezing in your chest when you breathe?

10.6   Do you have chest pain?

10.7   Do you have night sweats?

10.8   Do you have bronchitis more than once a month?

11 *Cardiovascular system*

11.1   Do you know your blood pressure?

11.2   Do you have palpitations?

11.3   Do you have pain, or tightness, in your chest when sitting still? On exertion?

11.4   Do you have difficulty in breathing on exertion? When lying down? Just sitting still?

11.5   Do you have to rest during or after climbing two flights of stairs?

11.6   Have you ever been told that you had a heart murmur?

11.7   Do your ankles or feet swell?

11.8   Do you have cramps in your legs when walking? At night?

11.9   Do you have varicose veins? Cold or blue feet?

12 *Gastrointestinal system*

12.1   Is your appetite good? Poor? As usual?

12.1a   Have you lost your interest in eating lately?

12.2   Do you have any difficulty swallowing?

12.3   Do you have heartburn?

12.4   Do you feel bloated after eating?

12.5   Do you have excessive belching?

12.6   Do you have nausea? Vomiting?

12.7   Have you ever vomited blood?

12.8   Do you have pain in your stomach? After eating?

12.9   Do you have pain elsewhere in your abdomen?

12.10   Do you have abdominal pain when you move your bowels?

12.11   What is the frequency, consistency, color, of your stools?

12.11a   Are you constipated more than twice a month?

12.11b   Do you have diarrhea?

12.11c   Are your bowel movements ever black?

12.11d   Have you ever seen fresh blood in your feces?

12.12   Do you have hemorrhoids?

12.13   Have you ever had jaundice?

13   Genitourinary system

13.1   Do you have burning when you urinate?

13.2   Do you urinate more than five or six times a day?

13.3   Do you have to get up at night to urinate? How many times?

13.4   Do you have a constant feeling that you have to urinate?

13.5   Do you sometimes lose control of your urine?

13.6   What is the color of your urine?

13.6a   Have you ever seen blood, pus, in your urine?

13.7   Have you ever passed a stone?

13.8   For the male patient:

13.8a   Do you have any difficulty in starting your urine flow?

13.8b   Have you noticed that your urine stream is weak and slow?

13.8c   Do you have any burning or discharge from your penis?

13.8d   Are there any swellings or lumps on your testicles?

13.8e   Are your genitals painful or sore?

13.8f   Do you have difficulty with erection?

13.9   For the female patient:

13.9*a*   At what age did your menstruations begin?

13.9*b*   What is the interval between periods? The regularity, the duration of your periods?

13.9*c*   Is the flow normal? Excessive? Slight? How many pads do you use per day? Per period?

13.9*d*   Are the menstruations associated with pain? For how many days?

13.9*e*   Do you feel bloated and irritable before your periods?

13.9*f*   Do you bleed between your menstruations?

13.9*g*   What was the date when your last menstrual period began?

13.9*h*   Do you use birth control pills? Other contraceptive methods?

13.9*i*   Do you have any excessive discharge from your vagina?

13.9*j*   If the patient is menopausal: When did your periods cease? Have you had any vaginal bleeding since your menopause? Do you have hot flushes?

13.10   Do you have pain with sexual intercourse?

13.10*a*   Do you consider that your sexual reactions are normal?

14   *Musculoskeletal system*

14.1   Do you have stiff or painful joints? Back? Muscles? Arms or legs?

14.2   Are your joints ever swollen?

15   *Skin*

15.1   Do you have any skin problem? Itching? Rash? Eczema?

15.2   Have you noticed any changes in coloration of your skin?

15.3   Have you noticed any lumps under your arms? In your groins?

15.4   Do you have excessive perspiration?

15.5   Do you bruise easily? Do you have difficulty in stopping a small cut from bleeding?

15.6   Have you ever been told that you had anemia?

16 Neurologic system

16.1 Do you have vertigo? drowsiness?

16.2 Do you ever faint or feel faint?

16.3 Have you ever had convulsions?

16.4 Do you have any muscular weakness? Paralysis?

16.5 Do you have any loss of sensation, tingling, numbness, in your fingers, toes, limbs?

16.6 Have you noticed any tremor, clumsiness, or awkwardness of your hands or feet?

16.7 Has your handwriting changed lately?

16.8 Do you consider yourself nervous?

54

Personal and Social Profile

1 Marital history

1.1 Are you single? Married?
- At what age were you married?
- How old is your husband (wife)?
- Is he (she) in good health?
- Have you been married more than once?
- divorced? • separated?
- widowed? Since when? What was the cause of the death of your husband (wife)?

1.2 Do you have children? How many? Age(s)?

1.2a Are they in good health?

1.2b Were complications encountered at birth?

1.2c What were your children's weights at birth?

1.2d If remarried: Do you have children by second or subsequent marriage?

1.2e Do you have children who live with you?

1.2f Do you have any particular problems with them?

1.3 If no pregnancies: Why?

1.3a Have you used contraceptive measures? Which one(s)? Do you still use them?

2 Home conditions

2.1 For the female patient who is a housewife: Are you satisfied with your present housing?

2.2 Have you changed domicile recently? How often? Why?

2.3 Do you do your own housekeeping?

2.4 Do you live in a house? An apartment? How many rooms?

2.5 How many people are living in your house, your apartment?

2.6 Besides your husband (wife) and children, are there other persons living with you?

3 Education

3.1 What is your level of education? Elementary school? High school? College?

3.2 Did you have to interrupt your education? Why?

4 Employment

4.1 What is your present occupation? Since when?

4.2 Are you satisfied with it? If not: Why?

4.3 Is the physical activity you have on your job heavy? Limited?

4.4 How many hours a day do you work?

4.5 How long have you been with your present company?

4.6 In case of unemployment: How long have you been unemployed? For what reason?

4.7 What were your past occupations?

4.7a Why did you take different jobs?

4.7b Do you have any difficulty in holding an occupation?

4.8 Do you think you are being (have been) exposed to occupational hazards? Dusts? Chemicals? Paints? Radiation?

5 Military service

5.1 Have you ever served in the armed forces? When? Where? How long?

5.2 Were you rejected? Deferred? For what reason?

5.3 Were you ever sick while in the service? What kind of disease? Venereal disease?

5.4 If served: Honorably discharged? If not: why?

6 Travels

6.1 Have you ever lived or traveled in foreign countries? In tropics? When? For how long?

6.2 Did you contract any disease while there? What kind of disease?

7 Dietary habits

7.1 What is your usual weight?

7.1a When did you weigh yourself last?

7.1b What was your weight at age 25? Your maximum adult weight? Minimum adult weight? When?

7.2 Do you follow a weight-reducing diet? On your own? Prescribed by a physician?

7.3 Do you avoid eating certain foods? Which ones? Why?

7.3a What happens if you eat these foods?

7.4 Do you skip any meals? Why?

7.5 Do you have snacks between meals? Before retiring? During the night?

7.6 Do you drink coffee? Tea? How many cups daily?

7.7 Do you drink beer? Alcohol? Wine? How much a day? For how long?

7.7a Do you drink by yourself? With other people? At home? In bars? In the morning upon awaking?

7.7b Have you ever been drunk? How many times?

7.7c Do you need to take a drink when you have to face unpleasant situations?

7.7d Does your drinking make you miss (affect) your work?

7.7e Have you ever been hospitalized because of drinking?

8 Tobacco, medication, and drugs

8.1 Do you smoke? How many cigarettes, cigarillos, cigars, pipefuls, a day? For how long?

8.1*a*   Do you inhale?

8.1*b*   How long have you been smoking at your present rate?

8.2   Do you use any medications? Rarely? Frequently? Regularly?
   • On your own? Prescribed?
   • How long? Why? How many a day?

8.2*a*   Specifically, do you take tranquilizers? Sleeping pills? Aspirin? Other analgesics? Pep pills? Vitamins? Laxatives? Contraceptive pills? Ulcer remedies? Antihypertensive drugs? Insulin? Corticosteroids? Anticoagulants?

8.3   Have you ever used marihuana? Hashish? Heroin? LSD? Similar drugs? For how long?

9   General and psychologic information

9.1   How many hours do you sleep on the average?

9.1*a*   Do you have difficulty falling asleep? Staying asleep?

9.1*b*   Do you wake up very early in the morning?

9.1*c*   Do you take sleeping pills?

9.2   Do you take vacations? How many weeks a year? Where?

9.2*a*   When did you last have at least 2 weeks' vacation?

9.3   Do you exercise regularly? If not: Why?

9.3*a*   Are you actively engaged in sports? Which ones?

9.4   What do you do with your spare time?

9.4*a*   Do you have any special interests or hobbies?

9.4*b*   How much time do you give to them?

9.5   Do you have any pets? Dogs? Cats? Birds?

9.5*a*   Do they look healthy?

9.6   Do you generally feel better at your job? At home?

9.7   Have you ever sought (or wanted) psychiatric advice or care? Why?

9.7*a*   Do you have periods of excessive depression?

9.7*b*   Have you ever seriously considered or attempted suicide? Why?

9.7*c*   Do you have any anxieties regarding personal, marital, familial, professional, financial matters?

9.8   Do you have any sexual problems?

9.9   Do you have any problem you would like to discuss?

Glossary of Clinical Manifestations

The following is a list of the main symptoms and signs of frequently occurring diseases and syndromes.

Aldosteronism, primary
   hypertension
   potassium depletion
   hypokalemic alkalosis
   muscular weakness
   polyuria
   ECG: U waves

Ankylosing spondylitis
   low back pain
   sciatica
   hip involvement
   iridocyclitis
   aortic regurgitation
   cardiac conduction abnormalities
   peripheral arthritis

Aortic aneurysm
   cough
   dyspnea
   dysphagia
   hoarseness
   chest pain
   back pain
   aortic regurgitation
   left ventricular failure

Aortic regurgitation
   palpitations
   orthopnea
   paroxysmal nocturnal dyspnea

Aortic regurgitation (*continued*)
   angina pectoris
   nocturnal angina
   diaphoresis
   congestive heart failure

Aortic stenosis
   exertional dyspnea
   angina pectoris
   exertional syncope
   orthopnea
   paroxysmal nocturnal dyspnea
   pulmonary edema
   bacterial endocarditis

Bronchiectasis
   chronic cough
   expectorations
   hemoptysis
   recurrent bronchial infections
   chronic sinusitis
   cor pulmonale

Carcinoid syndrome
   flushing
   diarrhea
   abdominal pain
   peptic ulcer

Carcinoid syndrome (*continued*)
  bronchoconstriction
  pulmonic stenosis
  tricusipid stenosis and regurgita-
    tion
  ectopic hormone production
    syndromes

Cirrhosis of the liver
  fatigue
  anorexia
  jaundice
  spider angiomas
  gynecomastia
  testicular atrophy
  palmar erythema
  hepatomegaly
  splenomegaly
  ascites
  esophageal varices

Colitis, ulcerative
  lower abdominal pain
  bloody diarrhea
  fever
  weight loss
  arthritis
  ankylosing spondylitis
  uveitis, iritis
  erythema nodosum
  pyoderma gangrenosum
  colonic strictures
  "toxic dilatation"
  carcinoma of colon
  liver disease
  thrombophlebitis

Colon, cancer
  changes in bowel habits
  increasing constipation

Colon, cancer (*continued*)
  alternating constipation and
    diarrhea
  abdominal pain
  tenesmus
  bleeding
  weight loss

Colon, irritable
  abdominal pain
  alternating constipation and
    diarrhea
  small stools
  gaseous distention
  flatulence

Cushing's syndrome
  trunkal obesity
  "buffalo" hump
  "moon" facies
  weakness
  hypertension
  hirsutism
  amenorrhea
  cutaneous striae
  bruising
  edema
  polyuria, polydipsia

Cystitis
  frequency
  urgency
  dysuria
  fever

Diabetes insipidus
  polyuria
  excessive thirst
  polydipsia

Diabetes mellitus
  polyuria
  polydipsia
  polyphagia
  fatigue
  complications
    angina pectoris
    myocardial infarction
    hypertension
    stroke
    intermittent claudication
    neuropathy
    retinopathy
    nephropathy
    infection
    female: vulvar pruritus
    male: impotence

Endocarditis, infective
  fatigue
  fever
  weight loss
  arthralgia
  embolic phenomena
  petechiae
  splinter hemorrhages
  Osler's nodes
  clubbing
  cardiac murmurs
  splenomegaly

Felty's syndrome
  rheumatoid arthritis
  splenomegaly
  neutropenia

Folic acid deficiency
  diarrhea
  flatulence

Folic acid deficiency (*continued*)
  cheilosis
  glossitis
  mental changes

Glomerulonephritis, acute
  edema
  hematuria
  reduced urine output
  loin pain
  malaise
  nausea
  headache
  hypertension
  congestive heart failure
  renal failure

Goodpasture's syndrome
  hemoptysis
  dyspnea
  glomerulonephritis

Heart failure
  left ventricular failure
    fatigue
    dyspnea
    orthopnea
    cough
    paroxysmal nocturnal dyspnea
    acute pulmonary edema
    hemoptysis
    Cheyne-Stokes respiration
    cardiomegaly
    gallop rhythm
  right ventricular failure
    fatigue
    cyanosis
    systemic venous congestion

Heart failure (*continued*)
    hepatomegaly
    edema
    hydrothorax
    ascites
    pericardial effusion
    oliguria
    cardiac cachexia

Hemochromatosis
  diabetes
  hepatomegaly
  skin pigmentation
  arthropathy
  palmar erythema
  gynecomastia
  cardiac involvement
  loss of libido
  testicular atrophy

Hepatitis, viral
  fever
  anorexia
  nausea, vomiting
  malaise
  arthralgias, myalgias
  dark urine
  clay-colored stools
  right upper quadrant pain
  jaundice
  splenomegaly

Huntington's chorea
  choreic movements
  dementia
  (dominant autosomal)

Hypercalcemia
  anorexia
  nausea, vomiting
  constipation

Hypercalcemia (*continued*)
  hypotonia
  lethargy
  muscle weakness
  hypercalciuria
    nocturia
    polyuria
    polydipsia
  nephrolithiasis

Hyperkalemia
  cardiac arrhythmias
  ECG: high-peaked T waves
  muscular weakness
  flaccid quadriplegia
  respiratory paralysis

Hyperparathyroidism
  (hypercalcemia)
  renal colic
  fatigue
  polyuria, polydipsia
  weight loss
  vomiting
  bone pain
  pathologic fracture
  neurologic abnormalities
  pruritus
  peptic ulcer
  pancreatitis
  hypertension
  pseudogout
  band keratopathy
  (metabolic acidosis)
  associated endocrinopathies
    pituitary tumors
    gastrinoma
    insulinoma
    pheochromocytoma

Hyperparathyroidism (*continued*)
    medullary carcinoma of the
      thyroid

Hypertension, arterial, complications
  exertional dyspnea
  pulmonary edema
  angina pectoris
  myocardial infarction
  congestive heart failure
  intermittent claudication
  visual impairment
  cerebral vascular accident
  nocturia
  renal failure
  hypertensive encephalopathy

Hyperthyroidism
  goiter
  exophthalmos
  tremor
  intolerance for heat
  hyperdefecation
  emotional instability
  palpitations, tachycardia
  excessive sweating
  loss of weight
  increased appetite
  muscular weakness
  thyrotoxic myopathy
  oligomenorrhea or amenorrhea
  atrial fibrillation

Hypoglycemia
  acute epinephrine release
    sweating
    tachycardia
    tremor
    nervousness
    hunger

Hypoglycemia (*continued*)
  central glucopenia
    faintness
    headache
    mental confusion
    convulsions
    coma

Hypokalemia
  muscular weakness
  flaccid paralysis
  hyporeflexia
  myoglobinuria
  ECG abnormalities
  decreased renal concentrating
    ability
      polyuria, polydipsia
  paralytic ileus
  (metabolic alkalosis)

Hypoparathyroidism
  tetany
  convulsions
  mental confusion
  papilledema
  cataracts
  cutaneous moniliasis
  alopecia

Hypopituitarism
  oligomenorrhea or amenorrhea
  loss of libido
  male: impotence
  decreased tolerance to cold
  hypoglycemic episodes
  hypotension
  loss of axillary, pubic hair
  atrophy of breasts and genitalia
  adrenal crisis

Hypothyroidism
  intolerance to cold
  delayed reflexes
  dry skin
  brittle, sparse hair
  constipation
  lethargy
  hoarseness
  periorbital puffiness
  bradycardia
  menorrhagia
  diminished hearing

Intracranial mass lesions
  headache
  mental changes
  vomiting
  papilledema
  diplopia, hemianopsia
  ataxia, hemiplegia
  convulsions
  systolic hypertension
  bradycardia

Leriche syndrome
  occlusion of terminal aorta
  hip, thigh, buttock claudication
  impotence

Lung, cancer
  cough
  hemoptysis
  atelectasis
  pleural effusion
  dyspnea
  chest pain
  hoarseness
  superior vena cava syndrome
  dysphagia

Lung, cancer (*continued*)
  pericardial effusion
  superior sulcus (Pancoast) tumor
  Horner's syndrome
  extrapulmonic manifestations
    clubbing, hypertrophic
      osteoarthropathy
    neurologic lesions
    adrenal hyperfunction
    inappropriate antidiuresis
    hypercalcemia
    carcinoid syndrome

Malabsorption
  steatorrhea
  diarrhea
  weight loss
  muscle wasting
  abdominal distention
  peripheral neuritis, paresthesias
  anemia
  glossitis
  edema
  bone pain
  bleeding tendency

Mediterranean fever, familial
  fever
  abdominal pain
  peritonitis
  pleuritis
  arthritis

Menière's disease
  paroxysmal vertigo
  tinnitus
  progressive hearing loss

Mitral regurgitation
  fatigue

Mitral regurgitation (*continued*)
  exertional dyspnea
  orthopnea
  right-sided heart failure
  atrial fibrillation

Mitral stenosis
  dyspnea
  pulmonary edema
  atrial arrhythmias
  hemoptysis
  pulmonary and peripheral emboli
  pulmonary infections
  bacterial endocarditis

Myasthenia gravis
  diplopia, ptosis
  facial weakness
  difficulty in chewing
  dysarthria
  dysphagia
  generalized weakness
  easy fatigability

Myocardial infarction, complications
  pulmonary edema
  arrhythmias
  cardiogenic shock
  congestive heart failure
  embolism
  hypoxia
  rupture of papillary muscle
  mitral regurgitation
  aneurysm of left ventricle
  Dressler's syndrome
    fever, pericarditis, pleuritis
  cardiac rupture
  shoulder-hand syndrome
  pericarditis

Obesity, complications
  skin infections
  osteoarthritis
  diabetes mellitus
  varicose veins
  cholelithiasis, cholecystitis
  obesity-hypoventilation syndrome
  atherosclerosis
  hypertriglyceridemia
  hypertension
  coronary artery disease

Pancreas, carcinoma
  weight loss
  abdominal pain
  jaundice
  migrating thrombophlebitis
  depression

Peptic ulcer, complications
  hemorrhage
  gastric outlet obstruction
  perforation
  penetration

Pericarditis, acute
  chest pain
  friction rub
  ECG changes

Pericarditis, constrictive
  edema
  ascites
  exertional dyspnea
  elevated venous pressure
  hepatomegaly
  paradoxic pulse
  small quiet heart
  ECG changes

Pericarditis, constrictive (*continued*)
  protein-losing enteropathy
  nephrotic syndrome

Pernicious anemia
  fatigability, weakness
  sore tongue
  distal paresthesias
  anorexia
  diarrhea
  weight loss
  palpitation
  dyspnea
  subacute combined degeneration
  mental changes

Pheochromocytoma
  paroxysmal or permanent
    hypertension
  headache
  excessive perspiration
  palpitations
  tremor
  weakness
  hyperglycemia
  weight loss
  postural hypotension

Polyarteritis nodosa
  fever
  weakness
  weight loss
  myalgia
  arthralgia
  mononeuritis multiplex
  pericarditis, pleuritis
  abdominal pain
  renal involvement
  hypertension
  cutaneous involvement
  asthma (allergic granulomatosis)

Prostate, obstruction
  frequency
  hesitancy
  urgency
  slowing of the stream
  pain
  hematuria
  anuria

Pulmonary embolism
  sudden dyspnea
  substernal discomfort
  tachycardia
  syncope
  ECG changes

Pulmonary infarction
  pleuritic chest pain
  hemoptysis
  dyspnea
  pleural friction rub
  pleural effusion
  tachycardia
  fever
  x-ray densities

Reiter's syndrome
  arthritis
  urethritis
  conjunctivitis
  mucocutaneous lesions

Rheumatoid arthritis, extraarticular
    manifestations
  subcutaneous nodules
  keratoconjunctivitis sicca
  aortic insufficiency
  pleuritis
  diffuse pulmonary fibrosis

Rhumatoid arthritis (*continued*)
  nodular pulmonary lesions
  arteritis

Systemic lupus erythematosus
  arthralgia, arthritis
  fever
  skin eruptions
  renal involvement
    acute nephritis
    nephrotic syndrome
  pericarditis
  myocarditis
  pleuritis
  myalgia
  anorexia, nausea, vomiting
  abdominal pain
  psychosis, convulsions
  lymphadenopathy

Tamponade, cardiac
  dyspnea
  orthopnea
  tachycardia
  venous distention
  positive hepatojugular reflux
  hypotension
  small quiet heart
  paradoxic pulse
  clear lung fields

Thoracic outlet syndrome
  pain, numbness, weakness in arm
  Raynaud's phenomenon

Tuberculosis, pulmonary
  cough, sputum
  hemoptysis
  pleural chest pain, dry pleurisy

Tuberculosis (*continued*)
  fatigue
  fever
  night sweats
  weight loss

Uremia
  nausea, vomiting
  pruritus
  hypertension
  heart failure
  pericarditis
  drowsiness
  peripheral neuropathy
  muscle cramps
  anemia
  bleeding tendency
  pancreatitis
  infection
  coma

Wegener's granulomatosis
  rhinorrhea
  sinusitis
  chronic otitis media
  cough
  hemoptysis
  dyspnea
  pleurisy
  renal involvement

Zollinger-Ellison syndrome
  gastrinoma of pancreas
  intractable ulcer disease
  gastric acid hypersecretion
  diarrhea
  associated hyperparathyroidism